Using Nursing Research

PROCESS, CRITICAL EVALUATION, AND UTILIZATION

Using Nursing Research

PROCESS, CRITICAL EVALUATION, AND UTILIZATION

FIFTH EDITION

Patricia Ann Dempsey, RN, PhD

Professor Emerita of Nursing
New Mexico State University
Las Cruces, New Mexico

Arthur D. Dempsey, EdD

Associate Professor (Retired)
Florida International University
Miami, Florida

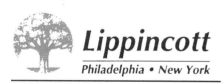

Lippincott
Philadelphia • New York

Visit us at http://www.nursingcenter.com

Acquisitions Editor: Margaret Zuccarini
Marketing Manager: Missy Mulqueen
Production Editor: Jennifer D. Weir
Editorial Assistant: Helen Kogut

351 West Camden Street
Baltimore, Maryland 21201-2436 USA

227 East Washington Square
Philadelphia, PA 19106

The publisher is not responsible (as a matter of product liability, negligence or otherwise) for any injury resulting from any material contained herein. This publication contains information relating to general principles of medical care which should not be construed as specific instructions for individual patients. Manufacturers' product information and package inserts should be reviewed for current information, including contraindications, dosages and precautions.

Printed in the United States of America

First Edition, 1982
Second Edition, 1986
Third Edition, 1992
Fourth Edition, 1996

Library of Congress Cataloging-in-Publication Data

Dempsey, Patricia Ann.
    Using nursing research: process, critical evaluation, and
utilization / Patricia Ann Dempsey, Arthur D. Dempsey.—5th ed.
        p.   cm.
    Rev. ed. of: Nursing research. 4th ed. c1996.
    Includes bibliographical references and index.
    ISBN 0-7817-1790-6
    1. Nursing—Research.   I. Dempsey, Arthur D.   II. Dempsey,
Patricia Ann.   Nursing research.   III. Title.
    [DNLM: 1. Nursing Research.   WY 20.5 1999]
RT81.5.D46   1999
610.73'072—dc21
DNLM/DLC
for Library of Congress   99-16519
                                                                CIP

The publishers have made every effort to trace the copyright holders for borrowed material. If they have inadvertently overlooked any, they will be pleased to make the necessary arrangements at the first opportunity.

To purchase additional copies of this book, call our customer service department at **(800) 638-3030** or fax orders to **(301) 824-7390**. International customers should call **(301) 714-2324**.

99 00 01 02 03
1 2 3 4 5 6 7 8 9 10

FOR OUR FAMILY

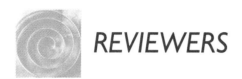

REVIEWERS

Patricia A. Calico, DSN, RN
Chair, Baccalaureate Nursing Program
Midway College
Midway, Kentucky

Mary Jane Hamilton, PhD, MS, BSN
Professor of Nursing
Texas A&M University—Corpus Christi
Corpus Christi, Texas

Anne M. Larson, PhD, MS, BA
Associate Professor of Nursing
Midland Lutheran College
Freemont, Nebraska

Penny Powers, RN, PhD
Department Head, West Virginia Nursing
South Dakota State University
Rapid City, South Dakota

Sally Preski, RN, CNS, PhD
Associate Professor
Texas A&M University—Corpus Christi
Corpus Christi, Texas

Roselena Thorpe, RN, PhD
Professor and Chairperson
CCAC—Allegheny Campus Nursing
    Department
Pittsburgh, Pennsylvania

Dianne R. Wasson, MSN, RN
Assistant Professor
Trinity College of Nursing
Moline, Illinois

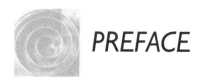

PREFACE

Like the four previous editions of Nursing Research, this fifth edition provides basic research principles and techniques to prepare the beginning research student to participate in nursing research. The book is carefully designed and sequenced to guide students through three processes basic to education in nursing research: (1) the research process, (2) the process of critical evaluation of quantitative and qualitative research for scientific merit, and (3) the process of utilizing the results of valid research in the practice setting.

AUDIENCE

The text is appropriate for all basic undergraduate research students, including RNs, who are enrolled in a basic research course that prepares them to be competent consumers of research and to begin to participate in research utilization in the practice setting. It is our conviction that students exposed to the research process for the first time find their learning is facilitated and their anxiety is reduced when they are guided through the research process and the research utilization process in a systematic manner and provided with activities to reinforce their learning.

The text is also a useful resource for master's and doctoral level nursing students wishing to review basic principles of quantitative and qualitative research and critical evaluation techniques. Practicing nurses will find the text useful to further refine their skills in critical evaluation of both types of research and in sharpening their basic utilization skills.

Although a chapter on quantitative data analysis is provided for review purposes, the text presumes that the reader has either completed, or is currently enrolled, in a basic introductory course in statistics.

SEQUENCING OF CHAPTERS

Because of the increasing importance of qualitative research in nursing, we have written this edition with the express purpose of providing integrated coverage of the basic principles of quantitative and qualitative research throughout the text. Students are introduced to the quantitative and qualitative research traditions in Chapter 2; each of the following chapters is carefully designed and sequenced to provide students with the basic principles of both research approaches. To enhance the development of essential critiquing skills, Chapter 3 provides students with the format most usually found in a published journal article; subsequent chapters are presented in the order the journal material most often appears. As each step in the research process is introduced throughout the text, step-by-step guidelines for critical evaluation of quantitative and qualitative studies guide students through specific parts of a journal article. Complete guidelines for evaluating a quantitative study are included in Appendix F and for evaluating a qualitative study are included in Appendix G. Examples of quantitative and qualitative research proposals and published research reports are also included as Appendices.

● MAIN PARTS OF THE TEXT

The text is organized into three main parts: Part I, Becoming Acquainted With Nursing Research; Part II, Applying the Research Process to Nursing Problems; and Part III, Using the Results of Research to Improve Nursing Practice.

In Chapter 1, the basic concepts related to research in general and nursing research in particular are discussed. The chapter also provides a brief overview of the historical development and future trends of nursing research in the United States. Chapter 2 presents the quantitative and qualitative traditions of scientific inquiry and Chapter 3 presents an overview of the research process and the format in which a published journal article usually appears.

In Part II, Applying the Research Process to Nursing Problems, chapters are sequenced according to the steps in the research process and in the order they most often appear in a journal article. In Chapter 4, the selection and statement of the research problem and review of relevant literature are discussed. Chapter 5 discusses research frameworks and hypotheses. Chapter 6 presents the topic of populations and sampling in relation to subject/participant selection, followed by Chapter 7 that focuses on the critical area of ethical considerations for protecting the rights of the human subjects who participate in research. Chapter 8 presents an overview of the qualitative research methods most often used by nurse researchers. Chapters 9, 10, and 11 are devoted to quantitative research: Chapter 9 discusses the quantitative research methods most frequently found in nursing literature, Chapter 10 presents quantitative data collection methods, and Chapter 11 provides a basic review of quantitative data analysis. Chapter 12 focuses on the communication and critical evaluation of quantitative and qualitative research findings, the final step in the research process.

Part III, Using the Results of Research in Nursing Practice, focuses on principles and techniques for utilizing the results of research to improve nursing practice. Chapter 13 discusses current issues regarding the utilization of research-based knowledge and provides specific techniques and activities to prepare the baccalaureate graduate to begin to participate in research utilization in the clinical setting.

● *KEY FEATURES*

- Each chapter includes an outline and student objectives for the chapter.
- Key terms are listed at the beginning of each chapter. Each key term is defined as it is introduced within the context of the material in the chapter.
- All key terms are defined in the Glossary. Students may find it useful to examine the definitions in the Glossary before reading each chapter.
- Guidelines for critical evaluation of quantitative and qualitative studies, based on the material in each chapter, are outlined and discussed. Application activities are designed to help the student to systematically critique published research.
- A summary of the main ideas is included at the end of each chapter.
- Application activities for each chapter are carefully designed to reinforce the material in the chapter.
- Suggested readings for each chapter are designed to guide students who wish to augment their knowledge.
- Appendix materials include a quantitative and a qualitative research proposal, examples of published quantitative and qualitative research reports, and comprehensive guidelines for critical evaluation of both types of research reports.

We are excited about presenting the material in this edition of our textbook and it is our sincere hope that nursing students, as well as practicing nurses, find the research arena as exciting and challenging as we have throughout the years.

P.A.D.
A.D.D.

ACKNOWLEDGMENT

Special acknowledgment and appreciation are due to Judith F. Karshmer, Professor of Nursing, and Joanne D. Hess, Associate Professor of Nursing, New Mexico State University, for their valuable suggestions during the development of the manuscript.

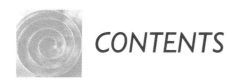

CONTENTS

CHAPTER **10**

QUANTITATIVE DATA COLLECTION   189

CHAPTER **11**

QUANTITATIVE DATA ANALYSIS   213

CHAPTER **12**

COMMUNICATING RESEARCH FINDINGS   237

PART **THREE**

USING THE RESULTS OF RESEARCH TO IMPROVE NURSING PRACTICE   249

CHAPTER **13**

UTILIZING THE RESULTS OF RESEARCH   251

APPENDICES

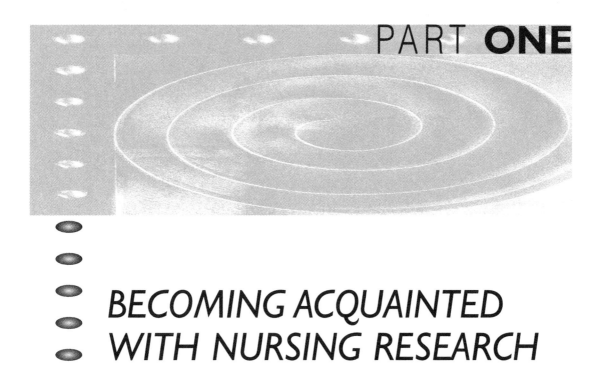

PART ONE

BECOMING ACQUAINTED WITH NURSING RESEARCH

*T*he material in Part I presents the nature of research and nursing research. In Chapter 1, the basic concepts related to research in general and nursing research in particular are discussed. The chapter also provides a brief overview of the historical development and future trends of nursing research in the United States. Chapter 2 presents the quantitative and qualitative traditions of scientific inquiry, and Chapter 3 presents an overview of the research process and the format in which a published journal article usually appears.

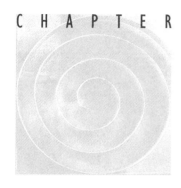

The Nature of Research and Nursing Research

OBJECTIVES   *On completion of this chapter, the student will be able to:*

1. Explain the four major characteristics of the scientific method.
2. Identify limitations of the scientific method.
3. Distinguish between basic and applied research.
4. Describe the nurse's role in research.
5. Discuss the historical development and future of nursing research.
6. Define key terms.

KEY TERMS   Applied research   Nursing research
                Basic research   Order
                Confounding variable   Phenomena
                Control   Population
                Data; datum   Research
                Deductive reasoning   Sample
                Empiricism   Science
                Generalizability   Scientific method
                Inductive reasoning   Variable

● BECOMING ACQUAINTED WITH NURSING RESEARCH

Now that you are beginning your experience with research—particularly nursing research—it is important to understand what research is and what research is not. Many people associate the word "research" with animal experiments conducted in the laboratory, the discovery of new drugs or treatments in medical science, or the many scientific experiments that have been conducted in space. In reality, however, research has many different meanings and broad applications.

● WHAT IS RESEARCH?

There are as many different views of what research is as there are writers who offer such views. We have attempted to synthesize these views and offer the following description of what research is:

> **Research** is an orderly process of inquiry that involves purposeful and systematic collection, analysis, and interpretation of **data** (units of information) to gain new knowledge or to verify already existing knowledge. Research has the ultimate goal of developing an organized body of scientific knowledge.

The purpose of research is to gain new knowledge. This new knowledge is acquired by an orderly process of inquiry during which data are purposefully and systematically collected, analyzed, and interpreted.

● HOW DOES RESEARCH DIFFER FROM OTHER WAYS OF GAINING INFORMATION?

Before further defining what research is, let us determine what it is not. Research is not going to the library to collect existing information on a specific topic and then writing a review of the material, such as in a term paper or research project. This activity, involving the reorganization or restatement of knowledge that is already known, is sometimes referred to as "search" rather than research. To be considered research, it must contribute new knowledge by providing answers to new questions, solving new problems, or verifying existing knowledge. Communicating knowledge that already exists is not considered research activity unless new questions are answered, new problems are solved, or existing knowledge is verified. Research is conducted only after an extensive examination of materials related to the proposed question or problem has been carried out. This examination determines if the answer to the question or problem is available in present knowledge. If correct answers are readily available, there may be no need for new research unless the researcher suspects an error or decides to validate the results by replicating (repeating) research that has already been conducted.

Other ways of gaining information to increase our knowledge are authority, tradition, trial and error, common sense, our own personal experience, and insight.

Much of what we do in nursing is based on authority, which means an experienced person in charge has stated, "this is the way to do it." Although this method may or may not prove to be correct, the experienced person's authority lends credence to this information. Tradition—the notion that "we've always done it this way"—has played a major role in the development of nursing. Although tradition is often used to enhance authority, always accepting the traditional way, or "bowing to tradition," can lead us to continue old methods with no attempt to evaluate and change them. Trial and error is a method of gaining information or solving a problem by trying one method and if it fails trying another method until one succeeds. Through the attempts and failures, one discovers which methods work and which do not. Using common sense simply means using one's reasoned judgment to find a solution. Personal experiences are another method of gaining information. Through our experiences, we discover methods that we usually continue to use in the future. Finally, we have all experienced insight—that "aha" feeling when we discover a solution to a problem suddenly seen in a different light. These insights occur not by reasoning, but by viewing the problem from a different perspective.

Although these are all good methods we use every day to gain information, none of them has the characteristics of research—the purposeful and systematic collection, analysis, and interpretation of data.

● WHAT ARE THE PURPOSES OF RESEARCH?

Research can be conducted for several purposes: (1) finding answers to questions or solutions to problems, (2) discovering and interpreting new facts, (3) testing theories to revise accepted theories or laws in the light of new facts, and (4) formulating new theories. Research has as its ultimate aim the systematic development and refinement of an organized body of scientific knowledge that can be used to guide academic and practice disciplines.

● *WHAT IS SCIENCE?*

Science is a unified body of systematized knowledge concerned with specific subject matter obtained by establishing and organizing facts, principles, and methods. A goal of science is to develop theories that can describe, explain, and predict phenomena and that can ultimately be used to control phenomena. **Phenomena** are facts or events known through the senses (what we observe, hear, smell, touch, or taste) rather than by thought or intuition and that can be scientifically described.

Inductive and Deductive Reasoning

In developing systematized knowledge, investigators use both inductive and deductive reasoning. **Inductive reasoning** is the logical thought process of reasoning from particular facts (specific observations) to a general conclusion or conclusions: "it is a way of thinking that is loosely described as moving from the specific to the general" (Powers & Knapp, 1995, p. 86). Inductive reasoning begins with specific observations and moves to generalizations. **Deductive reasoning** is the logical thought process of reasoning from generalizations (general conclusions) to specific conclusions: "it is a way of thinking that is loosely described as moving from the general to the specific" (Powers & Knapp, 1995, p. 40). Deductive reasoning begins with generalizations and moves to specific observations.

Consider the following example in relation to the nursing process: When you use inductive reasoning in the nursing process, your client assessment consists of gathering specific facts and observations, putting them together, then reasoning from these observations and facts to a general conclusion, the nursing diagnosis. Conversely, you use deductive reasoning when you are given a client's specific nursing diagnosis and you reason from the general conclusion that has been made about the client (the nursing diagnosis) to the specific facts that make up the nursing diagnosis.

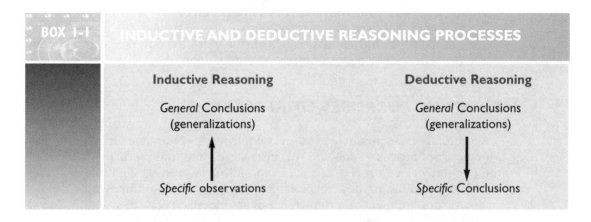

BOX 1-1   INDUCTIVE AND DEDUCTIVE REASONING PROCESSES

Inductive Reasoning	**Deductive Reasoning**
General Conclusions (generalizations)	*General* Conclusions (generalizations)
↑	↓
Specific observations	*Specific* Conclusions

● CHARACTERISTICS OF THE TRADITIONAL SCIENTIFIC METHOD

The **scientific method** is "an orderly, systematic, controlled approach to obtaining precise empirical information and testing ideas" (Doordan, 1998, p. 112). The scientific method is characterized by (1) order, (2) control, (3) empiricism, and (4) generalizability.

Order

Order means that the investigator follows a series of systematic steps that include: (1) identification of a problem to be investigated, (2) precise definition, measurement, and quantification of the phenomena related to the research problem, (3) collection and analysis of the data (information) that bears on the solution to the problem, and (4) formulation of conclusions regarding the problem being investigated. Following precise and systematic steps establishes confidence in the results of the investigation.

Control

Control of factors not relevant to the investigation is an essential requirement of the scientific method. **Control** is the process of eliminating or reducing the influence of confounding variables that could interfere with the findings of the research investigation. A **variable** is an attribute or characteristic that can have more than one value. Height, weight, hair color, and blood pressure are examples of variables. The investigator uses control measures to eliminate or reduce the influence of **confounding variables** (also termed extraneous variables or intervening variables)—variables that are outside the purpose of the study and could influence the results. For example, when investigating the relationship between the use of oral contraceptives and the occurrence of cerebrovascular accidents, the investigator must take measures to control for such confounding variables such as stress, diet, and smoking that could alter the outcome of the study.

Empiricism

Empiricism means that the evidence gathered from an investigation must be rooted in objective reality—that is, the evidence must be gathered directly or indirectly through the five human senses of sight, sound, smell, taste, and touch. Consequently, the empirical evidence resulting from a scientific investigation can be said to be based on objective reality rather than on the potential subjectivity of the researcher.

Generalizability

Generalizability, the final characteristic of the scientific method, means that the findings from a sample can be said to be representative of the entire population from which it was drawn. If the information gathered from a sample of a population can be said to be representative of the entire population from which it was drawn, the findings from the sample in a specific study can then be generalized to the entire population. Generalization requires that a specific population be delineated and that a sample be selected from this population. A **population** (N) is the total group of individual people or things meeting the designated criteria of interest to the researcher. From this designated population, a **sample** (n) is selected—that is, a smaller part of the population is selected in such a way that the individuals in the sample represent (as nearly as possible) the characteristics of the population. (Some authors prefer to use the symbol N to designate the sample and the symbol n to designate categories of the sample.)

Generalization enables an investigator to go beyond the results of the sample studied and apply the results to a broader group or population. For example, an investigator may want to investigate the effectiveness of stockinette caps on conservation of body heat in newborn infants. The population for the study was 150 infants from the newborn nursery of a private hospital. A sample of 30 of these infants was selected from this population in such a way as to ensure that they and their mothers were equivalent and normal subjects. Each infant was alternately assigned to one of two groups—those in one group wore stockinette caps and those in the other group did not. Temperatures of infants in both groups were measured at 5 minutes and 30 minutes after birth. The extent of temperature loss was recorded, and the differences in the mean (average) heat loss were reported. Findings of the study indicated no difference in the mean heat loss of babies in either group, resulting in the recommendation by the investigator that the routine use of stockinette caps to reduce heat loss in newborn infants was not warranted (Klingner, 1992).

The ultimate aim of this study was not merely to analyze the effect of stockinette caps on the 30 infants (the sample) who participated in the study, but rather to generalize these results to the entire population from which the sample was drawn. The ability to generalize permitted the investigator to formulate conclusions regarding the use of stockinette caps on the entire 150 newborn infants (the study population) and, potentially, on other newborns. The kinds of generalizations that result from such research studies contribute to the development of scientific theories, thus providing explanations and predictions of future events.

● LIMITATIONS OF THE SCIENTIFIC METHOD

The scientific method has a number of limitations involving not only the types of problems that can be investigated but also the measurement of phenomena. The scientific method cannot be used to answer moral or ethical questions such as: Should human cloning be practiced? Should assisted suicide be legal? As of yet, there are no precise measures of such psychological phenomena as anger and anxiety.

Other limitations include the ethical constraints that must be employed to protect the rights of subjects participating in research studies. Such ethical constraints often preclude the use of the scientific method to investigate certain problems. For example, it is not ethically acceptable to study the effect of a new drug by giving it to some people and withholding it from others if the drug has been shown to be necessary to sustain life. Ethical considerations for the protection of human subjects in research are discussed in Chapter 7.

⬤ THE QUANTITATIVE AND QUALITATIVE RESEARCH TRADITIONS

The characteristics of the scientific method (order, tight controls, empiricism, the ability to generalize findings and objectivity) are most often associated with the quantitative research tradition. Interpretation of the subjective meanings that individuals give to their own unique human experiences is the focus of investigators who employ the qualitative research tradition. These research traditions are discussed in the next chapter.

⬤ WHAT IS NURSING RESEARCH?

Nursing research is research that is conducted to answer questions or to find solutions to problems that fall within the specific domain of nursing—that is,

> The diagnosis and treatment of human responses to actual or potential health problems . . . The nursing profession remains committed to the care and nurturing of both healthy and ill people, individually or in groups and communities. *(American Nurses Association, 1995, p. 6)*

Nursing research focuses not only on the discipline of nursing but also on issues facing nurses themselves. It includes investigations of nursing practice, nursing education, and nursing administration.

The purpose of nursing research is "to test, refine, and advance the knowledge on which improved education, clinical judgment, and cost-effective, safe, ethical nursing care rest" (American Association of Colleges of Nursing, 1997, p. 1). Nursing research is conducted to develop and expand the organized body of scientific knowledge that is unique to the phenomena that are central to the discipline of nursing:

> Nursing science is a whole that is continuously changing through knowledge generation and research. The distinct nature of this knowledge has significant implications for nursing practice and in its contribution to the larger community of science. Nursing science-based practice is the imaginative and cre-

ative use of nursing knowledge to promote the health and well-being of all people. *(Barrett, 1997, p. 12)*

The ultimate goal of expanding the scientific knowledge base of nursing through research is to provide a scientific foundation for the delivery of optimal patient care: "Research-based practice is essential if the nursing profession is to meet its mandate to society for effective and efficient patient care" (American Nurses Association, 1994, p. 1).

BASIC AND APPLIED RESEARCH IN NURSING

Research may be classified by purpose—that is, as either basic research or applied research. This classification reflects the degree to which the findings can be applied to practical problems in the everyday world. **Basic research** (also called pure research) is primarily concerned with establishing new knowledge and with the development or refinement of theories. The findings of basic research may not be immediately applicable to practical problems, but they do provide a foundation of scientific knowledge for building further research. **Applied research** is also concerned with establishing new knowledge but is further concerned with deriving knowledge that can be immediately applied to solve practical problems directly related to clinical practice. Applied research has been referred to as "practical application of the theoretical."

An example of basic research that could contribute to nursing knowledge is the investigation conducted by McCarthy (1997). The purpose of this study was to determine if hypophagic tumor-bearing rats would alter their food intake in the same way as normal healthy rats when housed at a temperature below their thermoneutral zone and when anorexia was mediated by substances secreted by activated white blood cells. The results of the study indicated that physiologic responses affecting short-term food intake were intact in the 24 hypophagic tumor-bearing rats that were studied. Although the results of this basic research study cannot be immediately applied to clinical practice, they could provide the basis for further understanding of the physiologic processes involved in human tumor-based anorexia, providing a foundation for investigating such specific problems as weight loss and anorexia in caring for cancer patients.

The results of the applied research study "The Effect of a Social Support Boosting Intervention on Stress, Coping, and Social Support in Caregivers of Children With HIV/AIDS" (reprinted in Appendix C) provide an example of research that has the potential for application in specific practice settings. The results of the study indicated that seronegative caregivers participating in a social support boosting intervention showed substantially increased coping abilities. Nursing implications for the study "are to incorporate the social support network of the caregiver in the plan of care and recognize the complexity of the needs of the AIDS caregiver."

The distinction between basic and applied research often is not as clear-cut as we have described. Sometimes the results of basic research studies can be applied in a practical setting, and applied research studies can provide theoretical implications that may serve as the focus for basic research. The majority of research studies conducted in nursing have been applied research.

WHY SHOULD NURSES LEARN ABOUT RESEARCH?

One characteristic of a professional group is that it has a unique body of knowledge and skill. It is generally agreed that nursing is still in the process of defining what constitutes its unique body of knowledge and skill. Thus, it is important to encourage nursing research and to direct efforts toward the systematic investigation of questions related to the practice and profession of nursing. The guidelines for nursing research prepared by the American Nurses Association Cabinet on Nursing Research in 1985 remain timely today in establishing the role of research in improving nursing practice into the 21st century:

> The future of nursing practice and, ultimately, the future of health care in this country depend on nursing research designed to constantly generate an up-to-date, organized body of nursing knowledge. Society and its approach to health care are experiencing rapid change. . . . Thus, nursing research needs to proceed in orderly directions, generating knowledge built on previous information in order to provide the foundation for nursing education and practice in the twenty-first century. *(American Nurses Association, 1985)*

If nursing is to develop an organized body of scientific knowledge, there are several ways in which you as a nurse can participate:

1. Learn to evaluate nursing literature critically—this means developing the ability to read nursing literature critically as a means of discovering gaps in knowledge and evaluating the findings of research studies. This is such an important goal that throughout this text we present the principles and techniques of critical evaluation.
2. Learn how valid research results can be applied to nursing practice, and develop ideas about how scientific knowledge can be used in caring for patients. (The process of using research results for research-based nursing practice is discussed in Chap. 13.)
3. Begin to generate hunches and pose questions that could form the basis for future research.
4. Become involved in a research investigation that has the potential to contribute to new knowledge.

The American Nurses Association Council of Nurse Researchers in 1994 specifically defined elements of competence in research that are appropriate to nurses prepared in the various nursing education programs at the associate degree, baccalaureate, master's, doctoral, and postdoctoral levels:

> Nurses are responsible for assuming various research activities and roles as appropriate to their education. However, preparation for research is an evolving process along a continuum of learning. Only through the research contributions will the profession meet its mandate to society. *(American Nurses Association, 1994, p. 1)*

At the baccalaureate level, nurses are prepared to read research critically and to evaluate existing research to determine its readiness for use in clinical practice. Baccalaureate-prepared nurses are also prepared to understand the ethical principles involved in protecting the rights of human subjects and other ethical responsibilities incumbent on investigators. Education for research at the baccalaureate level also prepares nurses to participate in research activities by identifying clinical problems to be investigated, assisting experienced investigators to gain access to clinical sites, influencing the selection of appropriate methods of data collection, and collecting data and implementing nursing research findings. Finally, before mutual agreement to participate in data collection or other aspects of research, baccalaureate-level nurses are prepared to understand the research protocols of other disciplines (American Nurses Association, 1994, pp. 1-2).

● NURSING RESEARCH OVER THE YEARS

Although the emphasis on research in nursing has become a relatively strong movement only within the past 35 to 40 years, historically, nursing research has been emerging over a period of more than 100 years. The next section provides a brief overview of the historical development of nursing research in the United States.

When Florence Nightingale established her system of nursing and nursing education at the Nightingale School of Nursing in 1860, well over 100 years ago, she envisioned the development of a scholarly, humane, and scientific discipline. She used scientific inquiry, making use of her detailed records to formulate ideas for improving nursing and health care. She encouraged nurses to develop the habit of sound observation:

> In dwelling upon the vital importance of **sound** observation, it must never be lost sight of what observation is for. It is not for the sake of piling up miscellaneous information or curious facts, but for the sake of saving life and increasing health and comfort. *(Nightingale, 1859, p. 70* [emphasis in original])

If nursing education in the United States had followed the principles to which Florence Nightingale was dedicated, nursing research might have progressed more rapidly. However, nursing has continued to search for a specialized body of nursing knowledge throughout most of the 20th century.

The Years From 1900 to 1950

From about 1900 to 1946, nurses were "educated predominately in hospital-based programs in apprentice-type settings" (Abdellah & Levine, 1994, p. 3). In these hospital-based education programs, the emphasis was on nursing service provided by the students. Nurses learned as they cared primarily for sick individuals in hospitals and meticulously carried out the orders of authority figures, usually physicians. Because at that time most leaders in nursing had advanced preparation in the field of education, their research studies focused primarily on education for nursing rather than on the practice of nursing. The majority of these studies were concerned with the characteristics of the nursing students themselves as well as with their educational preparation.

Nursing literature from 1900 to 1950 does reflect nurses' concern for patient care. Articles were written by nurses about the care of patients with communicable diseases, hygiene and sanitation, asepsis, and high maternal and infant death rates. The first case studies appeared in the *American Journal of Nursing* in the 1920s. They were used as teaching tools for students as well as patient progress records to improve patient care.

By 1930, nursing literature began to reflect the need to distinguish nursing orders from medical orders and to evaluate the effectiveness of nursing procedures. During this period, the writers of articles began to express the need for student nurses to be relieved of excessive nursing service duties to benefit fully from their educational programs. In the late 1940s, after World War II, the concept of nursing expanded, reflecting the work of public health nurses. Nursing care began to expand from its focus on care of the hospitalized patient to include the care of the patient and family in a variety of settings, in cooperation with physicians and other health professionals, and the prevention of illness and the promotion of health. An awareness grew of the need for nurses to acquire knowledge of the social, behavioral, and natural sciences, as well as the humanities, to care for patients and their families.

The Years From 1950 to 1970

In the 1950s, recognition of the need to prepare nurses at the graduate level for leadership positions, advanced practice, and research contributed to the advancement of nursing research. To communicate the growing body of nursing research, the first issue of *Nursing Research* was published in 1952. *Nursing Research* continues to serve as an important resource devoted to the issues and problems associated with nursing research and to the publication of nursing research studies. In 1955, the American Nurses Association established the American Nurses Foundation, which supports and promotes research in nursing.

Nurses writing since the 1950s have reflected ideas about the conceptual development of nursing, nursing as a science, and the educational preparation needed for nurses to conduct research. From 1955 to 1965, researchers focused on student characteristics, selection and retention of students, and the educational process. Articles dealing with the quality of patient care began to appear in the literature. Research studies focused on long-term care and rehabilitation of patients and on problems of patients with chronic diseases such as heart disease, cancer, and strokes. Hospitals began to report experiences with intensive care and automation.

Before the 1970s, *Nursing Research* was the only major publication devoted to communicating the results of nursing research studies. Since that time, research reports and articles representing perspectives on the development of nursing as a science have been included in such journals as the *Western Journal of Nursing Research, Research in Nursing and Health, Advances in Nursing Science, Nursing Science Quarterly*, and *Scholarly Inquiry for Nursing Practice*.

The Years From 1970 to 1990

In 1970, the National Commission for the Study of Nursing and Nursing Education, funded by the American Nurses Association and additional private sources, published the findings of its independent investigation of the quality of nursing in the United States. The commission reported that nursing presented an "impoverished figure" in terms of research capacity and support (National Commission for the Study of Nursing and Nursing Education, 1970, p. 21). There was very little public or private funding for nursing research, and fewer than 500 U.S. nurses held earned doctoral degrees, the generally accepted level for research competence. Many of these had been prepared for educational administration or teaching, because there were almost no doctoral programs with specific preparation for research into clinical nursing practice or nursing intervention (Lysaught, 1981, p. 59). Thus, little research had been done on the actual effects of nursing intervention and care. The Commission summed up how this lack of research had hurt nursing practice:

> Lack of research leaves us without a body of facts or a set of probabilities to guide or assess the nursing care of a patient. Of necessity, nursing practice today consists of stereotyped techniques sprinkled liberally with personal idiosyncrasy. . . . Since we have not developed valid means for assessing the effects of varied interventions, it is almost impossible to define optimum nursing care. *(National Commission for the Study of Nursing and Nursing Education, 1970, p. 84)*

The Commission emphasized that nursing was still more of an art than a science. Nurse-patient interactions continued to be characterized by a combination of individual judgment, concern for the patient, and supportive care, rather than with procedures based on validated scientific knowledge. However, with the increased amount and complexity of knowledge concerning human health and response to illness, the art of nursing was no longer sufficient to ensure optimal patient care: "The aim of research should be to elevate the practice of nursing—not art **or** science, but art **and** science are needed to ensure the highest levels of humane and capable care" (National Commission for the Study of Nursing and Nursing Education, 1970, p. 125 [emphasis in original]).

By 1981, some of the recommendations of the Commission had been implemented. The 1981 Commission report optimistically predicted that the increase in the number of doctoral programs in nursing since the initiation of the National Commission's study should provide for a greater supply of nurses with "investigative skills for conceptual and theoretical inquiry into nursing that will extend the scientific base of all nursing practice" (Lysaught, 1981, p. 64). The report also pointed out the "dramatic increase" in federal funding for nursing research, generally related to the levels recommended in the Commission's 1970 report. However, the report noted that these funds "have often been used as pawns in political maneuvering, and the result is that planning and execution of research have often suffered through the vagaries of administrative and legislative battling" (Lysaught, 1981, p. 63).

In 1976 and 1981, and again in 1985, the American Nurses Association developed a statement of priorities for research in nursing, designed to guide nurse researchers in the study of areas of nursing that were crucial to the scientific advancement of the nursing profession.

In 1986, the National Center for Nursing Research was established as a part of the National Institutes of Health (NIH). The NIH is the nation's and the world's largest sponsor of biomedical research that supports both basic and clinical biomedical investigations. As a result, nursing research made a dramatic advance into the mainstream of health care science. Dr. Ada Sue Hinshaw summarized this historical milestone for nursing in remarks at her swearing-in ceremony as its first director:

> The establishment of the National Center for Nursing Research (NCNR) on April 18, 1986, by Secretary Bowen was an historic moment for the nursing profession. It provides a focal point from which to stimulate and facilitate the generation and testing of scientific knowledge to guide the practice of one of the country's largest health care professions. . . . The National Center's union with the National Institutes of Health is particularly significant for it brings nursing research into the mainstream of health care science. It allows for nursing research to be developed/conducted in collaboration with the other scientific disciplines in a complementary manner. . . . In turn, knowledge from nursing research can and will be incorporated in the broader base of health care science as a result of being developed and tested within this collaborative interdisciplinary environment. *(American Association of Colleges of Nursing, 1987, p. 1)*

The 1990s and Beyond 2000

In 1993, the National Center for Nursing Research was granted Institute status, becoming the National Institute of Nursing Research (NINR). As an institute within NIH, the NINR continues to support clinical and basic research, with the goal of establishing a scientific basis for the care of individuals across the lifespan—from management of patients during illness and recovery to the reduction of risks for disease and disability and the promotion of healthy lifestyles (National Institute of Nursing Research, 1997).

There have been major expansions in research related to clinical practice and growing concerns about ethical practices and the protection of human subjects. Nurses are increasingly studying nursing. They see an urgent need to investigate the organization and delivery of nursing care to patients. Predictions for the direction of nursing research into the 21st century indicate an increased concentration on both quantitative and qualitative research designed to investigate clinical nursing practice in all settings, more studies designed to validate already existing studies, continued evolution of nursing theories, more organizational activities to increase the use of research results in practice, and significant progress toward the goal of expanding the scientific knowledge base of nursing to provide a scientific basis for delivering optimal patient care.

● SUMMARY

Research is an orderly process of inquiry that involves purposeful and systematic collection, analysis, and interpretation of data (units of information) to gain new knowledge or to verify already existing knowledge.

Science not only is a unified body of knowledge concerned with specific subject matter but is also concerned with deriving systematized knowledge by establishing and organizing facts, principles, and methods about the subject matter of a discipline.

Scientists use either inductive reasoning (reasoning from particular facts [specific observations] to a conclusion) or deductive reasoning (reasoning from generalizations [general conclusions] to specific conclusions). The scientific method is characterized by order, control, empiricism, and generalizability.

Nursing research is research that is conducted to answer questions or to find solutions to problems that fall within the specific domain of nursing. Nurse researchers may conduct two types of research: basic research (also called pure research), primarily concerned with establishing new knowledge and with the development or refinement of theories, or applied research, which is concerned with establishing new knowledge and also knowledge that can be applied in practical settings without undue delay.

Nursing research has evolved over the past 100 years from focusing primarily on nursing education to developing a scientific knowledge base for the practice of nursing, with the goal of providing optimal patient care. The following application activities will help you evaluate your understanding of this material.

REFERENCES

Abdellah, F., & Levine, E. (1994). *Preparing nursing research for the 21st century.* New York: Springer.

Alligood, M. R., & Marriner-Tomey, A. (Eds.). (1996). *Nursing theory: Utilization and application.* St. Louis: Mosby.

American Association of Colleges of Nursing. (1987). *AACN Newsletter,* 13.

American Nurses Association Cabinet on Nursing Research. (1985). *Directions for nursing research: Toward the twenty-first century.* Kansas City: Author.

American Nurses Association. (1994). *Position statement on education for participation in nursing research.* Washington, DC: Author.

American Nurses Association. (1995). *Nursing's social policy statement.* Washington, DC: Author.

Barrett, E. (1997). What is nursing science? An international dialogue. *Nursing Science Quarterly, 10*(1), 10–12.

Doordan, A. M. (1998). *Research survival guide.* Philadelphia: Lippincott-Raven.

Klingner, S. J. (1992). The effect of stockinette caps on conservation of body heat in newborn infants. In P. Dempsey & A. Dempsey, *Nursing research with basic statistical applications* (3rd ed., pp. 227–243). Boston: Jones & Bartlett.

Lysaught, J. (1981). *Action in affirmation: Toward an unambiguous profession of nursing.* New York: McGraw-Hill.

Marriner-Tomey, A., & Alligood, M. R. (1998). *Nursing theorists and their work* (4th ed.). St. Louis: Mosby.

McCarthy, D. O. (1997). Short-term regulation of energy intake is intact in hypophagic tumor-bearing rats. *Research in Nursing and Health, 20,* 425–429.

National Commission for the Study of Nursing and Nursing Education. (1970). *An abstract for action.* New York: McGraw-Hill.

National Institute of Nursing Research. (1997). *Mission statement.* Washington, DC: Author.

Nightingale, F. (1859). *Notes on nursing.* Philadelphia: Lippincott.

Powers, B. A., & Knapp, T. R. (1995). *A dictionary of nursing theory and research* (2nd ed.). Thousand Oaks, CA: Sage.

BIBLIOGRAPHY AND SUGGESTED READINGS

D'Antonio, P. (1997). Toward a history of research in nursing, *Nursing Research, 46*(2), 105–110.

Kuhse, H. (1997). *Caring: Nurses, women and ethics.* Oxford: Blackwell.

Lusk, B. (1997). What values drive nursing science? *Reflections, 23*(3), 46–47.

Philips, J. R. (1996). What constitutes nursing science? *Nursing Science Quarterly, 9*(2), 48–49.

APPLICATION ACTIVITIES

1. List as many words as you can think of that describe the term "research."

2. Explain in your own words the difference between inductive reasoning and deductive reasoning.

3. Explain the relationship between a population and a sample.

4. Define the following terms in relation to the scientific method:

   a. Generalizability

   b. Empiricism

   c. Control

   d. Order

5. Define nursing research as you now understand it.

6. Locate a published article that is a report of a research study that interests you. Because not every article is a research article in the strictest sense, look for an article that has the following parts:

   a. Title (often long; usually identifies the research content)

   b. Author's name and affiliation

   c. Abstract (a short summary at the beginning of the article)

   d. Introduction and background

   e. Method or Methodology (discusses how the research was conducted)

   f. Results or Findings (reports what the study found)

   g. Discussion (interpretation of the results)

   h. References

   If you are not sure that you have found a research article, check with your instructor.

7. Using the above article, discuss how it fulfills the following criteria of research:

   a. The study is an orderly process of inquiry.

   b. The study involves purposeful and systematic collection of data.

   c. The study involves purposeful and systematic analysis and interpretation of data analysis.

    d. The study was designed to gain new knowledge (or to validate knowledge that already exists).

    e. The results of the study have the potential to contribute to an organized body of scientific knowledge.

8. What potential does the above study have for contributing to more scientifically based nursing practice?

9. Classify the above study by research purpose. Is it basic research or applied research? Why?

10. List at least three patient care problems that you believe could be researched from a nursing focus.

11. It has been stated that nurses should conduct their own research into the practice and profession of nursing. Do you agree or disagree with this statement? Justify your answer.

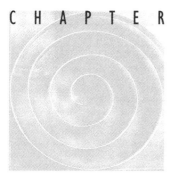

2

The Quantitative and Qualitative Traditions of Scientific Inquiry

OBJECTIVES   *On completion of this chapter, the student will be able to:*

1. Discuss philosophical approaches to nursing research and the nature of paradigms.
2. Discuss the philosophical assumptions of the positivist and naturalistic paradigms.
3. Describe the nature of quantitative and qualitative research.
4. Compare the major characteristics of quantitative and qualitative research.
5. Discuss limitations of the quantitative and qualitative approaches.
6. Define key terms.

KEY TERMS

Continuous data	Qualitative research
Dependent variable	Quantitative data
Discrete data	Quantitative research
Independent variable	Reliability
Naturalistic paradigm	Replication
Paradigm	Triangulation
Positivist paradigm	Validity
Qualitative data	

*I*n the previous chapter, the nature of science and scientific inquiry and the need for a scientific knowledge base in nursing were presented. This chapter examines the nature and function of the two major paradigms in nursing research: the positivist paradigm, associated with the quantitative research approach, and the naturalistic paradigm, associated with the qualitative research approach.

● PHILOSOPHICAL APPROACHES TO NURSING RESEARCH: THE NATURE OF PARADIGMS

In conducting scientific inquiry, the investigator is guided by the philosophical assumptions, goals, and purposes of a particular mode of inquiry known as a research paradigm. The term **paradigm** is sometimes used interchangeably with the term model. A paradigm is "similar to an action plan that describes work to be done in a discipline and frames an orientation within which the work will be accomplished" (Powers & Knapp, 1995, p. 118). A paradigm can be formally defined as "a way of looking at the world or a perspective on phenomena that presents a set of interrelated philosophical assumptions about the world. The perspective guides research and practice" (Doordan, 1998, p. 91). A paradigm has certain underlying basic assumptions that guide the inquiry (an assumption is a statement whose correctness or validity is taken for granted):

> The ontologic assumption asks the philosophical question, "What is the nature of reality?"
> The epistemologic assumption asks the question, "What is the relationship of the researcher to that being researched?"
> The axiologic assumption asks the question, "What is the role of values in the inquiry?"
> The rhetorical assumption asks the question, "What is the language of research?"

The methodologic assumption asks the question, "What is the process for the research?"

The answers that are given to these philosophical questions, as sets, provide the basic belief systems, the paradigms, for scientific inquiry: "they are the starting points or givens that determine what inquiry is and how it is to be practiced" (Guba, 1990, p. 18).

● MAJOR RESEARCH PARADIGMS

The two major paradigms for scientific inquiry in nursing are the positivist paradigm and the naturalistic paradigm. Each paradigm has "different philosophic premises, purposes, and epistemic roots that must be understood, respected, and maintained for credible and sound research outcomes" (Morse, 1994, p. 101).

The **positivist paradigm** (also termed the positivist-empiricist paradigm) traces its roots to the early 19th-century philosophical position of positivism: "a family of philosophies characterized by an extremely positive evaluation of science and scientific method" (Lincoln & Guba, 1985, p. 19). The paradigm embodies the traditional scientific method in its approach to research—that is, a scientific objective view of the world, "which assumes that reality can be objectively measured and observed, independent of historical, social, or cultural contexts" (Doordan, 1998, p. 95). In other words, there is a fixed objective reality "out there," and knowledge is considered reliable because it is objectively derived by the inquirer who does not bring personal values or subjectivity to the inquiry.

Another paradigm, the **naturalistic paradigm**, began as a countermovement to the positivist paradigm in the late 19th century. In this paradigm, "truth is seen as dynamic and seen in real historical, social, and cultural contexts" (Doordan, 1998, p. 84). In this perspective, the reality "out there" is subjective as mentally constructed by individuals. Findings of the inquiry are the result of the interaction between the inquirer and those being researched, and the researcher acknowledges that subjectivity and values are an inevitable result of the inquiry process.

● PHILOSOPHICAL ASSUMPTIONS OF THE POSITIVIST AND NATURALISTIC PARADIGMS

The Positivist Paradigm

In the positivist paradigm of inquiry, reality is seen as existing; the real world "out there" is driven by natural causes; reality is singular, objective, and apart from the researcher. "Reality is fragmentable into independent variables and processes, any of which can be studied independently of the others" (Lincoln & Guba, 1985, p. 37). This is the ontologic assumption. The researcher functions independently from that being researched and does nothing to influence the findings of the inquiry. This is the epistemologic assumption. Because objectivity is sought, values are to be held in check; the inquiry is value-free and unbiased (the axiologic assumption). In terms of the language of the inquiry (the rhetorical assumption), the researcher writes in a formal style and uses quantitative terms such as objectivity, cause-and-effect relationships, and generalization. Definitions are formulated at the beginning of the study and remain set throughout the study. The process for the research (the methodologic assumption) is by deductive reasoning. Discrete concepts are isolated and defined before the study. The research is characterized by a static design in that categories are isolated before the study; the inquiry is context-free—that is, the researcher keeps tight controls over the variables in the setting. The inquiry elicits primarily **quantitative data**—in other words, data characterized by numbers that are analyzed by statistical techniques. Finally, in the positivist tradition, the aim of the inquiry is to seek generalizations—that is, to extend the findings beyond the specific setting of the study.

The Naturalistic Paradigm

In the naturalistic paradigm of inquiry, reality is multiple and subjective as seen by the participants in the study; these constructed realities "can be studied only holistically" (Lincoln & Guba, 1985, p. 37). This is the ontologic assumption. The researcher interacts with that being researched, and it is this interaction process that creates the findings. This is the epistemologic assumption. The inquiry is subjective and value-laden; the researcher acknowledges the presence of values and biases as an inevitable result of the process (the axiologic assumption). In terms of the language of the inquiry, the researcher writes in a literary, informal style, using such qualitative terms as understanding, discovery, and meaning. Rather than defining the key terms before the study, the definitions may evolve during the course of the study. The process of the inquiry (the methodologic assumption) is by induction, and the emphasis is holistic—that is, on the entire phenomena as they emerge during the investigation. The inquiry is context-bound; the topic is studied within its setting. Rather than having a fixed design before the study, emphasis is on the emerging design; categories are identified during the inquiry process. The investigation elicits narrative information (words) that are analyzed for meaning. Rather than seeking generalizations, as in the positivist paradigm, the naturalistic paradigm seeks patterns within the specific setting.

Table 2-1 summarizes the philosophical assumptions of each of these paradigms. Because they come from different philosophical perspectives, the particular paradigm employed directs the entire process of the inquiry. The positivist paradigm is most often associated with quantitative research; the naturalistic paradigm is most often associated with qualitative research.

TABLE 2-1 *Philosophical Assumptions of the Positivist and Naturalistic Paradigms*

ASSUMPTION/ QUESTION	POSITIVIST PARADIGM	NATURALISTIC PARADIGM
• Ontologic/What is the nature of reality?	Reality exists: it is a single tangible reality, objective and apart from the researcher.	Reality is subjective, as constructed by the study participants.
• Epistemologic/What is the relationship of the researcher to what is being researched	Researcher is independent from what is being researched and does not influence the findings.	Researcher interacts with what is being researched; the interaction process creates the findings.
• Axiologic/What is the role of values in the inquiry	Inquiry is value-free and unbiased; objectivity is sought.	Inquiry is subjective and value-laden; researcher acknowledges that values and biases are present.
• Rhetorical/What is the language of the research?	Researcher writes in a formal style, using quantitative terminology. Definitions are set at the beginning of the study.	Researcher writes in a literary, informal style, using qualitative terminology. Definitions evolve during course of study.
• Methodologic/What is the process for the research?	Deductive reasoning processes	Inductive reasoning processes
	Focus in on specific, discrete concepts isolated before the inquiry.	Holistic; focus is on entire phenomena as they emerge during the inquiry.
	Context-free; tight controls over context (setting)	Context-bound; topic studied within its context (setting)
	Emphasis on fixed design	Emphasis is on emerging design; categories are identified during the inquiry process.
	Elicits primarily quantitative (numeric) information; numeric data analyzed by statistical procedures and techniques	Elicits primarily qualitative (narrative) information; narrative data are organized into categories/ themes and analyzed for meaning.
	Seeks generalizations	Seeks patterns within the specific setting

Sources: Creswell (1998); Lincoln & Guba (1985).

● THE NATURE OF QUANTITATIVE AND QUALITATIVE RESEARCH

Quantitative Research

Traditionally, **quantitative research** has been associated with the scientific method of inquiry, thus having the characteristics of the scientific method discussed in the previous chapter—order, control, empiricism, and generalization. In quantitative research, the study variables are preselected and defined by the investigator and the data are collected, quantified (translated into numbers), and then statistically analyzed, often with a view to establishing cause-and-effect relationships among the variables. The quantitative approach to research has its roots in the tradition of the "hard" or mathematically based sciences and reflects the rigor of the scientific research most often associated with such fields as physics and chemistry. The use of quantitative methodology for investigating human behavior has been most often associated with the disciplines of psychology and sociology.

Qualitative Research

In **qualitative research**, the investigator seeks to identify the qualitative (non-numeric) aspects of the phenomenon under study from the participant's viewpoint to understand the meaning of the totality of the phenomenon. Usually conducted in the natural setting, the in-depth narrative data "provide information about the subjective meaning of human experiences and phenomena" (Doordan, 1998, p. 101). Qualitative research has been associated with the social sciences and humanities. The use of qualitative methodology for investigating human behavior is frequently associated with the discipline of cultural (or social) anthropology.

DEVELOPMENT OF QUALITATIVE RESEARCH

Until the early 1960s, all of nursing research was quantitative research. The first qualitative studies in nursing appeared in the early 1960s, at the same time that the term "qualitative research" first appeared in the social science research literature (Abdellah & Levine, 1994). Up to that time, nursing research had been quantitative: "Even when these methods have failed to be as valid and reliable in nursing and other human sciences as they have been in the natural sciences, researchers in nursing have clung to them, feeling that their only claim to the title of scientist lay in the quantitative methods" (Omery, 1983, p. 62).

Although there is no doubt that the quantitative methods have resulted in significant contributions to understanding many of the phenomena in nursing, a growing number of nurse researchers are using the qualitative methods in their belief that the traditional scientific method imposes constraints on the study of humans:

> The (scientific) method's inherent nature . . . reduces the human being under study to an object with many small quantitative units . . . (and) gives no clue as to how to fit these small units back into the dynamic whole that is the living human being with whom the nurse interacts in practice. *(Omery, 1983, p. 62)*

Currently, although the majority of nursing studies continue to be quantitative, "with the advent of qualitative studies, a wealth of new and valuable insights has been generated, and more nurses are committed to knowing and understanding the use of qualitative research methods" (Morse, 1994, p. 100).

Quantitative and qualitative methods complement each other, and both approaches are needed to address the complex research problems of nursing. Because "the phenomena of interest to nursing include quantifiable and non-quantifiable, experiential phenomena, the discipline of nursing also embraces both quantitative and qualitative research" (Omery et al., 1995, p. 8). "The trend in the use of qualitative research in nursing appears to be upward, and the forecast for the 21st century is for continued and increasing usage" (Abdellah & Levine, 1994, p. 44).

QUANTITATIVE RESEARCH: AN OVERVIEW

Quantitative research can be described as a formal process of inquiry characterized by objectivity, tight controls over the research situation, the precise measurement and quantification of data, and the ability to generalize. Quantitative research methodology rests on the basic assumption that all of the traits or characteristics that make up the units of both human and non-human organisms, as well as nonliving objects, exist in some degree and can be measured objectively. In some cases there may be no trace of the trait or characteristic; in other cases there may be a small, moderate, or great amount of the characteristic. Because terms such as small, moderate, and great are too scientifically imprecise to be particularly useful in the quantification of data, the quantitative researcher establishes a numeric scale to determine the amount of the trait or characteristic that is present. For example, a researcher wishing to measure the amount of nicotine in an individual's blood serum might draw a sample of blood and subject the blood to analysis. There should be no nicotine in the blood of a nonsmoker; this level can be called the zero level. As the presence of nicotine is measured in moderate and heavy smokers, the researcher would then be able to establish a strict numeric scale that would quantify the amount of nicotine in the blood. Similarly, the blood-alcohol tests used by law-enforcement agencies provide numeric methods for determining if an individual is intoxicated as defined by the laws of a state.

The Nature of Variables

In accord with the scientific method discussed in the first chapter, the quantitative method requires that the research investigation be planned and carried out in a prespecified and systematic manner. The problem statement and the design of the research must be specific and detailed and set out before conducting the investigation. Preselected variables must be identified and described. In the previous chapter, a variable was defined as an attribute or characteristic that can have more than one value. In experimental research design, the **independent variable** is the variable that is purposely manipulated or changed by the researcher. When the independent variable is manipulated, the researcher proposes to examine the effect of this manipulation on the dependent variable or variables. The **dependent variable**, then, can be defined as the variable that changes as a result of the manipulation of the independent variable. For example, in the experimental study in Appendix C, the researchers proposed to determine the effect of a social support boosting intervention in caregivers of children with HIV. To manipulate the independent variable (social support boosting intervention), the researchers divided the study subjects into two groups—those who received the social support boosting intervention and those who did not. Their purpose was to examine the effect of the intervention on the group receiving the intervention (the experimental group) compared to those who did not receive the intervention. In this study, the effects of the intervention constitute the dependent variables; stress, coping, and social support were then measured.

Measurement and Quantification

Quantitative research also requires that there be precise definition, measurement, and quantification of the phenomena related to the research problem. In designing quantitative research, precisely developed instruments are used to measure the variables. These instruments must be both valid and reliable. The **validity** of a measuring instrument refers to its ability to measure what is purports to measure. The term **reliability** refers to the stability and consistency of a measuring instrument over time—that is, how well it will produce the same information each time it is used. For example, a scale is a valid instrument for measuring weight; a ruler is not. If the scale is reliable, you would expect it to have the same reading over time.

Quantitative research is characterized by the collection of quantitative (numeric) data. **Continuous data** can be located at some point along a continuum or scale and are characterized by fractional values of a whole unit. For example, 98.6° F, the traditional average body temperature, is a point on the Fahrenheit scale used to measure body temperature. **Discrete data**, in contrast, exist only in distinct units expressed as whole numbers that are precise and definite: six beds, five hospitals, six patients (not 6.5 beds, 5.66 hospitals, 6.25 patients).

Numeric measurement and quantification are characteristics that allow the quantitative researcher to be objective about the research. Such objectivity allows the researcher to be "outside" the research; that is, the researcher is not emotionally involved with the subjects of the research. Because the data gathered during the research are based on empirical evidence—that is, rooted in objective reality—the researcher is unbiased in the interpretation of the results.

Establishing Cause-and-Effect Relationships

Quantitative researchers who want to understand the how and why of events may seek to establish cause-and-effect relationships between the preselected study variables. If an outcome or outcomes can be predicted based on the investigation, then measures can be taken to control the outcome. The structure of the process becomes an if/then statement: for example, *if* a person is a heavy cigarette smoker, *then* can we predict that he or she has a higher risk of developing lung cancer than a person who is not a heavy cigarette smoker? If this is indeed a cause-and-effect relationship, lung cancer should then be controlled by stopping or significantly reducing smoking behavior.

The determination of cause-and-effect relationships between study variable requires manipulation of the independent variable(s) through experimentation with careful attention to confounding variables that may influence the outcome of the study. These ideas are discussed in greater detail in later chapters.

A further characteristic of the scientific method is generalization. Many quantitative research studies are conducted with the purpose of generalizing the results—that is, using the results from the study sample to draw conclusions about the larger population from which the sample was drawn. This requires that the design of the study and the statistical analysis of the data conform to the strict requirements for generalization that will be discussed in more detail in a later chapter.

Experimentation is not the only quantitative research strategy employed by quantitative researchers. Other strategies that will be discussed in a later chapter include quasi-experimental research (experiments that cannot be carried out with the rigor of true experiments); nonexperimental research, such as correlational research (that measures relationships); ex post facto research (analyzing events that have already occurred); and descriptive research (describing the characteristics of phenomena).

A major concern of quantitative researchers is replicability or repeatability. The term **replication** means repeating a study, using the same methods, to determine if the results will be the same as or similar to those of the original study. When a researcher obtains certain results, can another researcher use the same procedures and obtain the same or similar results? True quantitative research demands that the research be able to be replicated by other researchers and that such replication will yield the same or very similar results.

● QUALITATIVE RESEARCH: AN OVERVIEW

Qualitative research can be described as a formal process of inquiry, often conducted within a natural setting and characterized by a flexible, emerging design and the collection of primarily narrative data that provides insight and understanding of the meaning of phenomena from the participant's perspective.

Qualitative research has several distinct characteristics that can be contrasted with quantitative methods. Whereas quantitative researchers generally have only minimal contact with the subjects of the study, qualitative researchers frequently use themselves as the data-gathering instrument. This means that rather than using precisely developed data-gathering tools and instruments to gather data about their subjects' knowledge, interests, and backgrounds, qualitative researchers may spend long periods of time with the participants of their study, observing and recording their behaviors and interactions. The researcher keeps detailed notes about events that have been observed, interviews that have been carried out, and other salient facts that might have a bearing on the study. Because of the nature of qualitative research, the investigator gathers data in the setting where the activities are taking place.

In view of the potential mass of data that can be gathered, the qualitative researcher often deals with only a few members of the group being studied. This allows the researcher to focus intently on the study participants and to gather a great deal of information, which must then be analyzed in great detail. For example, if a qualitative researcher is interested in investigating the activities of student nurses as they learn and practice appropriate patient care, much of the research would take place in a clinical setting. The questions that students ask each other, as well as those asked by and of instructors, staff nurses, supervisors, physicians, patients, and any other individuals in the setting, would all be a part of the data gathered by the researcher. In addition to verbal interactions, the researcher would also gather data related to nonverbal cues, such as gestures, posture, and facial expressions.

While gathering data, qualitative researchers must make every possible effort not only to recognize their own value judgments but also to refrain from acting on them unless necessary. This can be difficult if activities are taking place that the researcher considers to be questionable or even dangerous. Qualitative researchers can experience feelings of conflict on this point because their nonintervention may be considered acceptance of the participants' activities. Clearly, in the hospital study mentioned earlier, the researcher would have to intervene if a nursing student was about to make a mistake in patient care that would endanger a patient.

In planning their research, qualitative researchers use essentially the same systematic series of steps in their research plan as quantitative researchers. The statement of the problem may not be as rigorously defined as in quantitative research, but few qualitative researchers go into the study setting without some notion of the general area they plan to investigate. Qualitative researchers also establish a plan for data collection. Because qualitative researchers are often their own data-collection instrument, the plan for collecting the data may include no more than the development and use of field notes. Some may choose to use audiotapes and videotapes to collect their data.

Like quantitative researchers, qualitative researchers establish a tentative plan to analyze their data and to formulate conclusions based on these data. Because **qualitative data** are words rather than numbers, the data analysis method does not depend primarily on statistical tests as in quantitative research, but rather on rich narrative descriptions from the perspective of the participants of the study, from which concepts and themes are developed. Qualitative researchers must be very careful to report accurately and completely on the data they have gathered and to gather sufficient data to warrant the conclusions that they formulate.

Generalization, the ability to use the findings of research on a sample to anticipate the actions of larger populations, is a major goal of quantitative research. However, because the primary purpose of qualitative research is to achieve understanding by eliciting meaning, qualitative researchers do not propose to generalize from their findings to larger populations: "Remember, generalizability is not the purpose of qualitative research but the purpose is rather to elicit meaning in a given situation and to develop reality-based theory" (Morse & Field, 1995, p. 6). However, given that any population, no matter how small, is a part of a larger population, some valid generalizations concerning the larger population may be formulated. That is to say, the nurses in one hospital are a part of a larger health care system, which includes the community, the state, and the nation. "As each level is explored, greater strength and depth will be added to the explanation of the social phenomenon under consideration" (Dobbert, 1982, p. 180).

Qualitative Research Methods

Included in qualitative methods are phenomenology, a philosophical-based research approach that proposes to understand the meaning of the "lived experience" of the whole human being; grounded theory that generates the theoretical underpinnings of the research by "grounding" (basing) the theory in the study data; ethnography that provides for in-depth investigation of a culture or cultures; historical research that deals with past happenings and how these affect the present; and action research, in which the researchers pursue action and research outcomes at the same time. Each of these is discussed in detail in Chapter 8.

⬤ COMPARISON OF THE MAJOR CHARACTERISTICS OF THE QUANTITATIVE AND QUALITATIVE APPROACHES

To help you further understand the quantitative and qualitative approaches to research, we have compared the major characteristics of these approaches as reported by various writers (Table 2-2). It is important to note, however, that in reality actual studies seldom exemplify all of these characteristics.

Goals or Purposes

A major goal of quantitative research is to test existing theory; generally, qualitative researchers aim to develop sensitizing concepts and to create theory rather than testing theory. Another major goal of quantitative research is to show relationships between specific and carefully defined preselected vari-

TABLE 2-2 *Major Characteristics of Quantitative and Qualitative Research*

	QUANTITATIVE RESEARCH	QUALITATIVE RESEARCH
• Goals or purposes	Test theory	Develop sensitizing concepts; create theory
	Show relationships between variables	Describe multiple realities
	Develop generalizations from findings Make predictions about phenomena; control phenomena	Develop insight and understanding from participants' perspective Discover uniqueness of meaning
• Reasoning process	Primarily deductive reasoning	Primarily inductive reasoning
• Focus	Concise and narrow	Complex and broad
• Design	Reductionist Structured, formal; detailed and predetermined	Holistic Flexible, evolving
	Static design; categories isolated before study	Emerging design; categories identified during research process
• Data collection instrument/tools/devices	Structured for precise measurement Questionnaires, rating scales, inventories; biophysiologic measurements	Researcher is key instrument of data collection. Field notes; audio and video recorders; film
• Researcher's relationship with study participants	Short-term contact	Intense contact
	Emphasis on objectivity	Emphasis on trust
	Researcher detached from participants	Researcher may spend much time with participants.
	Researcher an outsider, independent from what is being researched	Research may become an insider.
• Data analysis	Numbers are the basic elements for analysis of objective data.	Words (language) are the basic elements of analysis for subjective data.
	Use of counts and measures; statistical techniques	Develop themes and concepts; rich descriptions
	Data analysis occurs after data are collected.	Data analysis is ongoing throughout study.
• Reporting of findings	Formal style; objective	Rich narrative; expressive language

Sources: Abdellah & Levine (1994); Bogdan & Biklin (1998); Creswell (1994, 1998).

ables; qualitative researchers propose to describe multiple realities as they arise from the perspective of the participant during the study, with the aim of developing insight and understanding. A third goal of quantitative research is generalization of the study findings to a larger population; qualitative researchers aim to discover uniqueness of meaning in the situation. A further goal unique to quantitative researchers is to be able to predict outcomes to achieve control of phenomena.

Reasoning Process

The reasoning process in quantitative research is primarily by deductive logic; in qualitative research, inductive logic is employed.

Research Focus

The focus of quantitative research is concise and narrow, focusing on the accumulation of facts and causes of behavior and assuming that these facts do not change; qualitative researchers are concerned with a broader and more complex view of a changing and dynamic reality.

Research Design and Data Collection

Quantitative research design is characterized by reductionism. Quantitative design, determined before conducting the study, is structured, formal, detailed, and objective. Quantitative researchers identify and isolate specific variables for measurement and plan for such specific measuring devices as questionnaires, rating scales, and inventories to measure these variables. The design for qualitative research is holistic, focusing on the entire human experience. It is flexible and evolving; qualitative researchers identify categories as the study evolves and may act as their own data-collection instrument, using field notes and audiotapes and videotapes.

Quantitative researchers usually have short-term contact, if any, with their study subjects; the emphasis is on researcher objectivity and detachment from the subjects of the study. The quantitative researcher is an outsider who maintains a detached, objective view (at least hypothetically, unbiased). The qualitative researcher is an insider, with the goal of obtaining information by talking to and/or observing study participants who have had first-hand experience with the phenomena under study.

Data Analysis

Quantitative researchers employ numbers, counts, and measures and use statistical procedures to analyze their data. Words and the development of concepts and themes are the primary data-analysis method for qualitative researchers; the data are rich in description and analyzed from the perspective of the participant. Both quantitative and qualitative researchers may use computers to assist in the analysis of their data.

Reporting Study Findings

The findings of quantitative research studies are usually reported objectively and in a formal style. Qualitative researchers report their findings in expressive language, often quoting from the responses of the participants themselves: the task of the writer is "to portray the world of the site in terms of the constructions that respondents use, seeing the world 'through their eyes,' as it were, and expressing their constructions" (Lincoln & Guba, 1985, p. 365).

● LIMITATIONS OF THE QUANTITATIVE AND QUALITATIVE APPROACHES

Both the quantitative and the qualitative approaches have potential limitations, several of which will be discussed here.

Using the quantitative approach to answer nursing's questions about the experience of health and illness may not always satisfy the requirements of nursing as a holistic and relational practice discipline. Because quantification can reduce everything to numbers, quantitative research has the potential to produce data that may have little real world reality and may lack descriptive richness (Abdellah & Levine, 1994). It may be difficult to control extraneous variables and to establishing the validity and reliability of data-collection instruments.

Qualitative studies are criticized by quantitative researchers as being "soft" research, lacking in rigor and scientific objectivity: "The unstructured, free-flowing, and somewhat subjective aspects of qualitative methods are unfavorably compared to the mathematical 'purity' and objectivity of quantitative techniques" (Abdellah & Levine, 1994, p. 50). Qualitative methodology can be very time-consuming, both in the collection and in the analysis of data, potentially limiting the ability to study large populations.

● COMBINING QUANTITATIVE AND QUALITATIVE METHODS

Quantitative and qualitative research "are not incompatible, but can be complementary in carrying out nursing research that requires diversified approaches" (Abdellah & Levine, 1994, p. 50). Some nurse researchers have even recommended using both quantitative and qualitative methods in the same research study. The term for this study design is **triangulation**, "the use of two or more methods to simultaneously or sequentially examine the same phenomenon" (Morse & Field, 1995, p. 243). In using both quantitative and qualitative methods in the same study, "multiple methods of data collection enrich the perspectives that the researcher has on the phenomena" (Morse & Field, 1995, p. 164). For example, Morse used both qualitative and quantitative methods when examining parturition (childbirth) pain in the Fijian and Fiji-Indian women. She used ethnographic interviews to understand the cultural context of childbirth. Then, to confirm hypotheses regarding differences in the amount of pain attributed to childbirth in each culture, she used a psychological scale to measure the expected painfulness of parturition (Morse & Field, 1995, p. 165).

There is no doubt that both quantitative and qualitative research are compatible with each other in investigating nursing problems; indeed, each plays a unique role in contributing to the ongoing development of nursing knowledge. The important point to remember is that each of these research approaches has a different philosophical orientation and is guided by the underlying assumptions, goals, and purposes of a specific research paradigm.

● SUMMARY

Researchers may use either the quantitative or qualitative tradition of scientific inquiry in conducting scientific inquiry. The investigator is guided by the philosophical assumptions, goals, and purposes of a particular mode of inquiry known as a research paradigm. The philosophical assumptions of the positivist paradigm are associated with quantitative research; those of the naturalistic paradigm are associated with qualitative research.

In quantitative research, the study variables are preselected and defined by the investigator, the data are collected, quantified (translated into numbers), and then statistically analyzed, often with a view to establishing cause-and-effect relationships among the variables. In qualitative research, the investigator seeks to identify the qualitative (nonnumeric) aspects of the phenomenon under study from the participant's viewpoint to understand the meaning of the totality of the phenomenon.

Occasionally, nurse researchers combine quantitative and qualitative strategies in the course of their studies to triangulate or examine the phenomena under investigation from both perspectives. Both approaches provide valuable strategies for investigating nursing problems.

The following application activities for this chapter will help you to evaluate your understanding of this material.

REFERENCES

Abdellah, F., & Levine, E. (1994). *Preparing nursing research for the 21st century.* New York: Springer.

Bogdan, R. C., & Biklen, S. K. (1998). *Qualitative research in education* (3rd ed.). Boston: Allyn & Bacon.

Creswell, J. (1994). *Research design: Qualitative and quantitative approaches.* Thousand Oaks, CA: Sage.

Creswell, J. (1998). *Qualitative inquiry and research design.* Thousand Oaks, CA: Sage.

Dobbert, M. L. (1982). *Ethnographic research.* New York: Praeger.

Doordan, A. (1998). *Research survival guide.* Philadelphia: Lippincott-Raven.

Guba, E. (1990). *The paradigm dialog.* Newbury Park, CA: Sage.

Lincoln, Y. S., & Guba, E. G. (1985). *Naturalistic inquiry.* Beverly Hills, CA: Sage.

Morse, J. M. (Ed.). (1994). *Critical issues in qualitative research methods.* Thousand Oaks, CA: Sage.

Morse, J. M., & Field, P. (1995). *Qualitative research methods for health professionals* (2nd ed.). Thousand Oaks, CA: Sage.

Omery, A. (1983). Phenomenology: A method for nursing research. *Advances in Nursing Science,* *5*(2), 49–63.

Omery, A., Kasper, C., & Page, G. (Eds.). (1995). *In search of nursing science*. Thousand Oaks, CA: Sage.

Powers, B., & Knapp, T. (1995). *A dictionary of nursing theory and research* (2nd ed.). Thousand Oaks, CA: Sage.

BIBLIOGRAPHY AND SUGGESTED READINGS

Bailey, P. H. (1997). Finding your way around qualitative methods in nursing research. *Journal of Advanced Nursing, 25,* 18–22.

Bickman, L., & Roy, D. J. (1998). *Handbook of applied social research methods.* Thousand Oaks, CA: Sage.

Denzin, N. K., & Lincoln, Y. S. (Eds.). (1994). *Handbook of qualitative research.* Thousand Oaks, CA: Sage.

Dickson, G. L. (1995). Philosophical orientation of qualitative research. In L. Talbot, *Principles and practices of nursing research* (pp. 411–436). New York: Mosby.

Janesick, V. J. (1998). *"Stretching" exercises for qualitative researchers.* Thousand Oaks, CA: Sage.

Mitchell, G. J. (1996). Clarifying contributions of qualitative research findings. *Nursing Science Quarterly, 9*(4), 143–144.

Morse, J. M. (Ed.). (1997). *Completing a qualitative project.* Thousand Oaks, CA: Sage.

Munhall, P., & Boyd, C. (1993). *Nursing research: A qualitative perspective* (2nd ed.). New York: National League for Nursing.

Phillips, J. R. (1997). Beyond a decade of research: Moving to the white hole of unitary science. *Nursing Science Quarterly, 10*(1), 6–7.

Parse, R. R. (1996). Building knowledge through qualitative research: The road less traveled. *Nursing Science Quarterly, 9*(1), 10–16.

Sandelowski, M. (1995). On the aesthetics of qualitative research. *Image, 27*(3), 205–209.

Sandelowski, M. (1997). To be of use: Enhancing the utility of qualitative research. *Nursing Outlook, 45*(3), 125–132.

Streubert, H. J., & Carpenter, D. R. (1995). *Qualitative research in nursing.* Philadelphia: Lippincott-Raven.

Thorne, S., Kirkham, S. R., & MacDonald-Emes J. (1997). Interpretive description: A noncategorical alternative for developing nursing knowledge. *Research in Nursing and Health, 20,* 169–177.

○ ○

APPLICATION ACTIVITIES

1. Explain the following terms in your own words:

   a. Paradigm

   b. Quantitative research (associated with the positivist paradigm)

   c. Qualitative research (associated with the naturalistic paradigm)

   d. Triangulation

   e. Replication

2. List three differences between quantitative and qualitative research.

3. In the research study you selected for the Application Activity in Chapter 1, did the investigator use a quantitative research approach or a qualitative research approach? Describe three characteristics of the study that contributed to your decision.

4. Read the research article reprinted in Appendix C, "The Effect of a Social Support Boosting Intervention on Stress, Coping, and Social Support in Caregivers of Children With HIV/AIDS." Briefly describe why this study is an example of the quantitative approach to research.

5. Read the research article reprinted in Appendix F, "Nursing Students' Experience Bathing Patients for the First Time." Briefly describe why this study is an example of the qualitative approach to research.

6. Discuss the major differences in each of the above studies.

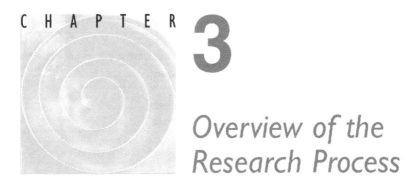

C H A P T E R 3

Overview of the Research Process

THE RESEARCH PROCESS
HOW IS THE RESEARCH PROCESS DIFFERENT
FROM THE PROBLEM-SOLVING PROCESS?
HOW IS THE RESEARCH PROCESS DIFFERENT
FROM THE NURSING PROCESS?

OVERVIEW OF THE RESEARCH PROCESS
EVALUATING PUBLISHED RESEARCH
SUMMARY

OBJECTIVES   *On completion of this chapter, the student will be able to:*

1. Explain the purpose of the research process.
2. List the steps of the research process.
3. Identify the three stages of the research process and discuss the function of each stage.
4. Compare the research process with the problem-solving process and the nursing process.
5. Discuss how the research process is used for planning both quantitative and qualitative studies.
6. Explain the purpose of conducting a research critique.
7. Define key terms.

KEY TERMS   Assumption   Research critique
                 Limitation   Research design
                 Pilot study   Research process
                 Problem-solving process   Research proposal

*I*n Chapter 2, the philosophical underpinnings and major characteristics of
the two approaches to nursing research—the quantitative approach and the
qualitative approach—were discussed. This chapter presents the basic components of the research process and describes the three stages of the research
process that are used in conducting a research study. Critical evaluation of
published research is also discussed.

● THE RESEARCH PROCESS

As you become acquainted with research terminology, you will see that both
quantitative and qualitative researchers use the term "research process." A
process is a method of doing something; a process has an identified purpose
and a series of steps to be followed to achieve a specified goal. The purpose of
the **research process** is to provide a guide for deriving systematic information
(new knowledge) concerning the phenomena of interest to the researcher. The
components of the research process are the steps the researcher follows in identifying the phenomena of interest and systematically gathering, examining, and
analyzing these phenomena with the goal of answering the research question.

● HOW IS THE RESEARCH PROCESS DIFFERENT FROM THE PROBLEM-SOLVING PROCESS?

Before we discuss the research process further, let's look at another process
that each of us uses every day of our lives—the **problem-solving process**. The
research process and the problem-solving process have different purposes,
processes, and goals. Problem-solving is a simpler process; its purpose is to
find an immediate solution to a practical problem in an actual setting. The
problem solver identifies a problem, collects information about the problem,
considers options, decides what to do to solve the immediate problem, then
may or may not look back to consider the effectiveness of the solution. The
basic purpose of research, on the other hand, goes far beyond solving the
immediate problem. Research provides new knowledge that is systematically
derived, is often capable of being generalized to a broader setting, could be

used to benefit a larger number of people, and contributes to the scientific knowledge base of a discipline.

For example, the nurse may decide that the application of a stockinette cap to a newborn infant would be an effective way to conserve body heat (problem solving). In contrast, a systematic research study (such as the study discussed in Chap. 1) that was designed to permit its results to be generalized could be conducted in relation to the same patient-care problem. The results would then be expected to contribute to scientific knowledge, thus benefiting a larger number of patients.

HOW IS THE RESEARCH PROCESS DIFFERENT FROM THE NURSING PROCESS?

Next, let's look at the relationship of the research process to another process that you have learned more recently—the nursing process. The focus of the nursing process is on a specific patient and family. Using the steps of the nursing process, the nurse identifies a clinical problem, assesses the problem, collects pertinent information related to the assessment, then interprets this information. The nurse then formulates a nursing diagnosis as a basis for planning interventions, implements the plan, then evaluates the process.

However, as familiar as you may become with the nursing process, there are distinct differences between the nursing process and the research process. Not only is the research process a more complex process than the nursing process, but the research process has its own distinctive terminology and rigorous methodology. Also, the nursing process focuses on outcomes designed primarily to improve the nursing care for a specific patient and family, whereas the research process has the broader focus of guiding researchers in formulating outcomes that have the potential to benefit larger numbers of people as well as contributing to the scientific knowledge base of nursing.

OVERVIEW OF THE RESEARCH PROCESS

Although your primary purpose for learning about research as a baccalaureate student is to develop your skills in critiquing published research and evaluating the findings for use in practice, it is also important that you understand the entire research process from the initial planning of a research study to the final reporting of the study results.

Steps of the Research Process

Although the number and order of the steps of the research process vary according to authors, the following are those most commonly included:

1. Formulate the research problem.
2. Review the related literature.

3. Identify a theoretical or conceptual framework (if appropriate).
4. State the research objectives/questions or hypotheses.
5. Describe the methodology for data collection.
6. Collect the data.
7. Analyze the data.
8. Interpret the results.
9. Formulate conclusions.
10. Communicate the findings.

Stages of the Research Process

It is helpful to consider the systematic steps of the research process as consisting of three sequential stages (or phases) that should answer the research question or solve the research problem:

1. Planning (conceptualizing the study).
2. Implementation (doing the study).
3. Communication (reporting the study).

STAGE I: PLANNING THE STUDY

The initial stage of the research process for both quantitative and qualitative researchers is the planning stage. It is during the planning stage that the **research design** (the overall plan for the study) is formulated. The research question, which the research will answer, is selected and refined into a problem statement, and the methodology for the study is formulated. Because the philosophical underpinnings for the positivist paradigm and the naturalistic paradigm guide the methodology for the research, the researcher must decide whether to conduct a quantitative or a qualitative study. This decision depends on the research question.

For a quantitative study, the research problem is usually narrow and quite specific; a qualitative study has a more general approach in that the topic may be broad and there may be little known about it. For both quantitative and qualitative studies, the problem to be investigated must be researchable and the answer not already known (unless the researcher's purpose is to replicate an existing study) so that the research can contribute to new knowledge. Appropriate methods must be available to investigate the problem. Consideration must be given to the availability of subjects (participants) expected to provide data for the study, as well as to the ethical implications of the research, especially as these pertain to the protection of the study participants' rights. The constraints of time and money imposed by the study are also important considerations in selecting the research problem.

Examples of general problem areas in nursing that might be selected by either quantitative or qualitative researchers include preoperative teaching of hysterectomy patients, adherence of diabetic patients with prescribed medication regimens, and family caregivers' ways of coping with the homebound elderly.

To place the problem in the context of what is already known, the quantitative researcher conducts a literature review—that is, reviews the literature related to the problem, citing references to pertinent publications and journal articles. Qualitative researchers may also conduct a literature review at this point or may plan to wait until they have collected some data, then use the emerging ideas and concepts to guide their literature search. The literature review serves to summarize existing knowledge in relation to the problem and helps the investigator to learn more about the problem area.

Next, quantitative researchers may use the information gained so far to identify a theoretical framework (or a conceptual framework). Using a theory (or theories) to guide the research allows the researcher to predict the outcome of the study. This is done by formulating a hypothesis—an educated guess—that will serve as a framework to guide the rest of the study. Testing the theory using the hypothesis then becomes the purpose for conducting the study. Not all quantitative studies are conducted to test hypotheses; some studies are designed to answer questions or to describe phenomena. The quantitative researcher then defines the major study variables so there will be no question about what the researcher means when using the terms. Because one of the purposes of qualitative research is to generate theory rather than to test theory, qualitative researchers do not usually design their studies within a theoretical framework.

The methodology for data collection describes the way that pertinent information will be gathered to answer the research question or describe the phenomena related to the research problem. Included in this step is a detailed discussion of the selection of subjects who will participate in the study, as well as a description of the procedures and techniques that will be used to collect the data. Qualitative researchers may discuss the setting for the study and the critical concern of gaining entry to the site.

The data-analysis component includes a plan for analyzing the data after they have been collected in a form that facilitates analysis. Quantitative researchers usually include "dummy tables" (tables that contain no data) in planning for data analysis to enable them to anticipate the statistical tests they will be using. Qualitative researchers often present a more general plan for data analysis.

Stating Assumptions and Limitations.   In the planning stage of a research study, it is customary for the investigator to state the assumptions and limitations for the study. **Assumptions** are statements based on logic or reason whose correctness or validity is taken for granted. The following statements are examples of assumptions:

Hospitals are for sick people.
Pain hurts.
Most people want to maintain themselves in a healthy state.

In most studies, assumptions are implied by the investigator and need not be stated explicitly. If they are significant enough to affect the study's course or its outcome, the investigator should state these assumptions explicitly so that others may evaluate their effect on the study.

Limitations of a study are restrictions identified by the researcher that may affect the outcome of a study but over which the researcher has little or no control. Important limitations should be anticipated in the planning stage and discussed in the report of the research to allow the reader to judge their effect on the study. Although all studies are limited in some way, limitations in quantitative studies are often related to inadequate methodology and to the use of small, unrepresentative samples—in other words, samples that do not reflect the characteristics of the population from which they were drawn. These limitations limit the generalizability of quantitative studies. Often, qualitative researchers cannot state the limitations for their studies during the planning stage of their research (that is, before conducting the study); limitations may not be known until the qualitative researcher is in place and gathering the data.

Writing the Research Proposal.   To structure the planning stage of a research study, both quantitative and qualitative researchers formulate a **research proposal**, a detailed written description of the proposed research study. Sometimes called a prospectus, the research proposal serves as a blueprint for the research project and must be completed before conducting either a quantitative or a qualitative research study. The written proposal communicates the problem being investigated and the procedures that will be used in the investigation.

A research proposal is written for several purposes. Having to sit down and write a proposal for the research study forces the researcher to think through various aspects of the study that might not otherwise have been considered. The plan can then be evaluated by others, who may improve it by suggesting something that has been left out or by considering whether or not the ideas would be workable in the actual study setting. The written proposal provides a guide to follow in carrying out the research. It saves the researcher from having to remember the many details already considered and the anticipated problems already solved. A well-thought-out proposal saves time, helps avoid mistakes, serves as a basis for writing the final report of the study, and should result in a higher-quality research study. Written research proposals are required for all academic research studies, such as theses and dissertations, and for all research submitted for funding by various government agencies and private organizations.

Both quantitative and qualitative researchers follow the research process to design their studies. We have reprinted a quantitative proposal (Appendix A) and a qualitative proposal (Appendix B). Both proposals were written by graduate nursing students. In reading these proposals, note that both follow the research process.

STAGE II: IMPLEMENTING THE RESEARCH PROPOSAL: CARRYING OUT THE STUDY

After a completed research proposal has been evaluated by those who can offer suggestions and has been revised, perhaps, to incorporate their suggestions, it must be approved by the appropriate institutional committees. This is very important, for it ensures the protection of the rights of the study subjects as well as conformity with the policies and procedures of the institution. Once this approval is given, the researcher is then ready to implement the written proposal. It is in the implementation stage of the research process that the actual collection and analysis of data for the research study take place. Before launching into the full study, the researcher may conduct a **pilot study**, a small-scale version of the actual study conducted with the purpose of testing and potentially refining the research plan.

In the implementation stage of the research process, the researcher follows the written proposal; if unexpected problems arise in the research situation, the researcher may decide to alter the procedures while still implementing the written proposal as closely as possible.

Although both quantitative and qualitative researchers follow the steps in the research process to design their research proposals, the progression through the process may be different when the studies are conducted. Quantitative studies follow the components of the process in a linear progression as far as possible. In this progression, they collect the data, then analyze the data and interpret the findings. Depending on the type of qualitative study being conducted, implementation may be circular—that is, data collection, data analysis, and interpretation may occur concurrently. As data collection proceeds, the qualitative researcher analyzes the data, grouping them into themes or categories, and continues to examine and interpret the data. The researcher then decides whether new data should be collected and may continue to collect data until no new categories emerge. Using inductive reasoning to build concepts and theory from the data, the qualitative researcher continuously examines and interprets the data and makes decisions about how to proceed with the remainder of the study based on what has already been identified.

Table 3-1 demonstrates the linear progression in quantitative research and the circular progression in qualitative research.

TABLE 3-1 *The Research Process*

1. Formulate the research problem.
2. Review the related literature.
3. Identify a theoretical or conceptual framework (if appropriate).
4. State the research objectives/questions or hypotheses.
5. Describe the methodology for data collection.
6. Collect the data.*
7. Analyze the data.*
8. Interpret the results.*
9. Formulate conclusions.
10. Communicate the findings.

*In qualitative studies these steps may be circular—that is, they may occur concurrently or go back and forth.

STAGE III: COMMUNICATING THE RESULTS OF THE STUDY

Researchers formulate conclusions and communicate their findings, both in writing and orally, so that others can have access to the new knowledge. Written reports range from formal, detailed reports to abridged reports for publication. In a report that is written to communicate the research to other investigators, the researcher should clearly discuss the purposes, procedures, findings of the research and recommendations for further study in sufficient detail to enable another investigator to replicate the study.

A research report may be written as a thesis or a dissertation to fulfill academic requirements. Research reports may also be written to fulfill the requirements of funding agencies. Researchers frequently share their studies by oral presentations at conferences and seminars and by participating in poster sessions (visual presentations).

Although researchers do communicate their research in books, research is most often reported as an article in a journal. You will become most familiar with research through articles that are published in journals. Although not all published articles follow this format, the following is a commonly used format for a journal article:

I. Preliminary information
  A. Title (often long; usually reflects the article content)
  B. Author(s)—name and affiliation
  C. Abstract—a short summary of the essential features of the article
II. Main text of the article
  A. Introduction and background
    1. Problem statement and significance of the study
    2. Literature review
    3. Identification of framework
    4. Research objectives, questions, or hypotheses
  B. Methodology (how the research was carried out)
    1. Research design
    2. Sampling and setting
    3. Methods of measurement
    4. Data-collection process
  C. Results (statistical and narrative report of results)
    1. Data-analysis procedures
    2. Results (findings) of the study
  D. Discussion (what the results mean)
    1. Interpretation of the findings
    2. Conclusions
    3. Limitations of the study
    4. Implications for nursing
    5. Recommendations for further research
III. References.

In your review of journal articles, you will find that articles have their own distinctive formats, often differing in the sections that are explicitly identified by the authors. Differences are due to the individual style of the author as well as to such specific requirements of the publisher as space limitations and manuscript style.

● EVALUATING PUBLISHED RESEARCH

The ultimate aim of conducting nursing research and communicating the results is to use this knowledge as a basis for scientific nursing practice. Because research-based practice is dependent on the findings of published scientific studies, each research study must be critically evaluated not only to assess its scientific merit but also to determine its readiness to be put into practice. A **research critique** is an objective and critical evaluation of the strengths and weaknesses of an entire research study. In conducting a research critique, both negative and positive aspects of the report should be evaluated. Because all research studies have weaknesses, the key to critical evaluation is not only to cite specific weaknesses but also to evaluate their impact on the entire study.

To provide you with the skills you will need to conduct a research critique, we have formulated basic guidelines that follow the research process. As each component of the research process is presented throughout the remainder of this text, specific critiquing guidelines will be discussed. Activities will provide you with the opportunity to apply these guidelines as you learn to critique published research reports. You will then be ready to learn about the exciting process of research utilization in the final chapter, where you will be provided with the practical skills needed to determine the readiness of research findings for use in clinical practice and to use the utilization process to develop a research-based protocol or procedure.

● SUMMARY

Both quantitative and qualitative researchers use the research process, which differs from both the problem-solving process and the nursing process. The research process may be viewed as consisting of three stages: the planning stage, the implementation stage, and the communication stage. In the planning stage, a research proposal, also called a prospectus, is developed. This includes the overall plan (design) for the study, as well as any assumptions and limitations of the study. The study is carried out during the implementation stage. During the communication stage, the results of the study are written and submitted for scrutiny by the research community. Because research-based practice is dependent on the use of research that has scientific merit, each research study must be critically evaluated for scientific merit before it is used in clinical practice.

The following application activities will help you to apply the material in this chapter.

BIBLIOGRAPHY AND SUGGESTED READINGS

Bogdan, R. C., & Biklen, S. K. (1998). *Qualitative research in education* (3rd ed.). Boston: Allyn & Bacon.

Chinn, P. L., & Kramer, M. K. (1995). *Theory and nursing: A systematic approach* (4th ed.). St. Louis: Mosby.

Crabtree, B., & Miller, W. (Eds.). (1992). *Doing qualitative research*. Newbury Park, CA: Sage.

Doordan, A. M. (1998). *Research survival guide*. Philadelphia: Lippincott-Raven.

Morse, J. M., & Field, P. A. (1995). *Qualitative research methods for health professionals* (2nd ed.). Thousand Oaks, CA: Sage.

Munhall, P. L., & Boyd, C. O. (1993). *Nursing research: Qualitative perspectives* (2nd ed.). New York: National League for Nursing Press.

Streubert, H. J., & Carpenter, D. R. (1995). *Qualitative research in nursing: Advancing the humanistic imperative*. Philadelphia: Lippincott.

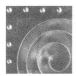

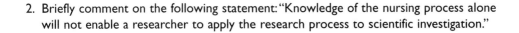

APPLICATION ACTIVITIES

1. List the steps in the research process and briefly discuss each step.

2. Briefly comment on the following statement: "Knowledge of the nursing process alone will not enable a researcher to apply the research process to scientific investigation."

3. Explain in your own words why both quantitative and qualitative researchers use the research process to derive scientific knowledge.

4. Read the research proposals in Appendices A and B so that you can see what information a research proposal contains and what a completed proposal looks like. Why do these two proposals represent the planning stage of the research process rather than the implementation stage?

5. Explain why the proposal in Appendix A is an example of a quantitative research proposal. List three characteristics of quantitative research that are included in this proposal.

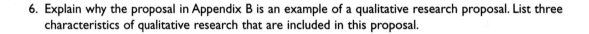

6. Explain why the proposal in Appendix B is an example of a qualitative research proposal. List three characteristics of qualitative research that are included in this proposal.

7. Explain the following terms in your own words:

   a. Assumption

   b. Limitation

   c. Pilot study

   d. Research design

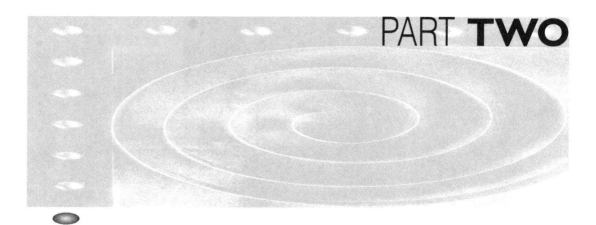

PART **TWO**

APPLYING THE RESEARCH PROCESS TO NURSING PROBLEMS

*T*he chapters in Part II focus on the application of the research process to nursing problems and are sequenced according to the steps in the research process and the order in which they most often appear in a published journal article.

In Chapter 4, the selection and statement of the research problem and review of relevant literature are discussed. Chapter 5 discusses research frameworks and hypotheses. Chapter 6 presents the topic of populations and sampling in relation to subject/participant selection. Chapter 7 discusses the critical area of ethical considerations for protecting the rights of human subjects who participate in research.

Chapter 8 presents an overview of the qualitative research methods most often used by nurse researchers. Chapters 9, 10, and 11 are devoted to quantitative research. Chapter 9 presents the quantitative research methods most often found in the literature, Chapter 10 discusses quantitative data-collection techniques, and Chapter 11 presents a basic review of quantitative data analysis.

Chapter 12 focuses on the communication and critical evaluation of research findings, the final step in the research process.

CHAPTER 4

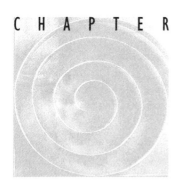

Problem Statement and Literature Review

OBJECTIVES   *On completion of this chapter, the student will be able to:*

1. Understand the process for selecting a researchable problem.
2. Identify the major sources of researchable problems.
3. Specify criteria to evaluate a researchable problem.
4. Discuss the purposes of a literature review.
5. Identify potential sources of research literature.
6. Define key terms.
7. Use evaluation guidelines to critique the problem statement and literature review components of published research reports.

KEY TERMS   CINAHL   Internet
                CD-ROM (Compact Disk-Read Only   Primary source
                   Memory)   Secondary source

The purpose of this chapter is to present the initial steps of the research process: selection and statement of the research problem and review of the related literature. Critical evaluation of these components of a published report is also discussed.

● HOW DO RESEARCHERS IDENTIFY RESEARCHABLE PROBLEMS?

Formulation of a researchable problem begins with the identification of a general problem area of interest to the researcher and the subsequent narrowing down of the topic to a very specific problem to be investigated. Selection of the problem to be investigated is an extremely important initial step in the research process and determines to a large extent the nature and quality of the research. Think of yourself as a nurse researcher. If you were asked to identify a research problem, it would be most helpful for you to think of the research problem as a question needing to be answered or as a situation needing a solution. First, you could look at your professional experiences and describe a situation that aroused your interest—even one that annoyed or irritated you—and led you to say to yourself, "Something ought to be done about this problem."

Examples of general problem areas of interest to nurse researchers might include preoperative teaching for mastectomy patients, discharge planning for premature infants, successful breast feeding in primiparas, or medication errors made by geriatric patients after discharge from the hospital. Once you had identified a general problem area related to your interests and experience, you would have to narrow it down to one specific problem that is manageable within the research process. A problem that is too broad can result in a study that is too general or too difficult to conduct; the results may be hard to interpret.

It is often helpful to state the problem as a question. For example, you could narrow down the general problem area of successful breast feeding in primiparas by asking, "What is the effect of teaching about breast feeding to primiparas?" You could then generate more specific problems: "Are there differences in comparable success with breast feeding in primiparas taught specific concepts and techniques related to breast feeding versus primiparas not exposed to such teaching?" or "What is the effect of individualized versus group instruction on successful breast-feeding practices in primiparas?" Or you could ask, "How do primiparas who perceive themselves as successful with breast feeding describe their experiences, and what meanings do they ascribe to these successes?"

It is well worth the time and effort it takes for a nurse researcher to select a problem specific enough to result in a manageable study. However, in their efforts to narrow down a general problem area, researchers need to be careful not to end up with a question so trivial that it is not worth the time and effort involved in researching it!

WHAT ARE THE SOURCES OF RESEARCHABLE PROBLEMS?

Major sources of researchable problems include: (1) the researcher's own professional background, personal interests, and experiences, (2) social and political issues, (3) the literature, and (4) theory.

The Researcher's Background and Interests

Nurse researchers are in an excellent position to identify researchable problems unique to nursing. For example, the research problem identified by the graduate student who wrote the quantitative research proposal to investigate compliance with universal precautions in pediatric settings (Appendix A) stemmed from her own clinical observation over a period of time. She noticed that nurses caring for pediatric patients were being careless in their compliance with universal precautions guidelines, especially by not wearing gloves for intravenous sticks. She also observed that the younger and sicker the child, the less likely the nurses were to adhere to universal precautions. She then formulated her research problem by asking a two-part question: What are the rates of compliance to universal precautions by registered nurses working with pediatric populations in hospital settings, and how are the age of the children and the size and type of hospital related to compliance?

Social and Political Issues

The researcher's interest in investigating social, political, and economic issues can also serve as sources for researchable problems. The impact of Medicare insurance revisions on health care for the elderly is an example of one such source.

The Literature

Another important source of researchable topics is the literature, particularly the nursing literature. Research studies reported in various nursing and related journals can provide ideas about the many researchable problems observed by other researchers. Most research studies raise additional questions or include recommendations for further study that can form the basis of new studies. A study that has already been conducted can be replicated—that is, repeating a study using the same methods to determine if the results will be the same as those of the original study. For example, if the research on the use of stockinette caps on newborns to conserve body heat that we discussed in Chapter 1 had been reported in the nursing literature, a researcher could replicate the study by conducting it again, following the original study as closely as possible.

Theory as a Source of Researchable Problems

Investigation of problems derived from theory can provide a meaningful contribution to scientific knowledge. Theory is not merely an accumulation of facts; theory provides an explanation of facts that can be used to explain or to predict certain phenomena. Research and theory are reciprocal in their relationship. Research can contribute to theory by confirming or failing to confirm some aspect of theory. An appropriate theory or theories can guide research by pointing to areas that need to be investigated and by providing a framework for designing a research study and for interpreting the findings of the study. The more that research is directed by theory, the more potential it has to make a meaningful contribution to the development and organization of a body of scientific knowledge for nursing. The role of theory in research is further discussed in the next chapter.

HOW DO RESEARCHERS EVALUATE A RESEARCH PROBLEM?

Having identified a potentially researchable problem, the researcher can ask the following questions to evaluate the proposed problem and decide whether it should be investigated through the research process:

1. Is the topic interesting?
2. Is the problem researchable?
3. Is it practical to conduct research on this problem?
4. Is this problem significant enough to warrant being researched?
5. Is it ethical to conduct research on this problem?

Is the Topic Interesting?

Because the researcher must become deeply involved in planning, implementing, and finally communicating the research study, the topic should be one that will sustain the researcher's interest over a prolonged period of time.

Is the Problem Researchable?

A researchable problem is one that is suitable for solution through research—that is, the problem can be investigated through the collection and analysis of data that exist in the real world. The meanings of the concepts must be clear and must be presented through tangible, observable evidence—that is, evidence obtained through direct observation or through other activities that will provide similar evidence relating to the meanings of the concepts linked to the problem. Examples of nonresearchable problems include ethical questions and problems requiring simple "yes or no" answers.

Is It Practical to Conduct Research on the Problem?

A research problem is practical if it is possible for the researcher to carry out the necessary research-related activities. Once the researcher finds a topic of interest within his or her area of expertise, the following questions should be considered:

1. Are appropriate methodology and resources available in terms of suitable measuring instruments or equipment?
2. Are subjects (participants) available and willing to participate in the study?
3. Will the researcher have the cooperation necessary to complete the research?
4. What is the cost involved in conducting this study?
5. What is the approximate time needed to complete this study?

Qualitative researchers, in particular, must be willing to commit to extensive time in the field.

Is the Problem Significant Enough to Warrant Being Researched?

Even though a topic may be interesting in itself, the researcher must consider whether it is sufficiently significant to warrant a research study. A good nursing research problem should have practical and/or theoretical significance. Its solution should contribute to the improvement of nursing care or to the advancement of nursing as a profession. The National Nursing Research Agenda (NNRA), developed by the National Institute of Nursing Research, can provide valuable guidelines for selecting significant research problems. In 1992, NNRA panel members developed the following basic criteria as guidelines for choosing problems and issues for research and as considerations for future funding. Priority areas are those in which:

- The area represents a significant and costly current and/or future health care problem.
- There are gaps in the state of the science underlying the problem or issue.
- Nursing can make a unique contribution to solving the problem through the development of new basic, clinical, or systems knowledge.

- The area of science underlying the problem or issue has potential for the development of new knowledge because it is on the cutting edge of science (NINR, 1998, p. 2).

Based on these guidelines, the most recent NNRA priorities (1998) not only address present needs but also anticipate future health challenges. These priorities can be categorized according to three major themes:

Chronic Illness or Conditions, represented by symptom management of chronic neurologic conditions, rehabilitation issues in traumatic brain injury, and improving quality of life for transplantation patients);
Behavioral Changes and Interventions, consisting of research into extending advances in cardiovascular risk factor management to special populations; and
Responding to Compelling Health Concerns, with an emphasis on end-of-life care *(Grady, 1998, p. 43).*

Is the Research Ethical?

Finally, the researcher must evaluate the ethical implications of the problem to protect the rights of the subjects who would participate in the study. Obtaining informed consent from participants, protecting them from harm, and maintaining anonymity and confidentiality are major considerations that will be further discussed in Chapter 7.

● SELECTING THE RESEARCH APPROACH

The selection and statement of the research problem—the initial step in the research process—is extremely important and determines the nature and quality of the research study. The researcher must then decide whether to conduct a quantitative or a qualitative study: "Whether certain 'problems' are better suited for qualitative or quantitative studies is open to debate. However, the *nature of the problem* is an important factor, albeit only one on the list" (Creswell, 1994, p. 10).

In designing quantitative studies to establish cause-and-effect relationships or to compare variables, there may be a substantial body of literature on which the researcher can build. Also, theories may exist that need to be tested or verified.

In designing qualitative studies, where there may be little information on the topic and the variables may be largely unknown, qualitative researchers focus on the context that may shape studies and facilitate understanding of the phenomenon being studied. Also, in many qualitative studies a theory base does not guide the study because those available are inadequate or incomplete, or simply do not exist (Creswell, 1994, p. 10). For the qualitative researcher, "the project starts with a single idea or problem that the researcher seeks to understand, not a causal relationship of variables or a comparison of groups. Although relationships might evolve or comparisons might be made, these emerge late in the study after we *describe* a single idea" (Creswell, 1998, p. 21).

● *REVIEW OF RELATED LITERATURE*

Once a researcher has identified a potential research problem, the next step in the research process is to review the literature related to the problem. The literature review provides the researcher with the opportunity to determine how much pertinent material is available concerning the potential study and helps to put the problem in the context of what has already been done. Quantitative researchers can usually locate many research articles that have a bearing on the study. Conversely, qualitative researchers may find that little or no research has been done regarding their phenomenon of concern, even when the phenomenon has been studied before.

Why Review the Literature?

There are four primary reasons for reviewing the literature. The first is to determine what has already been done that relates to the problem. This helps to avoid the duplication of previous studies and also helps to develop a framework for the problem that relates it to completed studies. Because one of the aims of research in nursing is to develop theories of nursing, the literature search may provide a framework of theory within which to investigate the problem. The role of theory in research is discussed in detail in the next chapter.

Second, the literature review provides ideas about the kinds of studies that need to be done. Reviewing the literature may stimulate the researcher to develop new insights into reported research or to formulate new problems to be investigated. Previous investigators often make suggestions regarding problems that need further investigation.

Third, a search of the literature may reveal research strategies, specific research procedures, and information regarding measuring instruments that have been found to be productive as well as nonproductive in studying the problem selected. Capitalizing on the successes as well as the errors of other researchers helps the researcher to profit from their experiences.

Finally, the literature review serves to guide the researcher in discussing the results of the study in terms of agreement or nonagreement with other studies. Results that contradict findings of other studies can suggest further studies to resolve such contradictions.

The critical evaluator of research has a different goal for reviewing the literature than that of the researcher. Because research-based nursing practice requires that there be sufficient scientific evidence to warrant the development of a protocol or procedure to address a clinical problem, the literature relating to the problem must first be identified. Each study relevant to the problem must then be critically evaluated for scientific merit and for applicability to the clinical problem. If the results of the studies prove to have a sufficient research base that is relevant to the problem and could guide practice, a research-based protocol or procedure to address the clinical problem can then be developed. This task is addressed in the final chapter of this text.

Recommendations for Locating Pertinent Materials for the Literature Review

It is very important to become familiar with the available library resources before beginning a literature review. The initial time spent in becoming familiar with these will ultimately save much valuable time. It is helpful to get a written guide explaining the resources and services of the library and the procedures that need to be followed. Participating in a guided tour of the library to learn to use the library to its fullest extent can be most helpful.

It is preferable to obtain reference materials from primary sources rather than secondary sources. A **primary source** provides first-hand information or ideas obtained from the original material. For example, each of the research articles reprinted in the appendices is an example of a primary source of information in that the authors of these studies have provided a first-hand report of their own research. A **secondary source** provides a second-hand source of information—that is, someone else's interpretation of the original material. Primary source materials minimize the error and distortion that may be characteristic of secondary source materials.

To find appropriate literature on a specific topic, you may want to start with the on-line catalog of the library or libraries you are using. Often, the library will have the topic you have selected listed under the subject heading in the catalog. This allows for the relatively easy process of searching for a topic. Sometimes the subject selected does not appear in the catalog. At that point, a synonym for the topic should be tried. Usually, after a few synonyms are used, titles of books concerning the topic or its synonym should appear. Consulting with a reference librarian can aid you in expanding or narrowing your search. Once you have established the subject or subjects you can locate pertinent books on the shelves. Occasionally, a researcher may find that a library does not have an on-line catalog but uses the older, traditional card catalog that must be searched by hand.

Books, however, are seldom the most recent sources for information on a topic. Because of the amount of time it takes to write, edit, and publish a book, the materials presented may be slightly dated or may even be out of date.

Books should be evaluated on the basis of:

1. Publication date. Generally, more recently published materials are preferable, unless the book is a classic or seminal work that has been cited by many other authors.
2. Author. An author who has written on the same topic many times may be a recognized expert in the field and may prove to be a useful source of information.

3. Publisher. There are many publishers of books world-wide. A variety of scholarly publishers, such as university presses, focus on research-based books. Some publishers, called "vanity press" publishers, accept payment from the author to publish the book. If the author has paid to have the book published, publication information will indicate that it was published by the author. This could mean that the author has been unable to find another publisher; thus, one might question the quality of the material contained in the book.

Periodicals often contain the most current ideas relating to research; as with books, some periodicals are more reputable than others. Newspapers and magazines displayed at the checkout counter of the grocery store or in the magazine section of bookstores tend not to be scholarly in focus or in quality. Although they may occasionally have a summary of useful research, they typically lack bibliographies or citations that can lead to other sources of information. This is not true of all magazines, however. *Scientific American* and a number of other science-based popular magazines do publish materials that are intended for a wide audience and can prove useful for the researcher.

Publications in scholarly journals that are the domain of specialists in a field are most helpful. Because of the increasing number of nurse researchers in the past decades, there has been a significant expansion of journals that publish nursing research. These journals include but are not limited to:

Advances in Nursing Science
Applied Nursing Research
Clinical Nursing Research
Computers In Nursing
Image: Journal of Nursing Scholarship
International Journal of Nursing Studies
Journal of Advanced Nursing
Journal of Nursing Administration
Journal of Nursing Education
Journal of Nursing Scholarship
Journal of Obstetric, Gynecological and Neonatal Nursing
Journal of Professional Nursing
Journal of Transcultural Nursing
Nursing Clinics of North America
Nurse Educator
Nursing Research
Nursing Science Quarterly
Research in Nursing and Health
Scholarly Inquiry for Nursing Practice
Western Journal of Nursing Research

Many of the above-listed journals are peer-reviewed. This means that each article is evaluated by one or more experts in the field before the editor of the journal accepts it for publication. Theoretically, at least, the peer-review process is designed to ensure that the article is not accepted for publication merely on the whim of the journal editor, but rather that publication is based on scholarly merit. Publishers of professional journals often use "blind reviewing," in which the reviewers do not know who wrote the article. The blind review process is designed to ensure that acceptance or rejection of an article is not based on any one person's prior knowledge of an author.

Printed Sources for Locating Relevant Literature

Indexes and abstracts can be helpful in identifying relevant references. Indexes are lists of books and articles, or the contents of a book; abstracts present the main ideas of articles and books.

The following indexes are useful in locating appropriate articles concerning a topic:

1. The *Cumulative Index to Nursing and Allied Health Literature*, published continuously since 1956, indexes approximately 250 English-language journals in nursing and allied health sciences, as well as selected articles from popular magazines and some biomedical journals from *Index Medicus*.
2. *Hospital Literature Index*, published quarterly by the American Hospital Association, selectively indexes approximately 600 English-language journals on health care administration and planning.
3. *Index Medicus*, a government publication under the auspices of the National Library of Medicine, surveys more than 2,600 international biomedical journals, of which several are nursing journals.
4. *International Nursing Index*, published quarterly by the American Journal of Nursing Company in cooperation with the National Library of Medicine, surveys approximately 200 domestic and foreign journals, in addition to nursing articles from more than 2,600 nonnursing journals.

The following abstracts are helpful:

1. *Dissertation Abstracts International* contains abstracts of doctoral dissertations in the humanities and social sciences, the sciences, engineering, and nursing.
2. *Psychological Abstracts*, published by the American Psychological Association, abstracts the international literature on psychology and related disciplines and contains categories related to nursing and nursing education.
3. *Sociological Abstracts* contains abstracts of the international literature in sociology and has sections on nursing.

The following indexes and abstracts are the other major sources commonly used by nurse researchers:

1. *Abstracts of Health Care Management Studies*
2. *American Journal of Nursing*: annual and cumulative indexes

   3. *Biological Abstracts*
   4. *Bioresearch Abstracts*
   5. *Bioethics Line*
   6. *Child Development Abstracts*
   7. *Education Index*
   8. *ERIC* (Educational Resources Information Center)
   9. *Excerpta Medica*
   10. *International Index*
   11. *Nursing Outlook*: annual and cumulative indexes
   12. *Nursing Research*: annual and cumulative indexes
   13. *Nutrition Abstracts*
   14. *Public Health, Social Medicine, and Hygiene*
   15. *Readers' Guide to Periodical Literature*
   16. *Research Grants Index*
   17. *Science Citation Index*

In addition to indexes and abstracts, compilations of measuring instruments can be very helpful in identifying relevant references and locating appropriate measuring instruments. Examining a measuring instrument used by a researcher and/or reading critical reviews of the measuring instrument may also be useful.

Accessing Computerized Literature

There are an increasing number of electronic indexes available that are valuable in locating relevant literature. These indexes are available on **CD-ROMs** (Compact Disk-Read Only Memory) located in many libraries. Because of the way the computer searches for words and the amount of information contained on a CD-ROM, a single word or topic request (such as primiparas or breast feeding) may result in thousands of references. To reduce the number of citations available, it is helpful to use a combination of words. Some indexes allow this to be done. Others require a Boolean expression (a system of logic used to give computers instructions). Boolean logic uses the connectors and, or, and not. If the topic is teaching primiparas about breast feeding, you might enter "primiparas and breast feeding." This instructs the computer to look for articles that contain both of these words. If the topic is primiparas but not breast feeding, "primiparas not breast feeding" might be entered. This instructs the computer to ignore articles that have both of these key words attached. If you are interested in both topics (primiparas and breast feeding), you would enter "primiparas or breast feeding." This instructs the computer to check for articles that have either primiparas or breast feeding as a key word.

Some searches may also include the use of the plus or minus signs. A plus sign between words means to include the second word in the search; it functions like "and" in this case. "Primiparas + breast feeding" would give the same information as "primiparas and breast feeding." The minus sign functions in the same fashion as the word "not." "Primiparas – breast feeding" would yield the same information as "Primiparas not breast feeding."

One of the major literature sources for nursing and health-related references is the computerized version of the *Cumulative Index to Nursing and Allied Health Literature* (**CINAHL**). This CD-ROM contains the same information as the printed resource but allows a much quicker search for articles than searching by hand. The system also allows the abstract of the article to be printed out.

MEDLARS (Medical Literature Analysis and Retrieval System) is the computerized literature retrieval service of the National Library of Medicine in Bethesda, Maryland. MEDLARS contains millions of references to journal articles and books in the health sciences published after 1965. MEDLINE (Medical Literature On-Line), the retrieval capability of MEDLARS, contains citations and selected abstracts from approximately 3,000 journals published in the United States and foreign countries. It has hundreds of thousands of references to biomedical journal articles published in the current year and the three preceding years. Other CD-ROM and on-line databases useful for nursing research include:

> AIDSLINE (AIDS Literature On-Line): AIDS literature source
> CancerLit (source for cancer literature)
> PAIS (Public Affairs Information Service): a database that covers literature in government, public policy, and foreign policy. Included are abstracts of journal articles, books, government documents, and documents of international organizations.
> PsycLIT (Psychology Literature): the electronic version of *Psychological Abstracts*.
> SOCIOFILE: citations and abstracts from journals and other sources concerning sociology and related social science disciplines in a variety of languages, including English.
> Dissertation Abstracts on Disc provides the same information as the printed version of *Dissertation Abstracts*.
> AB/INFORM: a database that is based on business journals. Information on health-related topics, such as health insurance or the health care industry, might be found in this database.
> ERIC is also available on CD-ROM.

CD-ROM–based databases are usually updated frequently (often quarterly) so that they provide current information.

On-Line Searches

The **Internet** has opened a large number of resources for both researchers and critical evaluators. The Internet, including the World Wide Web (WWW), is an international electronic network that allows computers to communicate regardless of where the machines are located. New sites are being added around the world on a daily basis. Each site has a specific address that, when entered into an appropriately equipped computer, tells this computer to connect with the computer located at that address. Because most of the information is transferred through telephone lines, this address can be thought of as a kind of telephone number.

Many institutions of higher learning have Web sites and provide access to the Internet for students and faculty. Some of these institutions also have a variety of bibliographic search materials available on-line. Because many library catalogs are available on-line, materials that were once difficult or almost impossible to obtain may be located by the use of the Internet. This is a great help for users of a local library when trying to find a specific book or article that is not available in that particular library; the interlibrary loan department can use the Internet to obtain not only books but also copies of articles. In some instances, there may be a charge for this service. One very useful site for obtaining information on books and journals is the Library of Congress (http://www.loc.gov).

Another excellent on-line source of indexed articles is the CARL (Colorado Association of Research Libraries [http://uncweb.carl.org]) database, which is available on line. This database provides abstracts of articles as well as the complete article (for a fee). CINAHL also has on-line access (for a fee) at http://www.cinahl.com. *Psychological Abstracts, Sociological Abstracts,* and *ERIC* are also available on-line. MEDLINE is also available through the National Library of Medicine (http://www.nim.nih.gov). All of the information and abstracts contained in the *Index Medicus* are available through this source. Copies of articles are available (for a fee) through *Loansome Doc*, a system that provides this service to hospitals and other medically related sites.

Other governmental sites from which to access information include:

National Institutes of Health: http://www.nih.gov
Centers for Disease Control and Prevention: http://www.cdc.gov
Food and Drug Administration: http://www.fda.gov
National Library of Medicine: http://www.nim.nih.gov

Many nursing organizations have Web sites that provide information not only about the organization itself, but also about any available publications, as well as links to other organizations that share common interests. Some of these organizations include:

Sigma Theta Tau: http://www.stti.iupui.edu
American Nurses Association: http://www.nursingworld.org
National League for Nursing: http://www.nln.org

A number of publishers put information concerning their books and journal offerings on-line. Sometimes they provide abstracts of books and articles and the index to the latest issue of a journal or journals. Others, such as the *Nursing Standard* (a British journal at http://www.nursing-standard.co.uk), provide complete copies of some of their articles on-line.

Many journals in nursing and medicine might be sources of articles for critical evaluation. Some are published independently by an organization, but many are published by a large publisher. The following publishers include many of the major journals for nursing research on their rosters:

Lippincott Williams & Wilkins *(Nursing Research, Journal of Obstetric, Gynecological and Neonatal Nursing)*
http://www.nursingcenter.com
Sage *(Western Journal of Nursing Research, Journal of Holistic Nursing)*
http://www.sagepub.com
Blackwell Science *(Journal of Advanced Nursing)*
http://www.blackwell-science.com
W. B. Saunders *(Applied Nursing Research)*
http://www.wbsaunders.com
John Wiley & Sons *(Research in Nursing and Health)*
http://www.interscience.wiley.com

In some instances the journal or material is wholly on-line and is not available through any other source.

You may also want to search for a topic using the Internet. There are a number of organizations that provide searches of the Internet by using what are called search engines. These include but are not limited to:

Yahoo: http://www.Yahoo.com
AltaVista: http://Altavista.digital.com
Hotbot: http://www.Hotbot.com
Lycos: http://www.Lycos.com
Magellan: http://www.McKinley.com
Excite: http://www.Excite.com
InfoSeek: http://www.Infoseek.com

When using one of these search engines, type in the word or phrase being looked for and the computerized search engine looks for this information, just as is done on a CD-ROM. As with a CD-ROM, care must be exercised to delineate the topic, or thousands of "hits" may be found. Also, search engines use different ways to search their databases, so one search engine may yield only a few items concerning a topic, while another may provide many more items. It is best to search for a topic using two or three search engines. These search engines may also allow the use of Boolean expressions.

Evaluating Sources of Information on the Internet

There are some important caveats when searching the Internet. Because of the Internet's vast size, there is no quality control exercised by editors and other fact checkers. This means that anyone with an opinion can make information available on the Internet. Care must be used to weed out unusable or inaccurate information.

A few things to look for are:

1. Is the author qualified? Are credentials presented, and can they be checked?

2. Is the sponsoring organization reputable? "Edu" at the end of an address means that the information is coming through an educational institution. "Org" means that the sponsor is a nonprofit organization. "Com" means a business enterprise is involved. "Net" means that the information is coming through a network provider. "Gov" means that the information is coming through a government source. There are also national endings that identify the country of origin. Even if the information comes from a credible source such as an educational institution, care must be exercised to determine the accuracy, objectivity, and depth of coverage of the information, because many individuals have access to the Web and are free to express their opinions and ideas.

3. Date of posting is also important. Sometimes the Internet provides the most recent information available to researchers and critical evaluators. Usually the search engine provides a brief statement of when the information was posted on the web in the summary statement that describes the topic. The more recent the information, the more useful it may be.

PROFESSIONAL MEETINGS AS A SOURCE OF INFORMATION

Another source for obtaining current research information is presentations at professional meetings. The problem faced by both the researcher and the evaluator of research is to discover where and when a relevant professional meeting is taking place and obtaining a copy of the presentations. The program for the meeting typically lists the title of the presentation and the name and affiliation of the presenter; it often includes an abstract of the presentation. If possible, obtain a program of the meeting to determine which presentations might be useful, and request that the presenter send you a copy of the presentation.

Many professional organizations post information concerning conferences and meetings on the Web. Sometimes this information includes the program and abstracts of the planned presentations and provides enough information to allow you to contact a presenter to obtain a copy of a presentation. *PapersFirst and ProceedingsFirst* are services sponsored by the Online Computer Library Center. These services provide copies of papers and proceedings from many professional meetings (for a fee) through participating libraries.

HINTS FOR RECORDING LIBRARY MATERIALS

Abstracting Selected References

When searching the literature as a critical evaluator of research, you should plan to photocopy all articles that you plan to quote directly to reduce citation errors. You should also plan to photocopy all tables and charts that you cite so that you have the complete information when writing the literature review.

After locating references pertinent to your topic, you should begin with the latest one, because it may contain additional references from previous research. Read the abstract of the article and/or the summary to see whether the article is pertinent to your topic. Then scan the article, noting the important points. If you decide not to photocopy the entire article, plan to use separate index cards (4 × 6 is a convenient size) to record useful information. A separate index card for each reference helps organize the materials when you are ready to write the literature review. The card should contain the following information:

1. The complete bibliographic reference in the format of the style manual required by your department. Doing this will save time when using the reference.
2. The complete call number for a source, in case you need to recheck it.
3. A coding system for each reference should be developed. Mark such factors as relevance to your study, type of article, and whatever else would be helpful for your research. For example, information on the relevance of references could be coded as R+ (very relevant), R (relevant), or R– (less relevant). Information concerning the type of reference could be coded as RS (research study) or V (an article expressing the author's viewpoint).
4. A summary of the reference on the card, listing its essential points and noting the important or unusual aspects of the article that will contribute to your study. If you quote directly from the article, copy the quotation word for word, noting that it is a direct quotation.
5. Note whether the reference is a primary or secondary source. If possible, check secondary sources for accuracy. For example, if an article states "so and so" as cited in "thus and such," you would be wise to find the actual article or book (if possible) to determine whether the citation was accurate.

Writing The Literature Review

After thoroughly investigating relevant references, both the researcher and the critical evaluator need to organize them to write the literature review. To refresh your memory, review the notes on each card, discarding irrelevant references. Include only those references that you used to substantiate your research. Next, make a tentative outline showing the relationships among the topics. Then analyze your cards, putting them into the appropriate categories of the outline. For each category, analyze the similarities and differences between the references. Summarize those references that state essentially the same thing—for example, "Smith (1998), Brown (1999), and Green (1998) report that . . ." Include studies that show results, even if they are contradictory to other studies.

When organizing the literature review, first discuss the references that are least related to the problem, progressing to the most relevant references. Conclude the review with a brief summary of the main points, general conclusions, gaps in the literature, and implications for the research.

● CRITIQUING THE PROBLEM STATEMENT AND LITERATURE REVIEW OF A RESEARCH REPORT

Points to Consider in a Quantitative Report

The initial section of a quantitative research report contains the introduction and background for the study. Early in this section, the research problem should be clearly identified and enough background information presented to acquaint the reader with the importance of the problem. The author should clearly indicate the rationale for selecting the research problem. The problem should not only be timely in terms of current trends in nursing but should also be significant enough that the results have the potential to benefit nursing practice and to contribute to nursing knowledge. Finally, the quantitative approach should be appropriate for the investigation.

Although it may not be explicitly titled as such, the literature review generally follows the discussion of the problem and serves to place the problem in the context of what is already known, as well as to identify important gaps in the literature. The organization of the review should be logical and should include relevant references that are well documented. References should be current unless pertinent classical references are cited. It is helpful to the reader if the review concludes with a brief summary of the literature and its implications for the research. Box 4-1 lists these points as evaluation guidelines.

Points to Consider in a Qualitative Report

The initial section of a qualitative research report contains the introduction and background for the study. The problem for the research—that is, the phenomenon of interest—should be clearly identified early in the report, with information presented to justify the rationale for conducting the investigation. The problem should be timely and significant enough to nursing so that the results have the potential to benefit nursing practice as well as contribute to nursing knowledge. The qualitative approach should be appropriate to the investigation. Because often little or no research has been done related to the specific phenomenon of interest in a qualitative study, the report may have a only a brief literature review or none at all, in which case the author may explain the exclusion of a literature review. Note that the qualitative reports in

---

BOX 4-1

GUIDELINES FOR EVALUATING A QUANTITATIVE PROBLEM STATEMENT AND LITERATURE REVIEW

Problem Statement
1. The problem is clearly identified.
2. Background information on the problem is presented.
3. Rationale for selecting the problem is clear.
4. The problem is timely in terms of current trends in nursing.
5. The problem is significant to nursing in that the results could benefit nursing practice and/or contribute to nursing knowledge.
6. The quantitative approach is appropriate for investigating the problem.

Literature Review
1. The review is relevant to the study.
2. References are well documented and current (unless relevant classical studies are cited).
3. The relationship of the problem to previous research is clear.
4. There is a range of opinions and varying points of view about the problem.
5. The review identifies important gaps in the literature.
6. Documentation of references is clear and complete.
7. The organization of the review is logical.
8. The review concludes with a brief summary of the literature and its implications for the problem.

Appendices E and F both have brief literature reviews. If the report has a literature review, the references should be relevant to the study, well documented, and organized in a logical manner.

Box 4-2 lists these points as evaluation guidelines.

● SUMMARY

Researchers use a variety of sources to identify researchable problems, including the researcher's background and interests, social and political issues, the literature, and related theory. A research problem is evaluated based on the following criteria: Is the topic interesting? Is the problem researchable? Is it practical to do research on this problem? Is this problem significant enough to warrant being researched? Is it ethical to conduct research on this problem?

BOX 4-2   GUIDELINES FOR EVALUATING A QUALITATIVE PROBLEM STATEMENT AND LITERATURE REVIEW

Problem Statement
1. The problem (phenonemon of interest) is clearly identified.
2. Background information on the problem is presented.
3. The rationale for selecting the problem is clear.
4. The problem is timely in terms of current trends in nursing.
5. The problem is significant to nursing in that the results could benefit nursing practice and/or contribute to nursing knowledge.
6. The qualitative approach is appropriate for investigating the phenonemena of interest.

Literature Review (if present)
1. The documentation of references is clear and complete.
2. The organization of the review is logical.
3. The review is relevant to the study.

Before embarking on their research, researchers review the related literature to determine where their investigation fits into already existing knowledge and to locate other research that may have been conducted. Critical evaluators of research who plan to use research-based findings to write a protocol or a procedure to address a clinical nursing problem also review the literature to locate research with scientific merit on which to base the protocol or procedure. Researchers and critical evaluators of research survey both print sources and computerized sources. On-line (Internet) searches are now both possible and desirable, but caveats concerning the validity and reliability of the results of such searches must be kept in mind. Effective methods of abstracting useful sources and writing the literature review should be used.

The following application activities should help you to evaluate your understanding of the material in this chapter and will assist you in developing your skills in locating relevant literature and evaluating published research.

REFERENCES

Creswell, J. (1994). *Research design: Qualitative and quantitative approaches.* Thousand Oaks, CA: Sage.
Creswell, J. (1998). *Qualitative inquiry and research design.* Thousand Oaks, CA: Sage.
Grady, P. (1998). News from NINR. *Nursing Outlook, 46*(1).
National Institute for Nursing Research. (1998). *Report of the priority expert panel on community-based health care: Nursing strategies, 1998.* Washington, DC: Author.

BIBLIOGRAPHY AND SUGGESTED READINGS

Edwards, M. J. A. (1997). *The Internet for nurses and other allied health professionals* (2nd ed.). New York: Springer.

Hebda, T., Czar, P., & Mascara, C. (1998). *Handbook of informatics for nursing and health care professionals*. Menlo Park, CA: Addison Wesley.

Joos, I., Whitman, N. I., Smith, M. J., & Nelson, R. (1997). *Computers in small bytes: The computer workbook* (2nd ed.). New York: National League for Nursing.

Lybecker, A. J. (1998). Surfing the net. *Maternal Child Nursing, 23,* 17–21.

Nicoll, L. H., & Oulette, T. H. (1998). *Computers in nursing: Nurses' guide to the Internet* (2nd ed.). Philadelphia: Lippincott-Raven.

Teasdale, K., & Teasdale, S. (1997). Nursing on the Internet. *Professional Nurse, 12*(3), 181–182.

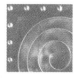

APPLICATION ACTIVITIES

1. Explain in your own words how researchers go about selecting a researchable problem.

2. Discuss three major sources of research problems.

3. Explain the difference between a primary literature source and a secondary literature source. Why are primary sources more reliable?

4. Identify a clinical nursing problem that could be improved if research findings were used—for example, teaching breast feeding to primiparas, pain assessment in postoperative infants, patient-controlled analgesia after hysterectomy, or the effect of preoperative teaching on postoperative compliance with treatment.

    My clinical nursing problem is:

5. Complete the following library search exercise designed to assist you in locating the literature relevant to the clinical problem you have just identified. If your library has CD-ROM search capabilities, use both textual references and the CD-ROM databases for your search. If you use computerized databases, you may be able to combine terms.

    First, you need to list as many key words as you can that might relate to your clinical nursing problem. For example, for the topic "teaching breast feeding to primiparas," the following key words could be related: primiparas, teaching, instruction, infants: feeding, infant nutrition, neonatal nursing, lactation, milk, bottle feeding, mothering, breast feeding.

Key words relating to my clinical nursing problem are:

a. Begin your library search by listing three complete references from the CINAHL concerning your clinical nursing problem. If you use the CD-ROM version, print out your references and their abstracts.

b. Go to the *Index Medicus, Excerpta Medica,* or MEDLINE and list two complete references related to your clinical nursing problem. If you use MEDLINE, print out your references and their abstracts.

c. List one complete reference from *Dissertation Abstracts* related to your clinical nursing problem.

d. Use *Psychological Abstracts,* PsychLIT, or Psychinfo-online to locate psychological studies related to your clinical nursing problem. List at least two complete references from this source. If you use the CD-ROM or on-line service, print out your references and their abstracts.

e. List at least one book that relates to your clinical nursing problem (include the author, title, publication date, and library call number).

f. Look in *Child Development Abstracts* to determine pediatric applications to your clinical nursing problem. List one reference if possible.

g. Are there any geriatric implications for your clinical nursing problem? List one reference if possible.

h. If there are references in the following indexes related to your clinical nursing problem, list one from each source:
   i. *Hospital Literature Index*

   ii. *International Nursing Index*

   iii. *Readers' Guide to Periodical Literature*

i. List at least three references from government documents related to your clinical nursing problem.

j. There are many other abstracts and indexes available that might provide additional reference citations related to your clinical nursing problem. List at least three abstracts and/or indexes related to your clinical nursing problem in addition to those you have already used, and cite one reference from each source.

k. If possible, enter the Internet and list at least two references from other libraries that relate to your clinical nursing problem. Identify the sources of these references.

l. Investigate audiovisual holdings concerning the broad area of nursing, and list the names of three films and/or videotapes.

6. In the following activity, you will begin to learn the process for critiquing published research reports to prepare you to use the utilization process that you will learn in Chapter 13.
   a. Select three of the research studies related to the clinical nursing problem that you used for your literature search. The three studies that you select should interest you enough to use them to learn the process of critical evaluation for the remainder of your research course.

   b. For each of the three reports, decide whether it is quantitative research or qualitative research.

   c. Use either the guidelines for evaluating the quantitative problem statement and literature review (see Box 4-1) or the guidelines for evaluating the qualitative problem statement and literature review (Box 4-2) to critique each article. (Note that complete guidelines for evaluating both types of reports are located in Appendixes G and H.)

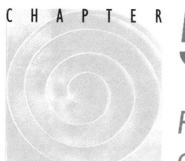

C H A P T E R

5

Research Frameworks and Hypotheses

OBJECTIVES   *On completion of this chapter, the student will be able to:*

1. Discuss concepts and constructs.
2. Identify models and conceptual models of nursing.
3. Discuss the functions of nursing theory.
4. Classify theories as broad-range, middle-range, or narrow-range.
5. Discuss how nursing theories are related to conceptual models of nursing.
6. Discuss the purpose of theory in a research study.
7. Describe the function of a framework in a research study.
8. Compare theory-linked research and isolated research.
9. Compare theory-generating research and theory-testing research.
10. List three ways of stating the purpose of a study.
11. Explain the purpose of a hypothesis in a research study.
12. Identify types of hypotheses.
13. Define key terms.
14. Use evaluation guidelines to critique the theoretical framework and purpose of published research reports.

KEY TERMS   Broad-range theories (grand theories)   Nondirectional hypothesis
Complex hypothesis   Operational definition
Concept   Proposition
Conceptual framework   Research hypothesis
Construct   Simple hypothesis
Direct definition   Statistical hypothesis (null hypothesis)
Directional hypothesis   Theoretical definition
Hypothesis   Theoretical framework
Isolated research   Theory
Middle-range theories (midrange theories)   Theory-generating research
Model   Theory-linked research
Narrow-range theories   Theory-testing research

*T*he purpose of this chapter is to present basic concepts related to the function of theoretical and conceptual frameworks in research, as well as an
overview of hypothesis formulation and testing. Critical evaluation of these
components in a published research report is also discussed.

● *USING THEORY IN RESEARCH STUDIES*

As you evaluate published nursing research, you will see terms such as theoretical framework and conceptual framework used in some, but not all, of
these studies. Several basic definitions should help you to understand terms
related to the use of theory in research studies.

Concepts and Constructs

A **concept** is an idea or a complex mental formulation of a specific phenomenon. For example, if you think of the word "table," what comes to your mind?
Is it a piece of wooden furniture that is round and has four legs? Or is it square
like a card table? Or is your table a food chart? Or is it a table of contents for
a book you are using in your nursing courses? Most likely, each person who is
asked to think about the concept of "table" will have a different idea or mental formulation of what this abstract phenomenon called "table" looks like.
Concepts range from being relatively concrete and more directly observable
and measurable (such as height and weight) to being relatively abstract (such
as wellness and self-esteem).

A **construct** is a highly abstract and complex concept—such as intelligence—that is deliberately invented (constructed) by researchers for scientific
purposes. A construct cannot be directly measured but must be indirectly

measured by noting the presence of indicators of the concept. For example, the more concrete concept of weight (in pounds) can be directly determined by reading the numbers on a scale. The more abstract and complex construct of intelligence cannot be as directly measured but must be inferred from such indicators of intelligence as verbal skills and mathematical reasoning on a standardized intelligence test.

Models and Conceptual Models of Nursing

A **model** is a symbolic representation of reality used to demonstrate the interrelationships among a set of concepts or phenomena that cannot be directly observed but that do represent reality. Examples of models include verbal models, which are worded statements; schematic models, which may be diagrams, drawings, graphs, or pictures; and quantitative models, which are mathematical symbols. Models may function to provide a sense of understanding as to how "theoretic relationships develop and are useful to illustrate various forms of theoretic relationships" (Chinn & Kramer, 1995, p. 216). Models may be presented as part of a theory or can be constructed to show links between related theories. "In nursing, a model is most often characterized as a conceptual model, a term that is used interchangeably with the term conceptual framework" (Powers and Knapp, 1995, p. 104).

Conceptual models of nursing include Dorothy Orem's Self-Care Model, Sister Callista Roy's Adaptation Model, Betty Neuman's Systems Model, Martha Rogers' Model: Science of Unitary Persons, and Imogene King's System Framework (Fitzpatrick & Whall, 1996). Each of these nursing theorists "developed conceptual models that helped direct theory development" (Marriner-Tomey & Alligood, 1998, p. 9).

Theories

Concepts are the major components or building blocks of theories. A **theory** is a set of logically interrelated statements that is "a creative and rigorous structuring of ideas that project a tentative, purposeful, and systematic view of phenomena" (Chinn & Kramer, 1995, p. 72). Note that a theory consists of ideas—theory is not reality—and that these ideas are created and structured by the theorist. It is important to note the tentative nature of theory and that theory cannot be proved: theory is "grounded in assumptions, value choices, and the creative imaginative judgment of the theorist" (Chinn & Kramer, 1995, p. 72).

The basic function of theory is to describe, explain, and predict phenomena. A specific type of theory—prescriptive theory—is intended to control or change phenomena by identifying a goal and specifying the specific procedures to attain the goal. A theory contains propositions. A **proposition** is a statement of a relationship between two or more concepts in the theory. The proposition is stated in such a way that a testable hypothesis or hypotheses can be derived from the abstract statements of the theory. A **hypothesis** is a statement of the predicted relationship between two or more variables in a research study.

Thus, concepts are the components of theory. A theory consists of propositions, which are the testable part of a theory from which research hypotheses can be derived.

Functions of Nursing Theory

Theory helps to provide knowledge to improve nursing practice by describing, explaining, predicting, and controlling the specific phenomena related to nursing:

> Nurses' power is increased through theoretical knowledge because systematically developed methods are more likely to be successful. In addition, nurses will know why they are doing what they are doing if challenged. Theory provides professional autonomy by guiding the practice, education, and research functions of the profession. *(Marriner-Tomey & Alligood, 1998, p. 3)*

Classification of Theory

Theory can be classified according to the range and specificity of the phenomena dealt with in the theory. The subject matter for a theory can range from being very broad and all-inclusive to being very narrow and limited.

Broad-range theories (also called grand theories) are "systematic constructions of the nature of nursing, the mission of nursing, and the goals of nursing care" (Meleis, 1997, p. 18). Broad-range theories in nursing deal with the scope, philosophy, and general characteristics of nursing. For example, a conceptualization of nursing's goal for high-level wellness for all individuals in society would be classified as broad-range theory. Although not all conceptual models can be classified as nursing theories, the following are examples of conceptual models that are classified as grand theories in nursing: Dorothea E. Orem's Self-Care Deficit Theory of Nursing; Martha E. Rogers' Unitary Human Beings; Imogene King's Systems Framework and Theory of Goal Attainment; and Betty Neuman's Systems Model (Marriner-Tomey & Alligood, 1998, p. 9).

Middle-range theories (also termed midrange theories) have a narrower focus than broad-range theories. "Middle-range theories are more precise than grand theories and focus on developing theoretical statements to answer questions about nursing" (Marriner-Tomey & Alligood, 1998, p. 11). Both middle-range and broad-range theories deal with a wide range of phenomena. However, unlike broad-range theories, middle-range theories do not deal with the entire range of phenomena of concern within a discipline. "When a theory is at the grand-theory level, many applications of that theory can be made in practice at the middle-range level by specifying such factors as the age of the patient, the situation, the health condition, the location, or the action of the nurse" (Alligood & Marriner-Tomey, 1997, p. 32).

Chinn and Kramer (1995) describe an example of middle-range theory: "A theory of pain alleviation represents a midrange theory for nursing; it is broader than a theory of neural conduction of pain stimuli but narrower than the goal of achieving high-level wellness" (p. 216). A theory of pain alleviation would be classified as a middle-range theory in that the phenomenon of pain is only one of the many phenomenon of concern within the discipline of nursing. Other phenomena include quality of life, incontinence, and uncertainty in illness. Examples of middle-range nursing theories include Nola Pender's Health Promotion Model; Madeline Leininger's Culture Care: Diversity and Universality Theory; and Ida Jean Orlando's Nursing Process Theory (Marriner-Tomey & Alligood, 1998).

Narrow-range theories (also called microtheories) deal with a limited range of discrete phenomena of concern to a discipline. They are the most specific and least complex of the types of theories, and their theoretical formulations are not extended to link with the total range of phenomena of concern within a discipline. A discrete theory of neural conduction of pain stimuli (as cited above) is an example of a narrow-range theory.

How Are Nursing Theories Related to Conceptual Models of Nursing?

The conceptual models of a discipline are broad conceptual structures or frameworks that provide a total perspective of the phenomena that are specific to that discipline. There is considerable agreement that nursing's metaparadigm (a specific type of paradigm) consists of the phenomena that are specific to the discipline of nursing. These central domain concepts are person, environment, health, and nursing. Nursing models can then be described as broad conceptual structures that provide a perspective of the total phenomena of nursing:

> What this means in terms of nursing practice is that the way nurses think about people and about nursing has a direct impact on how people are approached, what questions are asked, how information is learned and processed, and what nursing activities are included in nursing care. *(Alligood & Marriner-Tomey, 1997, p. 32)*

The propositions or relationship statements of theories are consistent with the model or the framework from which they are derived. Theories, also consisting of sets of concepts, are less broad than models and propose more specific outcomes: "When the nurse approaches people from the perspective of a certain nursing model and asks questions, processes information, and carries out activities in a certain way according to that model, a specific outcome is proposed based on the application of the theory of that model" (Marriner-Tomey & Alligood, 1998, p. 32).

The research proposal in Appendix A, "Compliance With Universal Precautions in Pediatric Settings," provides an example of a theory that has been derived from a model. The research study was developed within King's systems framework or model and its resultant theory of goal attainment. King developed her theory of goal attainment from her own systems framework. Two other theories that have been derived from King's systems framework are Frey's theory of social support and health and Sieloff's theory of departmental power (Alligood & Marriner-Tomey, 1997, p. 35).

In summarizing the relationship of nursing theory to nursing models, the following definitions are offered: "The conceptual models of a discipline provide different perspectives or frames of reference for the phenomena identified by the metaparadigm of that discipline" (Fawcett, 1993, p. 12–13). The different perspectives identified by the nursing paradigm are person, environment, health and nursing. Nursing theory can be defined as:

> an articulated and communicated conceptualization of invented or discovered reality pertaining to nursing for the purpose of describing, explaining, predicting, or prescribing nursing care. Nursing theory is developed to answer central domain questions. *(Meleis, 1997, p. 139)*

Although we have chosen to cite these particular definitions of nursing models and nursing theory, it must be noted that distinctions between the two are a debated issue and one on which not all authors agree.

What Is the Purpose of Theory in a Research Study?

Theory gives purpose and direction to a research study throughout the entire research process. Theory guides the research from the initial statement of the research problem through the analysis of the study data and provides a framework within which to analyze and interpret the results of the study. Analyzing the study results within the framework of the theory not only guides the researcher in organizing and giving meaning to the phenomena, but may also increase the applicability and generalizability of the study findings.

The following hypothetical—and very simplified—example should help to clarify the function of theory in a research study. The purpose of this hypothetical study is to describe the characteristics of 100 hypertensive male adults who do or do not adhere to their medication regimen. If the study is not designed within a theory, the report of the results, although interesting, has limited applicability and generalizability to other than the 100 hypertensive male adults receiving medications who participated in the study.

If, however, the research were formulated within the framework of a theory, such as Orem's theory of self-care, the applicability and generalizability of the findings could then be broadened. Consider the following example of the same study formulated within Orem's self-care theory. In describing her theory of self-care, Orem (1995) offered this definition of self-care:

> The practice of activities that maturing and mature persons initiate and perform, within time frames, on their own behalf in the interest of maintaining life, healthful functioning, continuing personal development, and well-being. *(p. 461)*

In our hypothetical study, formulated within Orem's self-care theory, the researcher was specifically looking for the relationship between adherence to medication regimens and self-care agency among the participants of the study. Self-care agency is defined by Orem as "the *complex acquired ability* of mature and maturing persons to know and meet their continuing requirements for deliberate, purposive action to regulate their own human functioning and development" (p. 461). In analyzing the study results within the framework provided by self-care theory, the researcher could now observe that study participants with enough self-care agency to adhere to their medication regimen could be viewed as having positive outcomes of good self-care: the ability to meet their own requirements for care that promotes health and well-being.

Thus, the knowledge gained from the study could now move from merely describing the 100 subjects of the study, as in the first design, to the broader area of describing hypertensive adult male's health and health care. Guided by the explanatory function of the theory, the researcher could now understand why the phenomena are occurring; the predictive feature could permit the ability to forecast what is most likely to occur in adult male hypertensive patients in the future. Providing we could assume that there is a prescriptive feature of self-care theory, caregivers could now be directed to assess systematically the self-care agency of medicated hypertensive adult males. They could then prescribe the enhancement of individual self-care agency, thereby potentially increasing adherence to the regimen and the attainment of positive outcomes of good self-care.

Research Frameworks

All research studies have a framework of background knowledge that provides the foundation for the study. This framework serves to organize the study by placing it in the context of existing related knowledge, as well as providing a context within which to interpret the results of the study. If a study is based on a conceptual model, the framework for the study is most often referred to as a **conceptual framework**; if a study is based on a specific theory or theories, the framework is most often referred to as a **theoretical framework**. The terms conceptual framework and theoretical framework are often used interchangeably.

Although all research studies have frameworks—that is, have conceptual underpinnings—not all researchers explicitly identify and describe their research frameworks, especially when the research is not based on a specific theory or conceptual model. In a study based on a single concept or more than one concept, each major concept should be identified, defined, and discussed by the researcher.

Isolated Research and Theory-Linked Research

Not all research studies are linked to the theory development process. Chinn and Kramer (1995) describe two types of research, isolated research and theory-linked research, that "reflect certain basic standards that have been established in order to obtain results that are considered reliable and valid or accurately representative of empiric reality" (p. 140–141).

Isolated research is research that is not linked to the theory development process. Our hypothetical study of hypertensive adult males' adherence to their medication regimen, when designed without a theoretical or conceptual framework, is an example of isolated research. The study focused on a specific problem and offered little potential for applying the results beyond the findings of the study. However, isolated research does have certain merits, according to Chinn and Kramer (1995): "The results of isolated research can provide new insights that prompt the researcher, or someone reading the report of the research, to speculate about larger implications of the research for the discipline, which in turn can lead to developing theory that has broader meaning for the discipline" (p. 141).

Theory-linked research, on the other hand, "is designed with reference or linkage to theory." Theory-linked research is designed to develop theory or to test theory, and "it is this quality that sets the stage for the study to contribute to the larger knowledge of the discipline" (Chinn & Kramer, 1995, p. 141). Theory-linked research is linked to the theory development process in one of two ways: the research is either theory-generating (designed to develop theory) or theory-testing (designed to test how accurately the theory depicts phenomena and their relationships). Box 5-1 depicts the two types of theory-linked research.

Theory-generating research is most often associated with the qualitative research approach. In a theory-generating qualitative study, the theory is "built up" from the data. The researcher does not begin with a theory or theories to test or verify; instead, "consistent with the inductive model of thinking, a theory may emerge during the data collection and analysis phase of the research or be used relatively late in the research process as a basis for comparison with other theories" (Creswell, 1994, pp. 94–95).

Theory-testing research is most often associated with the quantitative research approach, in which deductive reasoning is used to test the theory. "In quantitative studies one uses theory deductively and places it toward the beginning of the plan for a study. In quantitative research the objective is to

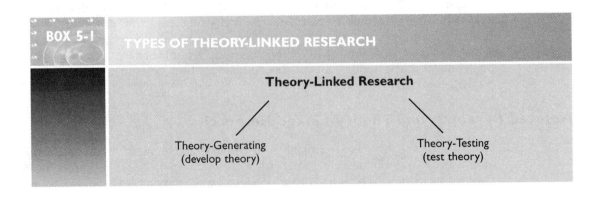

BOX 5-1   TYPES OF THEORY-LINKED RESEARCH

Theory-Linked Research

Theory-Generating
(develop theory)

Theory-Testing
(test theory)

test or verify theory, rather than to develop it" (Creswell, 1994, p. 87). The researcher tests a theory or theories by testing a hypothesis or research questions derived from the theory. Our hypothetical example using Orem's self-care theory was theory-testing research. The theory guided the research, and the researcher could test how accurately the theory depicted the phenomena and their relationships.

Theory and research are reciprocal in their relationship—that is, theory guides research and research tests (validates) the theory: "If you begin with a theory, research derived from the theory is used to clarify and extend the theory. If you begin with research, theory that is formed from the findings can be subsequently used to direct research" (Chinn & Kramer, 1995, p. 143).

Chinn and Kramer (1995) provide the following observation regarding the role of both theory-linked and isolated research in the development of nursing knowledge: "From a research point of view, both can be of excellent quality. Both types of research can ultimately contribute to knowledge, although isolated research is much more limited in the contribution it can make to a discipline" (p. 141).

How Do Researchers Choose a Theory?

Nurse researchers who use theories to guide their studies select theories that are unique to nursing as well as those borrowed from other disciplines. Selecting the most appropriate theory (or theories) depends on several considerations. Researchers must select a theory that has concepts and propositions that fit with the proposed study and one in which there are no contradictions between the theory and the variables selected for study. The theory should be one that provides a "best fit" with the proposed study and that can be useful in describing the relationship(s) between study variables.

We have already mentioned some of the nursing theories (conceptual frameworks) used by researchers. Examples of those from other disciplines include Selye's Stress Theory, Festinger's Cognitive Dissonance Theory, Lazarus and Folkman's Coping Theory, Kohlberg's Moral Reasoning Theory, and Bandura's Social Learning Theory.

● STATEMENT OF THE PURPOSE OF THE STUDY

After formulating the research problem and deciding on the research approach and the role of theory in the study, researchers then state the purpose of the study. For both quantitative and qualitative research, the purpose of the study is a single sentence or a short paragraph that summarizes the essence of the study.

The statement of the research study's purpose can be written in three ways: (1) as a declarative statement, (2) as a question, or (3) as a hypothesis. The form depends on the way the research question is asked and the extent of the researcher's knowledge about the problem. The statement of the purpose should include information about what the researcher intends to do to collect data (such as observe, describe, or measure some variable), information about the setting of the study (where the researcher plans to collect the data), and information about who the study subjects/participants will be.

The Purpose as a Declarative Statement

In our previously formulated research question designed to describe the relationship between the type of teaching and success in breast feeding by primiparas, the purpose of the study written as a declarative statement could read: "The purpose of this study is to describe the effect of structured individualized versus structured group instruction on successful breast feeding by primiparas in their home setting." Note that the statement includes information about what the researcher intends to do (to describe), the setting of the study (home setting), and the subjects of the study (primiparas).

The Purpose as a Question

Using the same research question, the purpose of the study written as a question could read: "The purpose of this study is to answer the question: Is there a significant relationship between a specific method of teaching about breast feeding and successful breast feeding by primiparas in their home setting?" Specific methods of teaching might include structured individual teaching, structured group teaching, and unstructured (incidental) teaching. The primiparas in the study could be interviewed regarding their perceptions of their own success with breast feeding and their satisfaction with the method of teaching to prepare them for breast feeding.

The Purpose as a Hypothesis

Using the same research question, the purpose of the study, written as a hypothesis, could read: "The purpose of the study is to test the following hypothesis: Primiparas who receive individualized instruction about breast feeding will have a significantly more successful breast-feeding experience in their home setting than primiparas who receive group instruction about breast feeding."

● MORE ABOUT HYPOTHESES

A hypothesis is a statement of the predicted relationships between two or more variables. A hypothesis can be thought of as the researcher's "educated or calculated guess" as to how the study variables are related. A hypothesis is the testable component of the propositions of a theory and is therefore derived from theory. A study may have more than one hypothesis (which are then referred to as hypotheses). In the statement of a hypothesis, an antecedent condition—called the independent variable—is related to the occurrence of another condition or effect, called the dependent variable. This can be shown as follows:

Condition X is related to the occurrence of condition Y
Independent variable (antecedent condition) = X
Dependent variable (effect) = Y
or
Method of instruction on breast feeding (group versus individualized) = X
Degree of success on breast feeding = Y

To test the hypothesis, the researcher purposely manipulates the independent variable and attempts to control all the other conditions. The effect on the dependent variable, which occurs presumably as a result of the manipulation of the independent variable, is then noted. In our example, the independent variable comes first in time and is "manipulated" by the researcher—that is, altered to be either individualized instruction or group instruction. The dependent variable is the phenomenon that occurs as a result of the researcher's manipulating the independent variable.

Formulating Hypotheses in Theory-Linked Research

In theory-testing research—that is, research designed to contribute to the process of theory development by testing a theory (or theories)—a hypothesis can be formulated only if the researcher has enough information from the propositions of the theory to predict the study's outcome and intends to test the significance of the prediction. A hypothesis serves to narrow the field of the research study and forces the researcher to be precise in stating the specific situation being studied. The hypothesis also guides the methodology for the remainder of the study—that is, the definition of key variables, the collection of relevant data to measure the variables, and the plan for analyzing the data. The hypothesis also serves as a framework for stating the conclusions of the study as a direct answer to the purpose of the study (which was to test the hypothesis). A well-formulated hypothesis must be consistent with existing theory and research findings. The hypothesis also must be a reasonable explanation or prediction of the situation being studied. Finally, the hypothesis must be testable; in other words, the researcher must be able to collect data that can be analyzed statistically to determine if the hypothesis should be supported or rejected. It is important to note that a hypothesis is not proved; it is either accepted (supported) or rejected (not supported).

Figure 5-1 depicts the function of a hypothesis in theory-testing research using deductive reasoning.

In theory-generating research, the purpose is to develop theory rather than to verify or test theory. Therefore, a hypothesis is not tested. Rather, in identifying and describing relationships among phenomena, researchers may

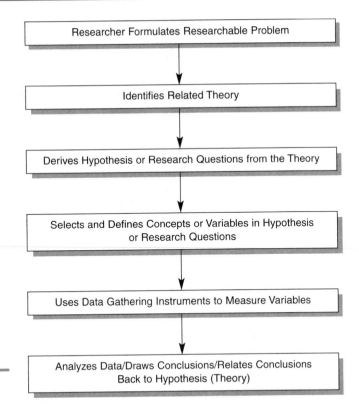

FIGURE 5-1. Deductive reasoning in theory-testing research.

use inductive reasoning to generate relationship statements or propositions, and a theory may emerge during data collection and data analysis.

Figure 5-2 depicts the process of using inductive reasoning in theory-generating research.

Formulating Hypotheses in Isolated Research

Not all research is designed to contribute directly to the theory-development process—that is, to verify theory through hypothesis testing or to generate theory that will contribute to the scientific knowledge base of nursing. Rather, researchers may design isolated research—that is, research that is not linked to the processes of theory development. In designing isolated research, researchers may or may not choose to formulate testable hypotheses; this decision depends on the purpose of their studies. When the purpose of the study is to test a hypothesis or hypotheses, these can be based on the personal or professional observations of the researcher or may be formulated as a result of reading the results of other research studies. In these cases, the hypotheses provide the same functions in guiding the study as in theory-testing research. However, because the hypotheses are not based in theory, the results of the study cannot be discussed in light of adding new knowledge to

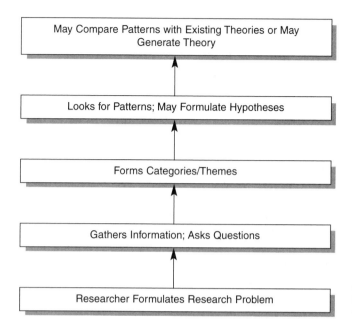

FIGURE 5-2. Inductive reasoning in theory-generating research.

a theory. Although isolated research cannot contribute directly to theory development, the results may serve as preliminary steps in contributing new insights that have the potential to contribute to theory development.

Types of Hypotheses

You will see the following terms used to describe different types of hypotheses: simple hypothesis and complex hypothesis; directional hypothesis and nondirectional hypothesis; research hypothesis and null hypothesis.

SIMPLE HYPOTHESIS AND COMPLEX HYPOTHESIS

A **simple hypothesis** is a statement of the predicted relationship between two variables—that is, a single independent variable and a single dependent variable. For example, "Primiparas who receive individualized instruction about breast feeding will have a more successful breast-feeding experience than primiparas who receive group instruction." The single independent variable is the method of instruction about breast feeding (individualized versus group); the single dependent variable is successful breast feeding. A **complex hypothesis** is a statement of the predicted relationship between three or more variables. This statement can express the relationship between the independent and dependent variables in several different ways:

1. The statement may have two (or more) independent variables and one dependent variable. For example, "Primiparas who receive instruction on breast feeding and instruction on anxiety-reduction

techniques will report a more successful breast-feeding experience than those who do not receive this instruction." The independent variables are instruction on breast feeding and instruction on anxiety-reduction techniques; the dependent variable is successful breast-feeding experience.

2. The statement can be composed of one independent variable and two (or more) dependent variables. For example, "Primiparas who receive instruction on breast feeding will report a more successful breast-feeding experience and less anxiety than those who do not receive this instruction." The independent variable is instruction on breast feeding; the dependent variables are successful breast-feeding experience and reduced anxiety.

3. The statement can be composed of two (or more) independent variables and two (or more) dependent variables. For example, "Primiparas who receive instruction on breast feeding and instruction on anxiety-reduction techniques will report a more successful breast-feeding experience and less anxiety than those who do not receive this instruction." The independent variables are instruction on breast feeding and instruction on anxiety-reduction techniques: the dependent variables are successful breast-feeding experience and reduced anxiety.

Table 5-1 shows these examples of simple and complex hypotheses.

DIRECTIONAL HYPOTHESIS AND NONDIRECTIONAL HYPOTHESIS

A **directional hypothesis** specifies the predicted relationship between the independent variable (or variables) and the dependent variables (or variables). For example, "Primiparas who receive instruction about breast feeding will report a successful breast-feeding experience." A **nondirectional hypothesis** predicts that a relationship exists between the independent and dependent variables but does not specify the direction of the relationship. A nondirectional hypothesis may be formulated when the researcher has no clear indication of the nature of the predicted relationship and plans to use the results of the study to describe whatever relationship exists. Note the "neutral nature" of the following nondirectional hypothesis: "Instruction in breast-feeding techniques for primiparas is related to the decision about whether or not to breast feed the baby." Rather than predicting the nature of the decision, the hypothesis merely states that a decision will be made.

In the research article reprinted in Appendix D, the hypothesis tested was "there is a relationship between the set of independent variables—age, gender, past painful experiences, temperament, medical fears, general fears, and child-rearing practices—and the set of school-age children's responses to venipuncture: pain location, pain intensity, pain quality, observed behaviors, and heart rate." The children's responses to venipuncture are all dependent variables. This is a complex hypothesis because it has more than one independent variable and more than one dependent variable. The hypothesis is also nondirectional: it predicts the existence of a relationship between the set

TABLE 5-1 *Examples of Hypotheses*

	INDEPENDENT VARIABLE(S)	DEPENDENT VARIABLE(S)
SIMPLE HYPOTHESIS		
Individualized instruction on breast feeding will lead to greater success in breast feeding for primiparas than group instruction on breast feeding	Method of instruction on breast feeding	Success in breast feeding
COMPLEX HYPOTHESIS		
1. Primiparas who receive instruction on breast feeding and instruction on anxiety-reduction techniques will report a more successful breast-feeding experience than those who do not receive this instruction.	Instruction on breast feeding and instruction on anxiety-reduction techniques	Report of successful breast-feeding experience
2. Primiparas who receive instruction on breast feeding will report a more successful breast-feeding experience and less anxiety than those who do not receive this instruction.	Instruction on breast feeding	Report of successful breast-feeding experience and reduced anxiety
3. Primiparas who receive instruction on breast feeding and instruction on anxiety-reduction techniques will report a more successful breast-feeding experience and less anxiety than those who do not receive this instruction.	Instruction on breast feeding and instruction on anxiety-reduction techniques	Report of successful breast-feeding experience and reduced anxiety

of independent variables and the set of dependent variables, but the researcher does not predict the direction of the relationship.

RESEARCH HYPOTHESIS AND STATISTICAL HYPOTHESIS

A **research hypothesis** states the expected relationship between the variables that the researcher expects as the study's outcome. It is stated in the declarative form. The **statistical hypothesis** is a statement of no statistically significant difference or relationship between the variables of a study. The statistical hypothesis is also referred to as the **null hypothesis** (H_0) because it is stated in the null (no difference) form. The statistical hypothesis may not reflect the outcome expected by the researcher and may be confusing to a beginning researcher. It is used as a part of decision-making procedures that are statistically based. The null hypothesis exists because statistical procedures are designed to test the null rather than the research hypothesis. For example, in the following research hypothesis, the researcher predicts the outcome of the study: "Primiparas who receive individualized instruction on breast feeding will have a more successful breast-feeding experience in their home setting than primiparas who receive group instruction on breast feeding." (Note that in the above example the research hypothesis is also a directional hypothesis.) The following statistical hypothesis, stated in the null (no difference) form, may not reflect the outcome that is really expected by the researcher: "There will be no significant difference in the breast-feeding experience in their home setting between primiparas who receive individualized instruction on breast feeding and primiparas who receive group instruction on breast feeding." Many researchers prefer to state the hypothesis in the null form because it reflects a more objective and scientific statement of the relationship between the variables. Also, the statistical procedures they plan to use to test the hypothesis may require the null form to determine whether an observed relationship is probably a chance relationship (due to sampling error, for example) or is probably a true relationship. The null form of the hypothesis, however, may not reflect the researcher's true prediction of the study's outcome. Statements in the null form can make it difficult to tie the hypothesis back to the background and theory of the research. Other researchers, therefore, prefer to use the research hypothesis, in which case the underlying null hypothesis is usually assumed without being explicitly stated.

One note: the success of a quantitative research study designed to test theory through hypothesis testing does not depend on the hypothesis being supported by the data. A well-designed and well-executed research study in which the hypothesis was not supported can add just as much to the knowledge base about the theory from which it was derived as a well-designed and well-executed study where the hypothesis was supported.

● DEFINITION OF TERMS

Key terms in the statement of the purpose of the study should be defined. Quantitative researchers define the terms of the study before data collection because they operate "within the deductive model methodology of fixed and set research objectives" (p. 107). On the other hand, qualitative researchers, "because of the inductive, evolving methodological design, may include few terms defined at the beginning of the plan; terms may be defined as they emerge from the data collection" (Creswell, 1994, pp. 107–108).

Research terms are defined directly, operationally, or theoretically.

Direct Definitions

A **direct definition** is the definition of a term as found in a dictionary.

Operational Definitions

An **operational definition** provides a full description of the method by which the concept will be measured or observed. This definition is stated in behavioral, observable, demonstrable terms by citing the operations (the manipulations and observations) necessary to produce the phenomenon. For example, in the previously described statement of the purpose of the study, "the purpose of this study is to describe the effect of structured individualized versus structured group instruction on successful breast feeding by primiparas in their home setting," the variables to be operationally defined include structured individualized instruction, structured group instruction, and successful breast feeding in a home setting. Structured individualized instruction might be operationally defined as "a one-to-one instructional relationship between the professional nurse and the primipara, where a planned teaching protocol is used consistently." Structured group instruction might be operationally defined as "instruction of several primiparas by the nurse, where a planned teaching protocol is used consistently." Successful breast feeding in a home setting might be operationally defined as "the duration of breast feeding (weeks or months)" or as "the degree to which difficulties with home breast feeding were identified as problematic on a questionnaire administered to the mother 6 weeks after delivery." A direct definition for primipara can be taken from a medical dictionary.

Theoretical Definitions

A **theoretical definition** of a variable uses the definition found in the specific language of the theory or conceptual model that serves as the framework for the study. For example, the study in Appendix D was guided by the Roy Adaptation Model of Nursing. For the purposes of her study, the author defined the variable of acute pain within this model, taking the following theoretical definition directly from Roy (1991): Acute pain refers to "discomfort which is intense but relatively short-lived and reversible." In our previously cited hypothetical study that proposed to determine the relationship between adherence to medication regimens and self-care agency among the study participants, formulated with Orem's self-care theory, we used Orem's definitions of "self-care" and "self-care agency." These are also examples of theoretical definitions.

A theoretical definition may also be termed a conceptual definition.

● CRITIQUING THE THEORETICAL FRAMEWORK AND PURPOSE OF A RESEARCH REPORT

Points to Consider in a Quantitative Report

Because a quantitative investigation is either theory-linked or isolated research, not all quantitative studies are conducted within a theoretical or a conceptual framework. Although there will be no discussion of a theoretical framework in an investigation that has been conducted as isolated research, it is important to evaluate whether it would have been more appropriately conducted as theory-linked research.

In a theory-linked investigation, the discussion related to theory should be near the beginning of the report. The discussion may be explicitly labeled as the theoretical (or conceptual) framework, or it may be presented as part of the literature review. The discussion should explain the theoretical background for the study in enough detail to allow the reader to understand its relation to the study variables and its role in guiding the remainder of the study. For example, the Roy Adaptation Model was used as the conceptual framework for the study in Appendix D. Note that this discussion is labeled as "Conceptual Framework," is placed very early in the study, and is followed by the "Review of Literature." Also note that in the study in Appendix C, the conceptual framework is not labeled as such and follows the literature review. In critiquing a research report, it is important to evaluate whether the theoretical framework is appropriate for the study.

Theory-linked investigations in quantitative research are most often theory-testing rather than theory-generating. In a study that is theory-generating, look to see if one of the purposes of the study is to generate theory. In theory-testing research, the theoretical framework must be appropriate for the research problem. The discussion should clearly relate the framework to the study question and should be useful for clarifying pertinent concepts and relationships.

The purpose of the study may also be termed the objectives or goals or aims of the study and may appear in the introduction with the problem statement or later in the report. The purpose statement should be appropriate for the study—that is, a declarative statement (or statements), research question (or questions), or statement of a hypothesis or hypotheses. The statement should be clear as to what the researcher plans to do, and where and from whom the data will be collected. In a hypothesis-testing study, each hypothesis must be logically related to the research problem, should specify an expected relationship among variables, and must be clearly and concisely stated.

Relevant terms must be defined either directly, operationally, or theoretically, and significant assumptions should be logical and clearly stated.

Box 5-2 lists these points as evaluation guidelines.

Points to Consider in a Qualitative Report

Because qualitative research is designed to generate theory, a qualitative investigation typically does not have a theoretical framework to guide the study. The purpose of the study should be clearly stated near the beginning of the report and should be clear as to what the researcher plans to do. Note that the authors of both qualitative reports in Appendices E and F have clearly stated the purpose of their studies on the first page of their reports. Any significant assumptions for the study should be logical and clearly stated. Box 5-3 lists these points as evaluation guidelines.

GUIDELINES FOR EVALUATING A QUANTITATIVE THEORETICAL FRAMEWORK AND PURPOSE

Theoretical or Conceptual Framework
1. Is the research isolated rather than theory-linked?

   Is this appropriate, or should the research have been theory-linked?

2. If the research is theory linked:

   Does the report describe a theoretical or conceptual framework?

   a. Is the framework appropriate for the research problem?

   b. Is the framework clearly developed?

   c. Is the framework useful for clarifying pertinent concepts and relationships?

Purpose of the Study
1. The statement describing the purpose is appropriate for the study: declarative statement, research question(s), statement of hypothesis or hypotheses.

2. The purpose statement is clear as to:

   a. What the researcher plans to do.

   b. Where the data will be collected.

   c. From whom the data will be collected.

3. If hypotheses are being tested:

   a. Each hypothesis is logically related to the research problem.

   b. Each hypothesis specifies an expected relationship among variables.

   c. Each hypothesis is clearly and concisely stated.

Definition of Terms
1. Relevant terms are clearly defined either directly, operationally, or theoretically.

Statement of Significant Assumptions
1. Significant assumptions are clearly stated and logical.

BOX 5-3

GUIDELINES FOR EVALUATING THE PURPOSE OF A QUALITATIVE REPORT

Purpose of the Study
1. The statement describing the purpose is clear as to what the researcher plans to do.
2. Significant assumptions are clearly stated and logical.

● *SUMMARY*

When using theory in research studies, a researcher may chose to use conceptual models of nursing, nursing theories, or theories borrowed from other disciplines. Theory gives purpose and direction to a research study throughout the entire research process. Theory can be classified as broad-range, middle-range, or narrow-range.

Theory-linked research is designed to develop theory or to test theory. Isolated research investigations do not have linkages to the theory-development process. Quantitative research is usually conducted to test theory; qualitative research is usually conducted to develop or generate theory.

Researchers develop a statement of the purpose of the study during the planning stage of the study to identify the direction for the research. The purpose of a quantitative study may be stated as a declarative statement, a question, or a hypothesis. A hypothesis is a statement of the predicted relationship between two or more variables. Types of hypotheses include simple hypotheses, which have only one independent and one dependent variable, and complex hypotheses, which have more than one independent and dependent variable. Hypotheses may also be stated in directional or nondirectional terms and as research hypotheses or as statistical (null) hypotheses.

The researcher must define the key terms in the purpose of the study, using a direct definition (found in a dictionary), an operational definition (a full description of the method by which the concept will be measured or observed), or a theoretical definition (the definition found in the specific language of the theory or theories used in the study). Points to consider in critiquing the theoretical framework and purpose of the study for both quantitative and qualitative research reports were discussed.

The following application activities will help you to evaluate your understanding of this material and will assist you in developing your skills in evaluating published research.

REFERENCES

Alligood, M., & Marriner-Tomey, A. (1997). *Nursing theory: Utilization and application.* St. Louis: Mosby.

Chinn, P. L., & Kramer, M. K. (1995). *Theory and nursing: A systematic approach* (4th ed.). St. Louis: Mosby.

Creswell, J. (1994). *Research design: Qualitative and quantitative approaches.* Thousand Oaks, CA: Sage.

Fawcett, J. (1993). *Analysis and evaluation of nursing theories.* Philadelphia: F. A. Davis.

Fitzpatrick, J. J., & Whall, A. L. (1996). *Conceptual models of nursing* (3rd ed.). Stamford, CT: Appleton & Lang.

Meleis, A. F. (1997). *Theoretical nursing: Development and progress* (3rd ed.). Philadelphia: Lippincott-Raven.

Marriner-Tomey, A., & Alligood, M. R. (1998). *Nursing theorists and their work* (4th ed.). St. Louis: Mosby.

Orem, D. (1995). *Nursing: Concepts and practice* (5th ed.). St. Louis: Mosby.

Powers, B. A., & Knapp, T. R. (1995). *A dictionary of nursing theory and research* (2nd ed.). Thousand Oaks, CA: Sage.

BIBLIOGRAPHY AND SUGGESTED READINGS

Barnum, B. S. (1994). *Nursing theory: Analysis, application, evaluation* (4th ed.). Philadelphia: Lippincott.

Brink, P. J., & Wood, M. (1994). *Basic steps in planning nursing research* (4th ed.). Boston: Jones & Bartlett.

Cody, W. K. (1997). Of tombstones, milestones, and gemstones: A retrospective and prospective on nursing theory. *Nursing Science Quarterly, 10*(1), 3–5.

Doordan, A. M. (1998). *Research survival guide.* Philadelphia: Lippincott-Raven.

Frey, M. (1996). Behavioral correlates of health and illness in youths with chronic illness. *Applied Nursing Research, 9*(4), 167–176.

Gaffney, F. K., & Moore, J. B. (1996). Testing Orem's theory of self-care deficit: Dependent care agent performance of children. *Nursing Science Quarterly, 9*(4), 160–164.

George, J. (1995). *Nursing theories: The base for professional nursing* (4th ed.). Norwalk, CT: Appleton & Lang.

Gigliotti, E. (1997). Use of Neuman's lines of defense and resistance in nursing research: Conceptual and empirical considerations. *Nursing Science Quarterly, 10*(3), 136–143.

Gioiella, E. C. (1996). The importance of theory-guided research and practice in the changing health care scene. *Nursing Science Quarterly, 9*(2), 47.

Good, M., & Morre, S. M. (1996). Clinical practice guidelines as a new source of middle-range theory: Focus on acute pain. *Nursing Outlook, 44*(2), 74–79.

Hammer, J. B. (1996). Preliminary testing of a proposition from the Roy Adaptation Model. *Image, 28*(3), 215–220.

King, I. (1997). King's theory of goal attainment in practice. *Nursing Science Quarterly, 10*(4), 180–184.

Nicoll, L. (Ed.). (1997). *Perspectives on nursing theory* (3rd ed.). Philadelphia: Lippincott.

Parse, R. R. (1997). Transforming research and practice with the human becoming theory. *Nursing Science Quarterly, 10*(4), 171–175.

Roy, C. (1997). Future of the Roy Model: Challenge to redefine adaptation. *Nursing Science Quarterly, 10*(1), 42–46.

Silva, M. C. (1981). Selection of a theoretical framework. In S. Krampitz &. N. Pavlovich (Eds.), *Readings for nursing research* (pp. 17–28). St. Louis: Mosby.

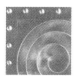

APPLICATION ACTIVITIES

1. Discuss three functions of nursing theory.

2. Explain the difference between broad-range theories, middle-range theories, and narrow-range theories.

3. Describe the purpose of theory in a research investigation.

4. Discuss how isolated research and theory-linked research differ in their relationship to theory development.

5. Define the following terms:

   a. Operational definition

   b. Hypothesis

   c. Direct definition

    d. Research hypothesis

    e. Statistical (null) hypothesis

    f. Theoretical definition

6. Read the following three hypotheses:

    a. Patients with slightly elevated blood pressure will have lower blood pressure after training
       in stress-reduction techniques.
    b. Nurses caring for AIDS patients have a higher level of anxiety than nurses caring for
       oncology patients.
    c. Primiparas whose husbands have received instruction in neonatal care have fewer adjustment
       problems with their infants than those whose husbands have not received such instruction.
       i. State the independent variable and dependent variable for each of these hypotheses.

    ii. State each hypothesis in the null form.

    iii. Write an operational definition for a term used in one of the null hypotheses you
         have just stated.

7. If you have done activity #6 in Chapter 4, you should have already critiqued the problem statement
   and literature review for the three articles related to the clinical area you are using to learn the
   process of critical evaluation. Now, to critique the theoretical framework and purpose in each of
   these studies, use the guidelines for evaluating a quantitative theoretical framework and purpose in
   Box 5-2. For a qualitative report, use the guidelines in Box 5-3. Evaluation guidelines are also given
   in Appendix G for a quantitative report and in Appendix H for a qualitative report.

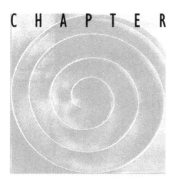

C H A P T E R 6

Subject Selection: Population and Sampling

SAMPLING
SAMPLING APPROACHES
DETERMINING SAMPLE
   SIZE

CRITIQUING THE SUBJECT SELECTION
COMPONENT OF A PUBLISHED
RESEARCH REPORT
SUMMARY

OBJECTIVES   *On completion of this chapter, the student will be able to:*

1. Discuss reasons for sampling.
2. Compare the characteristics of probability sampling with those of nonprobability sampling.
3. Identify the major methods of probability and nonprobability sampling.
4. Explain the reasons why qualitative researchers do not use probability sampling techniques.
5. List the major considerations in determining sample size in quantitative studies.
6. Define key terms.
7. Use evaluation guidelines to critique the subject selection component of published research reports.

KEY TERMS

Accidental sampling
Cluster random sampling
Convenience sampling
Diversity sampling
Event sampling
Expert sampling
Heterogeneity sampling
Judgmental sampling
Link-tracing sampling
Modal instance sampling
Multistage sampling
Network sampling
Nominated sampling
Nonprobability sampling
Power analysis

Probability sampling
Proportional sampling
Purposive sampling
Quota sampling
Random route sampling
Sampling frame
Simple random sampling
Snowball technique sampling
Stratified random sampling
Systematic random sampling
Target population
Theoretical sampling
Time sampling
Voluntary sampling

An essential consideration in the research design is the selection of the subjects who will provide the necessary data in relation to the purpose of the study. This chapter presents the important topic of sampling for both quantitative and qualitative research. Critical evaluation of this component of a published research report is also discussed.

SAMPLING

Because size, cost, time, or lack of accessibility often makes it impossible for the researcher to collect data directly from the entire group of interest, a study is often done on a smaller part of this group, called a sample. In Chapter 1, we defined the total group of interest to the researcher as the population, and the term sampling was defined as the process of selecting a number of individuals from the delineated target population in such a way that the individuals in the sample represent, as nearly as possible, the characteristics of the entire target population. Thus, the sample can be thought of as a miniature of the larger target population. A single unit or member of the target population is referred to as a population element or a sampling unit. A basic purpose for sampling in the quantitative research approach is to enable the investigator to use the sample's findings to generalize or extrapolate beyond the actual sampling units without having to study each element of the target population. The extent of this ability to generalize beyond the actual sampling units to the target population depends on the sampling approach used.

Selecting the Sample

In selecting a sample that would be representative of the target population, the investigator must first delineate the target population. A **target population** consists of the total group of people or objects meeting the designated set of criteria of interest to the researcher. The term target population does not necessarily pertain to human beings. For example, in nursing research, the target population may consist of people (such as patients or nursing students), organizations (such as hospitals or nursing homes), or objects (such as a population of patient records).

Following is an example of sample selection from a target population. A study proposes to investigate the effect of educational preparation on the political perceptions of all licensed nurses in Florida (the target population). This population of nurses would become the **sampling frame**—that is, the list of all of the members of the population from which the sample is taken. A sampling frame (list) should be comprehensive, up to date, and complete. Because it would probably not be feasible to collect data from all the licensed nurses in Florida (more than 250,000), a sample of these nurses would be selected for inclusion in the study. This would be done in such a way that they would be representative of all the licensed nurses in Florida. Such a selection could be accomplished by first obtaining a computer listing of all the licensed nurses in the state from the Florida Board of Nursing. The investigator would then select a fraction of the licensed nurses on the list in such a way that those selected for inclusion in the study would be representative of all licensed nurses in Florida. Each licensed nurse in the sample would then be a population element and a sampling unit.

● *SAMPLING APPROACHES*

Sampling theory distinguishes between two main approaches to sampling in research: probability sampling and nonprobability sampling. In **probability sampling**, the investigator can specify, for each element of the population, the probability that it will be included in the sample. Usually each element has the same probability of being included in the sample, but the basic requirement is that there exists a known probability that a given element will be included. The sampling units are selected at random (by chance), and neither the investigator nor the population elements have any conscious influence on what is included in the sample. **Nonprobability sampling**, on the other hand, involves the use of subjects who are both accessible and available; therefore, the investigator cannot estimate the probability that each element of the population will be included in the sample or even that it has some chance of being included.

The importance of the ability to estimate probability lies in the application of the study findings to the target population with a given degree of certainty.

Probability sampling has the advantage of permitting the investigator to generalize from the sample's findings to the target population with a given degree of certainty. This means that the sample findings do not differ by more than a specific amount from the expected findings if the investigator were to use the total population. In general, nonprobability sampling techniques do not permit generalization of the study findings from the sample to the population.

Selection of the sampling approach depends on the research problem and the purpose of the study. Not all studies are conducted with the purpose of being able to generalize from a sample to the entire population. The important point is that the sampling approach must be consistent with the problem being researched and with the purpose of the study. Probability sampling is associated primarily with the quantitative research approach; quantitative researchers use both probability and nonprobability sampling. Because of the nature of qualitative research, qualitative researchers use nonprobability sampling.

Probability Sampling Methods

The major methods for probability sampling include (1) simple random sampling, (2) stratified random sampling, (3) systematic random sampling, (4) cluster random sampling, and (5) random route sampling. The following discussion provides an overview of each of these sampling methods. Detailed procedures can be found in sources on more advanced research methodology.

Simple random sampling is a probability sampling procedure in which the required number of sampling units are selected at random from the population in such a manner that each population element has an equal chance (probability) of being selected for the sample. Each choice of a sampling unit must be independent of all other choices. One of the most acceptable methods for selecting a simple random sample is to use a table of random numbers, which can be either computer-generated or found in a statistics textbook. The numbers in a random-number table have been generated in such a way that there is no pattern. The same probability exists that any digit will follow any other digit, and each selection is an independent choice. To obtain a simple

---

BOX 6-1   PROBABILITY SAMPLING METHODS

Simple random sampling

Stratified random sampling

Systematic random sampling

Cluster random sampling

Random route sampling

random sample, first list each of the population elements, then assign consecutive numbers to each of these elements. Then, referring to a table of random numbers (Table 6-1), arbitrarily start at any point in the table and proceed in any direction to identify enough tabled numbers to associate with the population elements until the desired sample has been selected.

Rather than using a table of random numbers, it is also possible to select a simple random sample by drawing numbers from a box. The names of the target population elements are written on pieces of paper that are then folded, placed in a container, and mixed well. The first name chosen is assigned to the sample, but because the probability associated with subsequent choices is not constant, the slip should be replaced in the container each time a name is selected to approach random selection more fully. This procedure, called sampling with replacement, is not as rigorous as using a table of random numbers in that each choice of a sampling unit is not independent of all other choices; once a unit is chosen, it will not be included in the sample again.

One of the problems in using simple random sampling is the difficulty of obtaining or compiling a list of each of the population elements, either because they are not known or because, for a large population, the listing proves prohibitively long.

Stratified random sampling is a probability sampling procedure that is a variation of the simple random sample. The population is divided into two or more strata or groups with different categories of a characteristic. A simple random sample is then taken from each group. This procedure is used when the composition of the population is known with respect to some characteristic or characteristics. The variables (characteristics) chosen to stratify the population must be those that are important to the study. For example, a population of 500 human elements may be stratified on the basis of gender. Then half of the sampling units may be chosen from the female category and the other half from the male category by simple random sampling. This ensures that the sample will consist of equal allocations of males and females from each population stratum. A population may be divided into other strata or categories, such as age, educational background, occupation, ethnicity, and so on, depending on their importance for the study.

To ensure that the samples taken in a stratified random sample accurately reflect the composition of the population, researchers may choose to

TABLE 6-1 *Excerpt From a Table of Random Numbers*

57	87	89	93	27	86	05	14	21	98	04	67	95	16	47	11	37	31	34	21	87
22	50	14	55	00	34	33	21	24	47	14	30	62	50	67	96	51	49	40	43	80
44	48	62	90	52	60	28	86	51	92	99	77	98	26	64	77	32	29	20	34	47
55	69	81	45	58	72	83	83	80	73	19	77	80	33	14	76	93	40	93	76	82
83	55	52	48	67	21	15	87	46	87	92	06	03	21	27	71	07	68	15	05	64

use **proportional sampling**. This requires that the researcher be able to identify the percentage of the population that each stratum contains. The researcher then samples the population proportionately, based on these percentages. For example, if a researcher knew that the nursing staff of an agency was comprised of 20% LPNs, 30% RNs without a bachelor's degree, 46% RNs with a bachelor's degree, and 4% RNs with a master's degree, the researcher would sample the entire nursing staff in these proportions. Twenty percent of the sample would come from the LPNs, 30% from the RNs without a bachelor's degree, 46% from RNs with a bachelor's degree, and 4% from RNs with a master's degree.

Systematic random sampling is a probability sampling procedure in which subjects are randomly selected from the population at fixed intervals that are predetermined by the researcher. Before selecting the first element, the researcher determines how large the sample should be and decides on the size of the intervals. The first element is selected at random and subsequent elements are selected according to the intervals. Systematic random sampling is similar to random sampling in that the first population element is based on random identification. When the researcher knows the size of the population and it is not overwhelming large, the researcher may determine that a certain percentage of the population should be sampled. For example, if a population consisted of 200 nurses working in an urban hospital and a sample of 10% has been determined to be sufficient, the researcher would select the first individual's name at random from the nursing personnel list and then count down to the tenth name on the list to select the next person. This procedure would continue until 20 individuals had been selected. Thus, the researcher, using a table of random numbers, might select as the first subject the 87th person on the nursing personnel roster—then the 97th and 107th individuals would become subjects, and so on. If the list is exhausted before the available number of subjects have been selected, the researcher would continue to count from the beginning of the list. To ensure a completely random selection of subjects, the personnel list should be randomly ordered in the beginning to rule out biases that might be accidentally introduced if the list has been compiled in any specific order.

Cluster random sampling (also known as **multistage sampling**) is a probability sampling procedure that progresses in stages from larger sampling units to smaller sampling units. Cluster random sampling is most often used in large-scale studies in which the population is geographically spread out. The sampling unit is the cluster, consisting of groups, rather than individuals, all of whom have the same characteristic(s). A cluster could consist of nursing homes, hospitals, or home health agencies. For example, if the primary sampling unit (cluster) is a group of acute care hospitals, a random sample of these could be taken; then in subsequent sampling stages, a random sample of the various nursing units in each of these hospitals could be taken; then at the next stage, a random sample could be taken that consisted of the nursing supervisors on whom the actual measurements are needed for the study. Cluster sampling has the advantage of convenience and involves less time and money than large-scale studies while retaining the advantages of probability sampling.

Random route sampling is a probability sampling procedure that is useful in marketing research or other community-based research in which households, businesses, or other such premises need to be sampled. In random route sampling, the interviewer randomly selects an address, usually from a sampling frame, as a starting point and then identifies subsequent addresses by a predetermined random process, such as "across the street from the first address" or "left at the corner to the next odd-numbered address" and then calls on every *n*th address to conduct the required number of interviews. Although random route sampling is economical in terms of time and money, it can have the disadvantage of precluding the collection of data from a sample that is truly representative. For example, in conducting a marketing survey, selecting the sample from only one particular geographic area, such as either predominately wealthy or economically deprived, may not provide a truly representative sample of the population who might be targeted for the product being evaluated.

Nonprobability Sampling Methods

In nonprobability sampling, the investigator cannot estimate the probability that each element of the population will be included in the sample. Major procedures for nonprobability sampling include (1) convenience sampling, (2) quota sampling, (3) snowball sampling, (4) purposive sampling, (5) theoretical sampling, (6) voluntary sampling, (7) modal instance sampling, (8) expert sampling, (9) diversity sampling, (10) event sampling, and (11) time sampling. The following discussion provides an overview of these.

BOX 6-2   NONPROBABILITY SAMPLING METHODS

Convenience sampling

Quota sampling

Snowball sampling

Purposive sampling

Theoretical sampling

Voluntary sampling

Modal instance sampling

Expert sampling

Diversity sampling

Event sampling

Time sampling

Convenience sampling, also termed **accidental sampling**, is a nonprobability sampling procedure in which the sampling units are selected simply because they are available—they are in the right place at the right time that is convenient for the investigator's purposes. For example, in an investigation of the use of an emergency care facility during the night, the investigator might select an accidental sample consisting of any person presenting to the emergency facility between midnight and 6 a.m. during a specified 1-month period. Many nursing studies use convenience sampling because of the availability of already existing population groups.

Quota sampling is a nonprobability sampling procedure in which subjects are selected in such a manner that each stratum of the population is proportionately represented. To ensure that the sample does not become overloaded with subjects having certain characteristics, the investigator specifies a percentage for the inclusion of subjects in the sample so that the sample is proportionate to the characteristics of the population. For example, quota sampling may be used to ensure that a sample of males and females from certain age, ethnic, and occupational groups represents the proportions in which these characteristics occur in the population.

Snowball sampling, also known as **nominated sampling**, is a nonprobability sampling procedure in which study subjects are asked to provide referrals to other study subjects. In this method of sampling, investigators identify individual respondents whom they believe to have pertinent information related to their study. They then ask these individuals to name (nominate) others who might be able to provide further information; these respondents, in turn, are then asked to name other potential respondents. This sampling technique is also termed **network sampling** or **link-tracing sampling**.

Purposive sampling, also termed **judgmental sampling**, is a type of nonprobability sampling in which subjects are selected because they are identified as knowledgeable regarding the subject under investigation. The investigator establishes certain criteria thought to be representative of the target population and deliberately selects subjects according to these criteria. For example, in investigating the characteristics of undergraduate nursing students most likely to succeed in graduate programs, the investigator might ask persons who are knowledgeable regarding nursing education either to participate directly in the study or to recommend students to be selected for the study.

Theoretical sampling is a nonprobability approach to sampling most often associated with qualitative research, primarily the grounded theory method (to be discussed in the next chapter). As the study data are collected, coded, and analyzed, the researcher examines the emerging conceptual categories and themes and decides on further data-collection procedures that have the potential to contribute to the developing theory. The researcher may change the focus of the research questions, the locations where the questions are asked, or the participants in the study.

Voluntary sampling is a type of nonprobability sampling procedure in which volunteers either offer or are actively recruited to participate in a study.

A request for volunteers might be made through an international organization such as the Red Cross (for instance, for a study of couples in prenatal or neonatal classes) or through solicitation by advertisements in newspapers or journals. The use of volunteers has the potential to bias the results of a study because those individuals who did not choose to volunteer might have provided other perspectives than those of the volunteers.

Modal instance sampling is a type of nonprobability sample composed of subjects who represent the "typical case" that is constructed by the researcher for purposes of the study. The method draws its name from the mode, the most frequently occurring score or value in a set of measurements. Thus, the mode can be considered to be the typical case. For example, a researcher planning to use modal instance sampling could construct a profile of "the typical baccalaureate-prepared nurse" in a specific health care setting by using the combined qualities of age, education, and years of professional nursing experience. This information could be gathered through self-reports or by examining personnel records in the setting that was targeted for the research. In this instance, the researcher has chosen not to include other personal qualities such as gender, religion, or ethnicity. Using the modal instance technique, the researcher would then sample only those individuals who could be described as "the typical baccalaureate-prepared nurse" for purposes of the study.

Expert sampling is a nonprobability sampling procedure in which the researcher selects study participants based on the need to ascertain how experts in a field would react to or judge the phenomena of interest for the study. The researcher determines what constitutes the expertise needed for the study. For example, a sample of nurse midwifery educators with expertise in curriculum development specific to the preparation of nurse midwives could be selected for a study proposing to determine the effectiveness of two different nurse midwifery curricula.

Diversity sampling, also termed **heterogeneity sampling**, is a nonprobability sampling procedure used when the investigation requires that subjects with a wide variety of opinions and views be included in the sample. To achieve diversity sampling, the researcher would include individuals from all segments of the population without regard for representation of persons with these opinions and views as they occur proportionately in the population. Diversity sampling is particularly useful when the researcher wants to include outliers (individuals who are atypical of those who might otherwise be sampled) to elicit a broad range of opinions or views on the variables of interest. This type of sampling could be used in a community setting by including subjects from every stratum of the community.

Event sampling is a nonprobability sampling procedure in which the investigator is concerned only with sampling from those specific occurrences and/or events that are relevant to the study. For example, the research student who wrote the proposal "Compliance with Universal Precautions" (Appendix A) would collect her data about nurses using universal precautions only when they were working with children.

Time sampling is a nonprobability sampling procedure used by researchers who are concerned with collecting data on activities that take place at specific times of the day or night. For example, a researcher who wanted to observe what was happening during meal times in an intermediate care facility would collect data only at the times when meals were being served.

Both probability and nonprobability sampling have a respected place in research. The important factor in determining which sampling approach to use is consistency with the research problem and the purpose of the study.

● DETERMINING SAMPLE SIZE

Sample Size in Quantitative Research

The quantitative investigator whose objective it is to generalize the sample results to the population will need to sample from the target population and must decide how large a sample will produce sufficient data to allow for such generalizations. The decision as to the size of the sample is determined primarily by such considerations as the degree of precision required, the type of sampling procedure used, the homogeneity of the population, and cost and convenience. There are mathematical formulas and computer programs available for calculating an adequate sample size to permit generalization. For example, **power analysis** is a statistical procedure that allows the researcher to estimate how large a sample is needed to determine the likelihood of accepting a null hypothesis that should actually be rejected or determining that a relationship does not exist between variables when a relationship actually does exist. A general rule in probability sampling is to use as large a sample as possible within such constraints as time, cost, and accessibility. A sample should be large enough to achieve representativeness; the larger the number in the sample, the more likely it is to be representative of the population from which it was selected. In general, the larger the sample, the more generalizable are the study results; however, a large sample cannot correct for a poor sampling design. If the population is homogeneous, a smaller sample size may be adequate for generalization. Not all quantitative researchers design studies with the purpose of generalizing the results. Those who do not plan to do so are not as concerned with sample size and representativeness and often use nonprobability sampling procedures.

Sample Size in Qualitative Research

On the whole, qualitative researchers are not concerned with sample size. Unlike those quantitative researchers whose purpose in conducting studies is to generalize the results from the sample to the target population, most qualitative researchers are not interested in collecting data from a sample that is selected in such a way that it reflects the population being studied. Instead, because they propose to gain an in-depth understanding of the experiences of particular individuals or groups of individuals, qualitative researchers deliberately seek out their subjects (study participants) and determine their number and characteristics in relation to the in-depth understanding needed for their studies.

CRITIQUING THE SUBJECT SELECTION COMPONENT OF A PUBLISHED RESEARCH REPORT

Points to Consider in a Quantitative Report

Subject selection is described in the methodology section of a research report. If sampling techniques were used to select the subjects, the target population should be clearly described and the method for selecting the sample (either probability sampling or nonprobability sampling) should not only be described but should also be appropriate for the purpose of the study. The sample size should be adequate for the problem being investigated as well as for the number of variables in the study. Box 6-3 lists these points as evaluation guidelines.

Points to Consider in a Qualitative Study

The selection of the study participants should be clearly described. If sampling was used, the method and procedures for selecting the sample should not only be described but should also be appropriate for the study. Box 6-4 lists these points as evaluation guidelines.

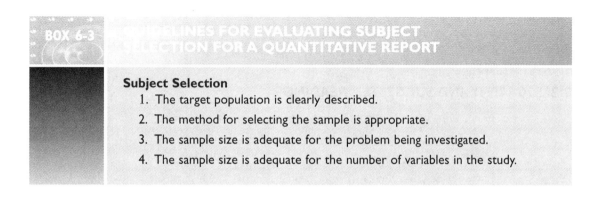

BOX 6-3   GUIDELINES FOR EVALUATING SUBJECT SELECTION FOR A QUANTITATIVE REPORT

Subject Selection
1. The target population is clearly described.
2. The method for selecting the sample is appropriate.
3. The sample size is adequate for the problem being investigated.
4. The sample size is adequate for the number of variables in the study.

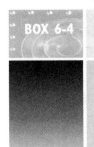

BOX 6-4

GUIDELINES FOR EVALUATING SUBJECT SELECTION FOR A QUALITATIVE REPORT

Selection of Subjects (Participants)
1. The selection of subjects (participants) is clearly described.
2. If sampling methods were used, are these clearly described? Are they appropriate for the study?

● SUMMARY

The method of selecting the subjects for a study must be consistent with the problem and the purpose of the study and involves identification of the target population. If sampling is indicated, the sample should be of sufficient size to be representative of the population and should provide sufficient data for analysis. The sampling approach (probability or nonprobability) must also be consistent with the research design. There are a number of probability sampling methods, including simple random sampling, stratified random sampling, systematic random sampling, cluster random sampling, and random route sampling. Nonprobability sampling methods that are often used in nursing research include, but are not limited to, convenience sampling, quota sampling, snowball sampling, purposive sampling, theoretical sampling, voluntary sampling, modal instance sampling, expert sampling, diversity sampling, event sampling, and time sampling.

Quantitative researchers may use power analysis to determine if a sample is large enough to be generalized to the population. Qualitative researchers are less concerned with sample size because they propose to gain an in-depth understanding of the experiences of particular individuals or groups of individuals. To achieve this, they deliberately seek out their subjects (study participants) and determine their number and characteristics in relation to the in-depth understanding needed for their studies.

The following application activities for this chapter will help you to evaluate your understanding of this material and will further assist you in developing your skills in evaluating published research.

BIBLIOGRAPHY AND SUGGESTED READINGS

Brink, P. J., & Wood, M. (1994). *Basic steps in planning nursing research.* Boston: Jones and Bartlett.
Coynes, I. T. (1997). Sampling in qualitative research. Purposeful and theoretical sampling; merging or clear boundaries? *Journal of Advanced Nursing, 26,* 623–630.
Doordan, A. M. (1998). *Research survival guide.* Philadelphia: Lippincott-Raven.
Dobert, M. L. (1982). *Ethnographic research.* New York: Praeger.
Faugier, J., & Sargeant, M. (1997). Sampling hard-to-reach populations. *Journal of Advanced Nursing, 26,* 790–797.
Patton, M. Q. (1990). *Qualitative research and evaluation methods* (2nd ed.). Newbury Park, CA: Sage.

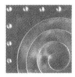

APPLICATION ACTIVITIES

1. Discuss three reasons why a researcher might decide to use sampling rather than to collect data from the entire population.

2. Explain the differences between probability and nonprobability sampling.

3. Describe three considerations in determining sample size for a quantitative study.

4. List and define three probability sampling methods.

5. List and define three nonprobability sampling methods.

6. Although a telephone book could be viewed as a sampling frame, depending on the purpose of the research, discuss at least two reasons why using a telephone book for a specific county would not be appropriate for selecting a simple random sample of voters in that county. What source would be more appropriate? Why?

7. Use the following procedure to select study subjects by simple random sampling:
   The desired sample size for a quantitative study is 20 subjects selected from a target population of 40 elements. Select the subjects to be included in the sample by following this procedure:
   a. List the elements (names) of the target population.

   b. Number the names consecutively from 1 to 40.

   c. Arbitrarily select a two-digit column from the excerpt of a table of random numbers in this chapter (see Table 6-1).

   d. When a number corresponds to a number assigned to a name on the list of the target population, assign that name to the sample.

   e. Skip any number that is not between 01 and 40, inclusive, and go on to the next number.

   f. Continue to select each two-digit number that corresponds to a list of names until 20 names have been assigned to the sample.

8. Use the guidelines for evaluating subject selection for a quantitative report (see Box 6-3) or the guidelines for evaluating subject selection for a qualitative report (see Box 6-4) to evaluate the subject selection component of each of the three research studies you have chosen to critique.

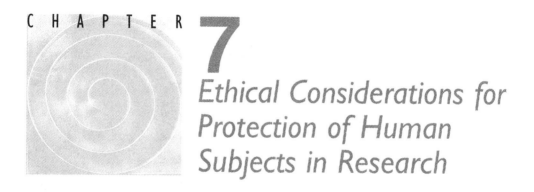

C H A P T E R 7

Ethical Considerations for Protection of Human Subjects in Research

OBJECTIVES   *On completion of this chapter, the student will be able to:*

1. Discuss the development of ethical codes.
2. Discuss the purpose of institutional review boards.
3. Identify the components of appropriate informed consent.
4. Discuss why some kinds of research cannot have prior informed consent.
5. Define key terms.
6. Use evaluation guidelines to critique ethical components in published research reports.

KEY TERMS   Anonymity   Institutional Review Board (IRB)
                 Confidentiality   Principle of beneficence
                 Debrief   Principle of justice
                 Human Subjects Review Board   Principle of respect for human dignity
                 Informed consent   Risk–benefit ratio

*T*he purpose of this chapter is to present basic material related to ethics in research. This is a crucial area for both quantitative and qualitative research and involves an understanding of ethical codes and guidelines for protecting the rights of human subjects who participate in research. Critical evaluation of the ethical components of a published report is also discussed.

● DEVELOPMENT OF ETHICAL CODES

Researchers working with humans must always remember that their subjects are real people with their own unique personalities and needs, not just numbers on a piece of paper. To this end, codes of ethics for human subject research have been developed to ensure the protection of the subjects' dignity and safety and the worthiness of research involving human subjects.

The Nuremberg Code (1949)

Ethical codes for the protection of the rights of research participants are based on the Articles of the Nuremberg Tribunal drawn up after the "doctor trials" following World War II. During these trials, Nazi doctors were accused of abusing human subjects incarcerated in concentration camps in the name of biomedical research. The defense that these individuals brought forward was that they were engaged in important research, regardless of the pain and suffering they caused in their helpless subjects. These articles served as the basis for the Nuremberg Code, which "became a prototype of many later codes intended to assure that research involving human subjects would be carried out in an ethical manner" (National Commission, p. 3).

The Nuremberg Code provided the first international standard against which to measure the individual rights of subjects participating in experimental and clinical research. This code includes the following points:

1. The voluntary consent of the human subject is absolutely essential.
2. The experiment should be such as to yield fruitful results . . . and not random or unnecessary . . .
3. The experiment should be based on . . . [prior knowledge] and the anticipated results should justify . . . the experiment.

4. The experiment should . . . avoid all unnecessary physical and mental suffering and injury.
5. No experiment should be conducted where there is an *a priori* reason to believe that death or disabling injury will occur; except . . . where the experimental physicians also serve as subjects.
6. The degree of risk should never exceed . . . the importance of the problem to be solved.
7. Proper preparations should be made and adequate facilities provided to protect . . . subject(s) against . . . possibilities of injury, disability, or death.
8. The experiment should be conducted only by scientifically qualified persons.
9. During the course of the experiment, the human subject should be able to bring the experiment to an end . . .
10. During the course of the experiment the scientist must be prepared to terminate the experiment if there is probable cause . . . that a continuation of the experiment is likely to result in injury, disability, or death to the experimental subject. *(Katz, 1972, pp. 305–306).*

The Declaration of Helsinki (1964)

In 1964 the World Medical Assembly adopted a code of ethics that has become known as the Declaration of Helsinki. This code was based on the Nuremberg Code and was revised in 1975 to provide further protection of human subjects.

The Belmont Report (1978)

In 1974 the National Research Act (Public Law 93348) created the National Commission for the Protection of Human Subjects of Biomedical and Behavioral Research. The Commission's task was to develop guidelines or principles for working with human subjects. A summary of these guidelines was published in 1978 in a document known as the Belmont Report (National Commission for the Protection of Human Subjects of Biomedical and Behavior Research). The Belmont Report set forth the following three basic principles for research on human subjects:

1. The **principle of respect for human dignity** (the right to self-determination and full disclosure): The report indicated that individuals should be treated as autonomous agents who are capable of self-determination that allows them to voluntarily take part in activities that may harm them when they are made fully aware of the potential dangers of such activities. The report also acknowledges that there are individuals who lack the capacity for self-determination (such as children and developmentally disabled individuals) who need protection.
2. The **principle of beneficence** (the right to freedom from harm and exploitation): Beneficence requires that each autonomous individual be treated in such a way that the researcher should do no harm

to the individual or, if risks cannot be avoided, that the benefits of research should be maximized while the possible harms should be minimized. Every effort must be made to maintain the well-being of the research subjects.

3. The **principle of justice** (the right to fair treatment and privacy): Justice requires that all participants have the right to privacy and respect and to be treated in a fair and equitable manner throughout the entire process of the research. Additionally, the resulting benefits of research must be equitably applied to all members of society rather than just to those who can afford them.

Codes of Federal Regulations for the Protection of Human Subjects (1981, 1991)

The U.S. government has provided a set of guidelines that researchers who receive federal funding for research must follow when using human subjects. These guidelines require that any agency receiving federal funding for research must establish a research review committee, known as an **Institutional Review Board (IRB)**, to ensure that the following conditions are met:

1. Risks to subjects are minimized by sound research procedures that do not expose subjects to risk unnecessarily. This means that research using human subjects should be so well thought out that the potential for unforeseen harm, either physical or psychological, should be minimized.

2. The anticipated benefits to subjects should outweigh the risks to the subjects, and knowledge to be gained should be of sufficient importance to merit any risks to which subjects might be subjected. This provision is termed the **risk–benefit ratio.**

3. The rights and welfare of the subjects must be adequately protected—that is, the researcher must terminate the research if subjects are being deprived of a procedure that might benefit them or are being subjected to one that is causing more harm than was anticipated.

4. The activity will be periodically reviewed by the IRB.

5. Informed consent has been obtained and appropriately documented. This condition is such an important area of concern that it will be discussed in greater detail in a later section of this chapter.

Institutional Review Boards

As a consequence of the need to conform to the federal guidelines previously discussed, all institutions sponsoring government-funded research on human subjects must have IRBs, also called **Human Subjects Review Boards**. The charge of the members of an IRB is to "review whether the benefits of proposed institutional research outweigh the risk and to ensure that investigators have explained the protocol sufficiently to all subjects to give informed consent" (Dabbs & Nolan, p. 101). Members of the IRB are charged with reviewing and monitoring the conduct of research to ensure that the following requirements are satisfied: (1) risks to subjects are minimized and risks are reasonable in relation to expected benefits (the risk–benefit ratio), (2) selection of subjects is equitable, (3) informed consent is obtained and appropriately documented, (4) provision for monitoring the safety and privacy of subjects is adequate (Dabbs & Nolan, p. 102). Although Federal guidelines do not dictate how IRB members are selected, they do mandate that the committee consist of at least five persons with varied backgrounds who have not only the competency to review research but also the diversity to promote respect for the welfare of human subjects. Members must also review the research in terms of the commitments of the institution and conformity to the standards of professional practice. "Although nurses are not explicitly included on IRBs, nurses are eligible because they possess the expertise to fulfill the membership requirements" (Dabbs & Nolan, 1997, p. 102). This means that IRBs should include nurses as well as other health professionals and that the nursing member has an equal voice in the deliberations of the review committee. Institutions that do not receive federal funding may also have research review committees for the protection of human subjects that function in much the same way as IRBs.

ANA Human Rights Guidelines for Nurses in Clinical and Other Research (1985)

Guidelines published by the American Nurses Association (ANA) in 1985 outline the responsibilities of nurses in practice, education, and research for safeguarding the rights of human subjects in research. The subjects of research include patients and outpatients, persons who are donors of organs and tissues, research volunteers, and volunteers with limited freedom— members of groups vulnerable to exploitation. This last category includes prisoners, residents of institutions for the mentally ill and mentally retarded, military personnel, and students.

This document details three basic human rights:

1. The right to freedom from intrinsic risk of injury: Subjects must be protected from physical, social, or emotional injury.
2. The right to anonymity: The identity of subjects participating in a study must not be disclosed, nor should the identity of individuals be recognizable through discussion or publication of the researchers' results, including photographs of the subject(s). If a subject's identity can be determined from the research, the researcher must have a signed consent from the subject in order to include the information that is gained from that subject's participation.
3. The right to privacy and dignity: Researchers should make every attempt to avoid invading their subjects' privacy and/or placing them in demeaning or dehumanizing situations.

The right to privacy also carries over to a patient's records. The Privacy Act of 1974 specifically denies the opening of records to unauthorized individuals. At times, however, a *bona fide* researcher needs to have access to existing records. Some states have established laws to protect the privacy of individuals, including access to medical records; other states have not developed such statutes. Many agencies have developed a prior consent form or release of information form that the potential subject signs as a routine part of obtaining whatever care is being provided. Without such prior consent, however, in many cases the IRB may grant access to records when the board is certain that patient confidentiality will be respected and that only authorized investigators will have access to the records.

ANA Position Statement on Ethics and Human Rights (1991)

The ANA's Position Statement on Ethics and Human Rights, published in 1991, expanded the organization's 1985 ethical guidelines statement. The following beliefs are stated:

1. Human beings deserve respect . . . and . . . deserve nursing services that are equitable . . .
2. Justice requires that . . . when differences among groups contribute to unequal . . . care, then remedial actions are obligated.
3. Justice applies to nurses as providers as well as recipients of care.
4. Because nursing care is essential, ... allocation of care cannot be . . . addressed when . . . individuals are excluded or when . . . limited access [is] borne by particular groups. *(ANA, 1991, p. 3)*

● CLASSIC EXAMPLES OF VIOLATIONS OF THE RIGHTS OF HUMAN SUBJECTS

Although the need for ethical codes and guidelines to protect the rights of research participants seems self-evident to most of us today, throughout the years there have been numerous examples of ethical misconduct on the part of researchers, resulting in blatant violations of these rights. The following research studies were conducted before federal regulations for the protection of human subjects in research were enacted. These studies, which are still being discussed in the research literature today, serve to emphasize the critical importance of ethical codes that are designed to protect the rights of human subjects in research.

The Tearoom Trade (1970)

A classic example of misconduct in human research that has generated a great deal of ethical controversy throughout the years is The Tearoom Trade, published in 1970 by Laud Humphreys. In this study, Humphreys reported on his observations of men engaging in homosexual activity in public restrooms. These restrooms were known as "tearooms" to the participants. To perform the observations for his study, Humphreys assumed the role of "watchqueen" or lookout, with the responsibility for warning of danger while the men performed homosexual acts. Later, by using the license plate numbers on cars parked outside the tearoom, Humphreys obtained the names and home addresses of the men. He altered his appearance and, claiming to be a health inspector, interviewed a number of the men in their own homes.

Although Humphreys received the prestigious C. Wright Mills Award for outstanding research on a critical social issue, his work generated bitter controversy. "When this study was published it resulted in a storm of controversy in the field of sociology, including fist fights in Humphreys' own department" (Korn, 1997, p. 10). In fact, some members of the faculty at the institution that awarded his Ph.D. degree attempted to void his degree because of the controversial nature of his research. His work also created a stir in various newspaper columns throughout the country.

The controversy generated by this study lingers today. A key ethical issue is the violation of the principle of respect for human dignity—the collection of data by covert means and the use of deception. Also violated was the subjects' right to informed consent—the subjects were not even aware they were participants in a research study. Another key ethical issue is the right to privacy that subjects have when participating in a study—did Humphreys adhere to this principle when he obtained the names and addresses of the individuals from the license plates of their automobiles parked outside the tearooms, or did he increase the possibility that they could be arrested? To his credit, Humphreys did safeguard the identities of the subjects who unknowingly participated in his study:

> Humphreys kept the master list of his subjects' names and code numbers in a locked box at a location only he knew, 1000 miles from the city in which he collected data. He even went to jail rather than reveal its whereabouts. Later he destroyed the list. During and after his research the identity of his subjects was absolutely protected. *(Reiss, 1978, p. 175, as cited in Mitchell, 1993)*

The Milgram Study (1974)

Milgram's classic study, Obedience to Authority, is another often-cited example of research that not only failed to protect the rights and welfare of subjects but also had a strong potential for negative consequences for the study subjects. In this study, subjects were told that they were involved in an experiment that proposed to measure the impact of punishment on a person's ability to learn. The subjects were to read a list of words to another person who, unbeknownst to the subjects, was the experimenter's confederate. If the confederate gave a wrong response, the subject was to "punish" the mistake by delivering an increasingly higher level of electric shock. The subject believed, incorrectly, that the confederate could receive a shock as high as 450 volts. Each subject was assured that no permanent damage would be done to the learner. However, the confederate, who did not receive any shock at any time, feigned great pain as the administered shocks increased in strength. When the subject protested about administering pain, he or she was told to continue by the experimenter—the voice of authority. A very high degree of obedience to authority was obtained, and the study demonstrated how ordinary individuals might engage in harmful activities if urged to do so by those perceived to have authority over them.

Although this study violated many of the ethical principles of research, it is to the credit of the researcher that each subject was **debriefed** (provided with information about the study after it was concluded) and was shown that the confederate—the "victim"—was not actually harmed and had, in fact, received no shocks. When this study was first published, it created an ethical controversy concerning the use of deception with study subjects, and it remains controversial today.

As a consequence of this and other studies requiring deception, many IRBs now demand that if the research design involves any form of deception, the researcher must provide a strong rationale for such deception and present a plan that allows adequate debriefing of the study subjects after the experiment's conclusion.

The Tuskeegee Syphilis Study (1932–1972)

By far the longest, and probably the most highly publicized, study that provides a glaring and tragic example of research that violated virtually all of the rights of the participants is the Tuskeegee Syphilis Study. Involving African-American males with syphilis, this experimental study was initiated in 1932 by the U.S. Public Health Service. The study was designed to investigate the long-term effects of untreated syphilis in a sample of semiliterate African-American men in Macon County, Alabama. Specific treatment for the disease was withheld from a sample of 399 African-American males who had been diagnosed as having syphilis. The research subjects thought they were receiving treatment for "bad blood," which the researchers mistakenly thought was a term recognized by the subjects as meaning syphilis. Their progress was compared to that of a control group of 201 African-American males who did not have the disease. The investigators then intended to follow the subjects through the rest of their lives to determine the long-term effects of untreated syphilis so that the natural course of the disease could be observed. Mortality rates were twice as high for the subjects with syphilis by the mid-1940s and continued to be higher than mortality rates for the control group. However, the U.S. Public Health Service did not provide the infected subjects with any form of treatment known to be effective until the research was publicly exposed in 1972—40 years after the experiment began. "The Tuskeegee Study had nothing to do with treatment; neither was any effort made to establish the efficacy of old forms of treatment" (Jones, 1993, p. 2).

In the years since the experiment was exposed, the U.S. government has made efforts to locate the remaining subjects and to provide them and their survivors with monetary compensation. On May 16, 1997, President Bill Clinton made a formal public apology to the eight remaining survivors and to the families of all of the men who were so ill used in this tragic episode in American history. In his apology, Mr. Clinton said:

> To Macon County, to Tuskeegee, to the doctors who have been wrongly associated with the events there, you have our apology . . . To our African-American citizens, I am sorry that your federal government orchestrated a study so clearly racist. That can never be allowed to happen again. . . . The United States government did something that was wrong—deeply, profoundly, morally wrong. It was an outrage to our commitment to integrity and equality for all our citizens.

Unfortunately, the consequences of the Tuskeegee Study linger. While there is a long history of racism in American medicine, an unintended consequence of this study is its reinforcement of African-Americans' distrust of the medical and public health systems. This has led to low participation by African-Americans in clinical trials and organ donation (Gamble, 1997).

● THE NATURE OF INFORMED CONSENT

The greatest concern in human subject research is the protection of the subject's right of self-determination by the assurance of **informed consent**. This means that the subject must be made fully aware of the study and voluntarily agree to participate in it. An example of the failure to obtain informed consent or of obtaining inadequate informed consent from human subjects can be shown in experiments using radioactive materials conducted by various U.S. government agencies during the 1940s, 1950s, and 1960s. There have been numerous investigations of these experiments. Some of the agencies that did obtain informed consent have been cited for providing inadequate information about the nature of their experiments and for failing to protect their subjects from harm. Clearly, this basic requirement of informed consent demonstrates that an investigator must not only plan for the present but must also consider the possibility of future re-examination when conducting experiments.

Essentially, the informed consent of subjects consists of the following six elements: (1) an explanation of the purpose of the study, (2) an explanation of potential risks and discomforts, (3) an explanation of potential benefits, (4) an acknowledgment that researchers will answer any questions the subjects may have concerning the study, (5) an acknowledgment that subjects can withdraw at any time, and (6) an assurance of anonymity and confidentiality.

1. Subjects must be given an understandable explanation of the purpose of the study. Subjects should also be told of the procedures and techniques that will be followed. In particular, experimental procedures and techniques should be identified. It can, however, be difficult to fulfill this requirement. Subjects' awareness of the nature of the

research, particularly an experiment, may affect the outcome. There are even those who suggest that a researcher cannot get a true random sample of a population because once the subjects consent to be part of an experiment, it automatically means that the subjects in the experimental study are different from those individuals who refused to participate in the study.

2. Each subject should be given an explanation of the potential risks and discomforts that may be encountered as a result of the study. Will the subject be exposed to a potentially harmful situation? Withholding medication or treatment may cause physical or psychological distress to the subject. Further, withholding treatment may actually expose the subject to physical risks. Each subject must know the hazards that he or she may face in consenting to participate in the study. The right of personal privacy and dignity for each subject must also be ensured.

3. Subjects should be told what benefits to expect. The benefits can be a broad explanation; they may be the basis for an appeal to the subject's altruism, or merely a simple explanation. The intent of many experiments is to improve the human condition. Each time a new treatment is tried, it is usually believed to be more effective than existing modalities. Subjects must also be told of alternative procedures that would be advantageous to them. For example, in the case of the use of an experimental drug, subjects must be aware that other, already proven drugs may aid in their treatment, while the experimental drug may do nothing for them. Subjects must also be informed if benefits are to be withheld from them.

4. Researchers must be willing to answer any questions the subjects may have about the procedures. Most subjects want to know not only what is happening to them but also why it is happening, and they must be informed if they request such information.

5. Subjects must be made aware that they can withdraw from the research investigation at any time without prejudice to their care. Researchers cannot compel or coerce subjects to remain in any investigation against their will.

6. Anonymity and confidentiality for every subject must be assured. **Anonymity** assures subjects that not only will their identity not be disclosed, but none of their responses will be linked to them. **Confidentiality** assures subjects that the researcher will safeguard their identities and their responses from public disclosure.

It is essential that the researcher be able to document that he or she has obtained the informed consent of the subject(s). Such consent is best obtained on a written form stating that the subject has willingly entered into the research and is aware of the procedures as well as the potential risks and benefits involved.

The following form might be used:

I [subject] do agree to participate in a research/experimental study concerning *[describe the nature of study]*. This project may expose me to risks and attendant discomforts. I am aware that *[describe the standard treatment]* might be advantageous to me in the treatment of my condition instead of the experimental treatment. However, *[describe the experimental treatment/procedure]* may benefit me. I am aware that my participation in this study will involve the following *[describe procedure for data collection]*. I may ask any questions about the procedures and treatments taking place and my questions must be answered honestly and fully. I am free to withdraw this consent and discontinue participation in this research study at any time without this decision affecting me in any way.

I understand that my responses will be kept confidential and not linked to me in any way.

Name and phone number of investigator   Signature of subject

In some instances, the subject may be paid to participate in the research study. The form may specify the amount to be paid and the duration of the experiment. The form may also specify whether there is any cost to the subject.

Oral consent is also valid but should be witnessed by a third party for the protection of both the researcher and the subject. If potential subjects are not able to give informed consent because of mental or physical disabilities or because they are below the legal age of consent, the researcher must secure the consent of a legally authorized guardian or next of kin.

On completion of a research investigation involving human subjects, the researcher has the obligation to remove any harmful after-effects, to debrief the subjects if necessary, and to follow through on any commitments that may have been made to the subject. This also includes the provision of any study results that have been promised to the subjects.

ETHICAL CONSIDERATIONS UNIQUE TO QUALITATIVE RESEARCH

Because the quantitative and qualitative research approaches differ in their relationship between the researcher and study subjects, the two major requirements that dominate the official guidelines for the conduct of research with human subjects—informed consent and protection of subjects from harm—may prove to be more difficult to implement in conducting qualitative research. However, there are certain ethical principles that the qualitative researcher must follow.

In quantitative research, the subjects have a very circumscribed relationship to the researcher. "[I]n qualitative research, on the other hand, the relationship is ongoing; it evolves over time. Doing qualitative research with subjects can be more like having a friendship . . ." (Bogdan & Biklen, 1998, p. 43). Because qualitative research may result in the development of friendships between researcher and subjects, it is incumbent on the researcher to ensure that these friendships result in respect for the rights of the subjects.

Also, in qualitative research, much of the research is done in such a way that there is no simple way to explain the nature of the research so that the subjects can be truly informed. A researcher who simply states to the research subjects that it would be interesting to see how people live their daily lives is not giving these subjects a great deal of information on which to base their informed consent.

As in quantitative research, qualitative researchers must be careful to keep their subjects' identities anonymous. Unless it is agreed to by both the researcher and the study subjects, the identities of the subjects should be protected so that the information "does not embarrass or in other ways harm them. Anonymity should extend not only to writing, but also to the verbal reporting of information" (Bogdan & Biklen, 1998, p. 460). Also, qualitative researchers must abide by the terms of any agreements made with their subjects and report their findings in an absolutely accurate manner.

In both quantitative and qualitative research, it is the researcher who ultimately bears the responsibility for conducting research in an ethical manner.

● POTENTIAL ETHICAL CONCERNS FOR FUTURE RESEARCH

Because of their potential for active participation in human subject research, nurses might well consider various ethical dilemmas that they may face in the future. The daily newspaper and television news reports abound with such dilemmas and will undoubtedly continue to do so. Included among the emerging ethical issues that may well involve nurses in human subject research are fetal tissue research, assisted suicide, and the cloning of human beings.

More and more, nurses will have the professional obligation not only to become knowledgeable participants in health care practice and research but also to involve themselves in institutional policy-making and the review of activities regarding research: "As patient advocates by virtue of their professional licenses, nurses in any role can and must take a lead in protecting human subjects' rights" (Pranulis, 1996, p. 474).

● CRITIQUING THE ETHICAL COMPONENTS OF A RESEARCH REPORT

In both quantitative and qualitative reports, adequate protection of the participants' rights must be described, including the process used to obtain informed consent and appropriate monitoring by an IRB or committee. Potential risks to the subjects should be described and evaluated by the author. Box 7-1 lists these points as evaluation guidelines for both quantitative and qualitative reports.

BOX 7-1   GUIDELINES FOR EVALUATING THE ETHICAL COMPONENTS OF A QUANTITATIVE REPORT AND A QUALITATIVE REPORT

Ethical Considerations

1. The procedure for obtaining informed consent is described.

2. Monitoring by an institutional review board or committee is described, if appropriate.

3. If the study poses any potential risks to subjects, does the researcher describe these risks and evaluate them?

SUMMARY

Protecting human subjects who participate in research is an extremely important consideration in any research situation. The development of modern ethical codes for research involving human subjects began with the Nuremberg trials immediately after World War II and continues to the present day. IRBs or research review committees have been developed in most health care settings to review potential research to guarantee that justice, beneficence, and respect for the dignity and privacy of research subjects are protected. The two major requirements for conducting research on human subjects—informed consent and protection of subjects from harm—are also examined by the IRBs before a research study can be undertaken. Finally, there are a number of potential ethical concerns, such as cloning and fetal tissue research, that will probably have an impact on nursing research in the future.

The following application activities for this chapter will help you to evaluate your understanding of this material and will assist you in developing your skill in evaluating published research.

REFERENCES

American Nurses Association. (1985). *Human rights guidelines for nurses in clinical and other research*. Kansas City: Author.

Bogdan, R. C., & Biklen, S. K. (1998). *Qualitative research in education* (3rd ed.). Boston: Allyn & Bacon.

Clinton, W. J. (1997). *Remarks by the president in apology for study done in Tuskegee*. Washington, DC: White House press release, May 16.

Dabbs, A. D., & Nolan, M. T. (1997). Nurses as members of institutional review boards. *Applied Nursing Research, 10*(2), 101–107.

Gamble, V. N. (1997). Under the shadow of Tuskegee: African Americans and health care. *American Journal of Public Health, 87*(1), 1773–1778.

Humphreys, L. (1970). *The Tearoom Trade: Impersonal sex in public places*. Chicago: Aldine.

Jones, J. H. (1993). *Bad blood* (2nd ed.). New York: Free Press.

Korn, J. (1997). *Illusions of reality: A history of deception in social psychology*. Albany: State University of New York Press.

Milgram, S. M. (1974). *Obedience to authority*. New York: Harper & Row.

Mitchell, R., Jr. (1993). *Secrecy and fieldwork*. Newberry Park, CA: Sage.

National Commission for the Protection of Human Subjects of Biomedical and Behavior Research. (1978). *The Belmont Report: Ethical principles and guidelines of research on human subjects*. Washington, DC: U. S. Government Printing Office.

Pranulis, M. F. (1996). Issues in clinical nursing research. *Western Journal of Nursing Research, 18*(4), 474–477.

Trials of war criminals before the Nuremberg Military Tribunals, volumes I and II: The Medical Case. (1948). Cited in J. Katz. (1972). *Experimentation with human beings* (pp. 305–306). New York: Russell Sage Foundation.

U.S. Department of Health and Human Services. (1981). Basic HHS policy for the protection of human research subjects. *Federal Register, 45*(46): Washington, DC: 8386–8391.

BIBLIOGRAPHY AND SUGGESTED READINGS

Bishop, A. H., & Scudder, J. R. (1996). *Nursing ethics: Therapeutic caring presence*. Boston: Jones and Bartlett.

de Raeve, L. (Ed.). (1996). *Nursing research: An ethical and legal appraisal*. London: Baillière Tindall.

Hall, J. K. (1996). *Nursing ethics and law*. Philadelphia: Saunders.

Kuhse, H. (1997). *Caring: Nurses, women and ethics*. Oxford: Blackwell.

Pallikkathayil, C. F., & Aaronson, L. S. (1998). Balancing ethical quandaries with scientific rigor: Part 1. *Western Journal of Nursing Research, 20*(3), 388–393.

Pallikkathayil, C. F., & Aaronson, L. S. (1998). Balancing ethical quandaries with scientific rigor: Part 2. *Western Journal of Nursing Research, 20*(4), 501–507.

Trials of war criminals before the Nuremberg Military Tribunals, Volumes I and II: The Medical Case. (1948). Washington, DC: U. S. Government Printing Office.

World Medical Assembly. (1975). *Declaration of Helsinki: Recommendations guiding medical doctors in biomedical research involving human subjects*. In R. J. Levine. (1986). *Ethics and the regulation of clinical research* (2nd ed., pp. 427–429). Baltimore: Urban & Schwarzenberg.

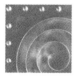

○ ○

APPLICATION ACTIVITIES

1. List three reasons why ethical codes to protect the rights of human subjects in research are necessary.

2. Explain the necessity for the following health care organizations to have IRBs or committees for the review of human subject research:

    a. A hospital

    b. A health department

    c. A hospice

3. How would these IRBs be similar, and how might they differ?

4. Read the informed consent at the end of the qualitative research proposal (Appendix B). Discuss how the researcher included the six elements of informed consent discussed in this chapter.

5. Read the quantitative research proposal (Appendix A). Discuss why informed consent of subjects was not required as a part of the study.

6. Discuss how the investigators met ethical criteria in the studies reprinted in:

   a. Appendix C

   b. Appendix D

   c. Appendix E

   d. Appendix F

7. Explain the following terms in your own words:

   a. Risk–benefit ratio

   b. Debriefing

   c. Anonymity

   d. Confidentiality

8. Use the guidelines for evaluating the ethical components in either a quantitative or a qualitative report (see Box 7-1) to evaluate this section of the three research reports you have selected to critique. Complete evaluation guidelines for both types of reports are in Appendixes G and H.

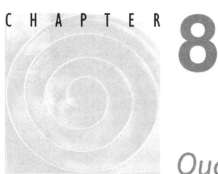

C H A P T E R

8

Qualitative Research Methods

THE MEANING OF VALIDITY AND RELIABILITY
QUALITATIVE RESEARCH METHODS
USING COMPUTERS IN QUALITATIVE
    DATA ANALYSIS

CRITIQUING THE DATA-COLLECTION
    AND DATA-ANALYSIS COMPONENTS
    OF A QUALITATIVE REPORT
SUMMARY

OBJECTIVES *On completion of this chapter, the student will be able to:*

1. Explain the meaning of validity in qualitative research.
2. Explain the meaning of reliability in qualitative research.
3. Discuss phenomenology.
4. Discuss grounded theory.
5. Discuss ethnography.
6. Discuss historical research.
7. Discuss action research.
8. Define key terms.
9. Use evaluation guidelines to critique the data-collection and
   data-analysis components of a qualitative research report.

KEY TERMS

Action research
Auditability
Audit trail
Confirmability
Constant comparative method
Credibility
Emic
Ethnographic research
Ethnomethodology
Ethnonursing

Ethnoscience
Etic
External criticism
Grounded theory research
Historical research
Internal criticism
Key informant
Phenomenology
Transferability

*I*n Chapter 2, the nature and major characteristics of the qualitative research approach were discussed. The purpose of this chapter is to introduce five of the many types of qualitative research methods: phenomenology, grounded theory, ethnography, historical research, and action research. Although some of these approaches are used more commonly than others, all of them, as well as additional approaches, can be found in the research literature. However, before addressing each of these, a brief discussion of validity and reliability is necessary. These are two of the most important characteristics associated with measurement in both the qualitative and the quantitative research approaches.

THE MEANING OF VALIDITY AND RELIABILITY

Both quantitative and qualitative researchers are concerned with establishing validity and reliability during their data collection. However, the meanings of the terms differ for qualitative and quantitative research because the selection of the sample, the data collection, and the data analysis are carried out differently.

Validity and Reliability in Quantitative Research

In quantitative research, the term validity refers to the extent to which a data-gathering instrument measures what it is supposed to measure—that is, the instrument is valid to the extent that it obtains data that are relevant to what is being measured. For example, a clinical thermometer is a valid instrument for measuring an individual's body temperature, but a sphygmomanometer is not valid for this purpose.

The reliability of a quantitative measuring instrument refers to the instrument's ability to obtain consistent results when it is reused. A measuring instrument is reliable if it consistently measures whatever it is supposed to measure in the same way each time it is administered. For example, when a paper-and-pencil test of intelligence is administered to an individual, the test should produce approximately the same results if it is administered again to the same individual. The more reliable a measuring instrument is, the more confident the researcher can be that the scores obtained would not fluctuate too greatly with repeated administration of the instrument.

Validity and Reliability in Qualitative Research

In qualitative research, the term validity "refers to the extent to which the research findings represent reality" (Morse & Field, 1995, p. 244). During every part of the data-collection process, the researcher must thoroughly check the information gathered to determine whether it "makes sense"—that is, whether it is compatible with other information that has already been gathered. For example, if a qualitative researcher interviews nurses in a hospital setting and they report that they always perform specific activities in a certain manner, but the researcher then observes that these activities are not being performed as reported, the researcher must attempt to reconcile the differences between the activities reported and the actual behaviors observed. The researcher should then include this information in reporting the validity of the research to ensure that, as much as possible, the findings represent reality.

In qualitative research, reliability is defined as "the measure of the extent to which random variation may have influenced stability and consistency of the results" (Morse & Field, 1995, p. 243). There are two specific concerns that must be addressed in determining reliability for a qualitative research study. The first is related to the extent to which the information gathered from the study participants is accurate. There is always the possibility that an informant may not have accurate information or may simply be lying. To reduce or eliminate these possibilities, the researcher should use a variety of informants, if possible, and ask the questions crucial to the research in several different ways to determine whether the responses are consistent. The second concern in determining reliability in qualitative research is related to the data-gathering instrument—often an interviewer or observer. If the data collector is careless or biased, the reliability of the study will be either substantially diminished or completely absent. A useful strategy for determining the reliability of a qualitative research study is related to the notion of replicability or reproducibility: the research report should give enough documentation of the questions asked and the responses obtained so that another researcher could go to the same or a similar setting and obtain similar responses by asking the same questions.

Determining validity and reliability is an extremely important consideration, and we have only touched on the notion to provide basic meanings for these terms.

● QUALITATIVE RESEARCH METHODS

Phenomenology as a Research Method

Phenomenological research is based on the philosophy of phenomenology espoused by Husserl and Heidegger, and others, that proposes to describe the meaning of the "lived experience" for individuals in order to understand "what it is like" from their perspective: thus, "human experience is inductively derived and described with the purpose of discovering the essence of meaning" (Morse & Field, 1995, p. 243).

Phenomenology is both a philosophy and a research method. When the philosophy of phenomenology is translated into a research setting, several processes must occur:

1. A person must communicate an experience or series of experiences to the researcher.
2. The researcher then attempts to translate the communicated experience into an understanding of the person's experience.
3. The researcher communicates his or her understandings to an audience in writing so that the members of this audience can then relate their understanding of this information to past and future experiences.

DATA COLLECTION

Because of the potentially large amounts of data to be gathered and analyzed, phenomenological research is usually based on written and/or oral data gathered from a very small number of study participants, often through the use of audiotapes and videotapes. These enable the researcher to analyze not only the words used by the participants in the study but also their inflections, pauses, and other pertinent characteristics of verbal responses. The nonverbal cues used by participants, such as gestures and physical stances, can also be recorded and analyzed.

DATA ANALYSIS

Because phenomenological research is based on the analysis and interpretation of other persons' experiences, the researcher must have special training to make valid analyses and interpretations of phenomenological data. Although there are several schools of phenomenological explanation, phenomenologists use either the hermeneutic (interpretive) method or the eidetic (descriptive) method for data analysis.

"Hermeneutics is an awkward word with a long tradition. It simply stands for the business of interpretation" (Addison, 1992, p. 110). Hermeneutic phenomenologists attempt to interpret the meaning of the lived human experience not only through the participant's perspective but also in light of sociohistorical influences.

In contrast to the hermeneutic interpretive approach to data analysis, eidetics is a descriptive approach to analyzing phenomenological data related to the human experience. Eidetic phenomenologists attempt to use their own reflection and insight to describe phenomena. To do this, they must be able to bracket—that is, they must identify their own preconceived opinions, previous knowledge, and assumptions regarding the phenomenon under study, deliberately set them aside, and remain neutral while analyzing the data.

The following two research studies are discussed as examples of the hermeneutic approach and the eidetic approach.

Pieranunzi (1997) used the heideggerian hermeneutic approach to phenomenology to determine psychiatric nurses' understanding of the meaning of power and powerlessness in the nurse–patient relationship. The purpose of the study was to discover some of the meanings inherent in psychiatric nursing practice. The specific question was, "What is the meaning of power and powerlessness as it occurs in the lived experience of practicing psychiatric nurses?" (p. 155). The researcher audiotaped and transcribed semistructured interviews to capture the nuances of the responses of 10 practicing psychiatric nurses. He then assembled a team to aid in the preliminary data analysis of the textual materials; additional analysis was conducted by his dissertation committee. Finally, the participants were contacted to review the results of the study and to provide feedback as to their accuracy. Although the researcher expected to find social issues, such as injustice and oppression within the system, predominating in the nurses' definitions of power and powerlessness, he elicited one major (constitutive) pattern, one theme, and three subthemes in his analysis. The constitutive pattern had to do with "the power of knowing," which the nurses used to understand and respond to patients intuitively (p. 158). The theme discovered was "power as connectedness in relationships," in which the nurses related to patients in ways that would change them both: "For these nurses, this is the essence of the art of nursing, perhaps the essence of nursing in its entirety" (p. 159). The first subtheme, "the personal versus the professional," indicated that for many nurses in this study, their most meaningful relationships, and the ones in which they felt "powerful," were deeply "connected and personal" (p. 160). The second subtheme, "the power of mutuality," means that the nurses were open to learn from their patients: "The notion that relationships with patients are not 'one-sided,' but enrich and constitute the nurse, was noted in the texts" (p. 160). In the third subtheme, "the contextualized nature of relationships," the nurses indicated that they felt their nursing practice influenced how they understood and functioned in relation to the external world (p. 160). Pieranunzi concluded that the results of this study would enable nurses to understand their practice better and would lead to strategies for empowerment of both nurses and the people they care for. He also observed that this use of "a hermeneutical data analysis approach has further shown the relevance of this method for knowledge generation in psychiatric nursing" (p. 155).

Kavanaugh (1997) used the eidetic phenomenological method in her study, "Parents' Experience Surrounding the Death of a Newborn Whose Birth

Is at the Margin of Viability." The purpose of her study was to describe the experience of parents "surrounding the death of a newborn weighing less than 500 g at birth" (p. 43). Eight parents (five mothers and three of their husbands) were interviewed 4 to 15 weeks after the death of the newborn. The investigator audiotaped the in-depth interviews with each parent. At least two interviews were conducted, the first face-to-face, and the others either face-to-face or by telephone. A total of 18 interviews were conducted. After the data were transcribed and analyzed, the parents were again contacted to validate the researcher's findings. Five themes were identified from the parents' descriptions of their experience: realization that the loss is occurring; initial response to the loss; decision making at the time of the loss; components of supportive relationships with others; and the adjustment at home. Kavanaugh concluded that the findings "demonstrate the unique experience of having a newborn who is born at the margin of viability and support the need for individualized, caring-based interventions for parents" (p. 43).

Grounded Theory Research

Grounded theory strategies were first reported by the sociologists Glaser and Strauss (1967) when they examined the politics of pain management in a hospital environment. Because there was little information available and no previously developed theory of pain management, they developed the grounded theory research method in an attempt to bridge what they perceived as a gap between theory and research. **Grounded theory** emphasizes the process of generating theory by systematically collecting and analyzing data concurrently; the theoretical formulations thereby remain connected to, or "grounded," in the data.

DATA COLLECTION AND DATA ANALYSIS

Grounded theory is characterized by the **constant comparative method**, in which data collection and analysis occur simultaneously so that all data being collected are compared to all data previously collected to determine their importance and position in the hierarchy of data analysis.

Grounded theory techniques for collecting and analyzing data rely heavily on "skilled observation and intensive interviewing combined with systematic detailed record keeping and simultaneous processes of data collection and analysis" (Powers & Knapp, 1995, p. 73). Data may also be collected by the use of questionnaires, from written records or any other available data, and from verbal and nonverbal communications, all of which are examined for their potential usefulness in the development of a theoretical framework. The data-collection and the data-analysis stages of the research process occur simultaneously. Data gathering is guided by an approach termed "theoretical sampling"—sampling on the basis of relevance for the evolving theory. Data are compared for similarities and differences and are arranged into categories; certain data fit into one category and other data fit into other categories. In the initial stages of the process, the categories may be too broad or may even prove to be incorrect and need to be revised. As more data are collected, an isolated datum (a unit of data) may be fitted into the appropriate category with greater ease. Using the constant comparative method of data analysis, each datum is constantly reviewed and compared to all of the other data. While using this strategy, the researcher begins intuitively to develop concepts regarding the data. When the categories are established and no new categories emerge, saturation is said to have occurred—that is, enough data have been collected and further data collection is considered to be redundant.

After the data are categorized based on similarity and dissimilarity and concepts emerge, the grounded theorist uses the inductive method of reasoning to generate a framework that could tentatively serve to explain the complex structure of the myriad of data that have been collected. A central hypothesis or theme may be formulated concerning a key or core variable(s) as well as a tentative theoretical formulation from which hypotheses may be derived that can then be tested through research. As these hypotheses are rejected or supported, the concept(s) most important to theory development emerge. Finally, the data are again compared to the emergent theory so that the theory can be tested and modified to conform with known data.

Baggs and Schmitt (1997) used grounded theory when they examined the concept of collaboration between resident physicians and nurses in an MICU in an urban university teaching hospital. The investigators interviewed 20 participants using semistructured, open-ended questions concerning the collaboration between physicians and nurses. The audiotaped interviews were then transcribed verbatim and entered into a computer, where the Ethnograph computer program was used to facilitate data management. The investigators coded and analyzed data during and after the data-collection process, as suggested by Strauss and Corbin (1990) as a grounded theory methodology. By coding their data into categories and subcategories, they found that the core of the process of collaboration for both groups was working together. They found two major antecedent conditions that had to occur before collaboration took place. The first was being available; this included being in the right place, having time, and having appropriate knowledge to share. The second antecedent condition was being receptive. This meant being interested in collaboration and having respect and trust for the other profession. The major outcomes of working together were described as improving patient care, feeling better in the job, and controlling costs. The researchers concluded: "The findings of the study pull together disparate concepts associated with collaborative practice and provide direction for future research" (p. 71).

Ethnographic Research

Ethnographic research, often referred to as participant observation, has long been the domain of the cultural anthropologist or ethnographer. In conducting **ethnographic research**, the primary purpose of the investigator is to formulate an in-depth description of a culture or subculture of the group being studied. Although the term "culture" can be defined in various ways, most definitions include patterns of behaviors and values shared by a group or groups. Such research requires that the researcher be physically present among the subjects during the data-gathering phase of the research process. The ethnographer attempts to describe the culture of a group from the perspective of the members—that is, how they view their own culture—through in-depth study that involves systematic observation of the group's activities, language, and customs.

Ethnographic methods may be used when the researcher must catalog all activities, or as many as possible, that are taking place in a social situation and then determine which activities are significant and which are trivial. This, essentially, is the technique used by cultural anthropologists or ethnographers. The cultural anthropologist as researcher often becomes a participant as well as an observer and attempts to elicit data by using both structured and unstructured interviews and observations. For example, there are various ways to examine beliefs about diseases and how to effect cures for these diseases. Groups of people in developed as well as underdeveloped countries practice various kinds of folk medicine to achieve cures. The cultural anthropologist's findings could be crucial for a nurse who must have a basic knowledge of these folk medicine beliefs and practices to communicate with a patient. How the illness experience is perceived and described by a subculture could also be a critical area for research. For example, the student who wrote the research proposal in Appendix B proposed to describe what living in a congregate setting is like from the perspective of the homeless person with AIDS. Additional examples of ethnographic studies for which participant observation could be used include disease classification among Spanish-speaking migrant workers, the root medicine still practiced in many areas of the rural South, the continuation of various healing activities of Native American groups, the introduction of herbal cures by different refugee groups, and the use of health foods and herbs in the population at large.

DATA COLLECTION

Systematic observation requires that the ethnographic researcher be in the field long enough to see deeply into the group being studied. The ethnographer may use unstructured interviews, structured interviews, observation, and available data or a combination of any of these. Ethnographic researchers employ a technique called key informant interviewing. **Key informants** are those individuals who are willing to participate in a study and whose positions or roles in a society or institution place them in a position to "know" what is really taking place. The researcher must identify such individuals and gain their trust to have opportunities to interview them. Interviews are recorded and transcribed, and researchers keep careful notes on observations that are made during and immediately after the observations. The procedures for observing and recording data are reported so that other field workers can attempt to replicate the study. Systematic observation is methodical; that is, strategies for observation are carefully laid out before the study. Even with such strategies in place, the researcher must be flexible enough to change methods of observation (and document such change) if the study setting requires it.

Levels of Participant Observation.   In collecting the data for ethnologic research, there are four levels of participant observation available to the researcher: (1) the complete observer; (2) the partial participant; (3) the observer as participant; and (4) the full participant.

The first level is that of a complete observer. If a researcher is working with a group of individuals whose language is not adequately understood, or if discourse must be conducted through an interpreter, the researcher will be primarily an observer.

At the second level of participant observation, the researcher may become a partial participant. This could take place where the observer has a degree of fluency in the language and a great deal of knowledge concerning the group being studied. For example, a researcher working in a community health setting might well fulfill this role. If the researcher is not a nurse, doctor, or member of the support staff of the research setting where the research is being conducted, the researcher might help with appropriate activities and still remain nonjudgmental. Thus, the researcher can look for a variety of patterns of behaviors, social interactions, rituals, and other activities that may be considered routine by the participants in the study.

The third level of participant observation is that of the observer as participant. In this instance, the researcher, as a member of the group, plays a dual role—first as a participating member of the group, with all of the rights and duties required of such a member, and second as an announced observer, where the group members are aware that they are being observed. For example, a critical care nurse could describe the variety of activities and interactions that occur between the various staff members in the critical care unit of a hospital. Some of the interactions would clearly be related to social and role expectations rather than professional interactions required to care for patients. Here the line between participant and observer is very narrow. Individuals within the group would know they were being observed, yet the observer would be able to perform the role of participant competently.

Finally, there is the role of full participant. The researcher conceals any intent to do research, and the subjects are not necessarily aware of the researcher's purpose. This was the method used by Humphreys to collect the data for his research on the tearoom trade (discussed in Chap. 7) when he assumed the role of full participant by posing as lookout in the tearooms while observing homosexual acts. As discussed previously, there are major ethical questions involved in conducting this type of research. Given the nature of informed consent required of subjects in a research setting, a study designed to collect data that requires total concealment of the researcher may be very difficult to conduct.

The researcher who uses any of the types of participant observation is limited as to the number of individuals with whom contacts can be made. The first contacts may be with marginal individuals who need social contacts and/or approval and whose information may be unreliable. Therefore, the researcher must be very careful that the data gathered are accurate and valid. A study of witchcraft beliefs might be extremely hard to document, for example, because of respondents' fear that they might be accused of witchcraft, or that they would become victims of witchcraft if they tell of known witches. Rapport and trust are crucial if the researcher is to obtain any kind of valid information.

DATA ANALYSIS

The ethnographer analyzes data continuously as they are gathered and sorted so that common themes emerge. Comparison of information received from informants and from other appropriate sources is used to ensure the accuracy (reliability) of the researcher's conclusions.

Ethnographers often refer to the analysis of their study as being either in the etic tradition or the emic tradition. **Etic** refers to the interpretation of data as an outsider looking in. **Emic** refers to the interpretation of the data from an insider's point of view.

Look at the ethnographic study in Appendix E. The researchers examined how high-risk pregnant women felt about being confined to bed for a minimum of 7 days, either at home or in the hospital. This became a "focused ethnography" based on the experiences of the women. The investigators tape-recorded interviews using leading questions, wrote field notes at the end of each interview, and asked the participants to keep a diary of their experiences during the bed rest. After transcribing the information, the investigators used the Qualpro computer software package to manage the data. They then coded the information and reached an acceptable agreement rate in determining the themes that emerged from the study.

In another study "Community Caring: An Ethnographic Study Within an Organizational Culture," Davis (1997) used ethnographic techniques to define the culture and common concerns shared by the staff members of a hospital-based ambulatory program for cardiac health and rehabilitation located in a community hospital close to a large city. Because of the need for organizations such as hospitals to aid in building healthy communities and to become more responsive to the health needs of the communities they serve, the researcher determined that studying the culture of the hospital might lead to ways to improve the development of models of health care that could be integrated into the community. The researcher recruited eight participants: a physician, a physical therapist, three nurses, the department director, a former patient, and a staff member of the community rehabilitation program. The researcher interviewed the participants, reviewed records and other documents, and observed exercise and educational classes, then used field notes and a log to record the data as they were being gathered. The data were continuously analyzed across sources and methods during the study to gain adequate descriptions. The researcher used the Ethnograph computer program to aid in managing and organizing the data. Five major themes emerged: different perspectives of communities; reciprocal relationships and teams; education and prevention; shared values; and understanding community needs (p. 92). The author concluded that new relationships must be developed between health organizations and the communities they serve.

ETHNOGRAPHIC SUBSTRATEGIES USED IN NURSING RESEARCH

The ethnographic orientation has been used in formulating a series of related orientations that use the prefix ethno-, such as ethnopharmacology, ethnobotany, ethnomusicology, and a host of others. The term ethno comes from Greek and means a "nation or group"; therefore, a researcher studying a topic with the ethno- prefix is studying a part of a specific group's culture. This section will focus on three of these substrategies used in nursing research: ethnomethodology, ethnoscience (also known as cognitive anthropology), and ethnonursing.

Ethnomethodology. **Ethnomethodology** (literally, "people's methods") has its roots in phenomenology in that it attempts to understand how people see, describe, and explain the world in which they live. The specific focus of ethnomethodolgy is on the tacitly held knowledge that people use to function in a familiar situation. This leads to explanations of the "common sense" or "taken-for-granted" (everybody does it this way) understandings that individuals hold. Ethnomethodologists propose to study how people "do" everyday things, such as invite laughter, initiate telephone conversations, and deal with the unexpected disruptions in the daily flow of their lives (Powers & Knapp, 1995).

Ethnomethodologists gather data by observing the behaviors, conversations, and remarks of their study's participants. By taking notes and organizing them to define common practices and speech shared by the participants, ethnomethodologists can base their explanatory systems on analysis of the speech and activities of groups rather than attempting to understand the perceptions of individuals, as is done in phenomenology. For example, when a group of friends gather in an informal setting, their dress, speech, and behaviors would be much different than if they were in a formal setting, such as attending a wedding or a funeral. These individuals share a common knowledge of appropriate behaviors for each social situation. Sometimes these behaviors or behavioral expectations are codified (as in the written rules of etiquette). In other situations, such as a picnic or swimming party, the rules of behavior are known to the participants but are not made explicit until they are analyzed by an ethnomethodologist. In these situations, such variables as age, gender, and male/female ratios would very much affect the "common rules" of shared behaviors.

The ethnomethodologist analyzes the data by using the "indexicality" of behavior and language used in a situation. The term indexicality means how previous activities and language are used to explain what is taking place. Friends meeting each other in an informal situation often do not use complete sentences to discuss or share information. A series of fragmented sentences might well be the total conversation, such as:

A: "How's—"

B (before A finishes the sentence): "Well, and—"

A: "Better than before she—"

B: "I'm so glad now that the wait is over."

Most of us have heard "conversations" such as this and often carry on similar conversations. The speech is said to be indexed: it has referents to individuals and actions known only to the participants in the conversation. The rules of interaction and discourse are known by the individuals in the situation. It is the ethnomethodologist's task to examine situations and formalize the implicit understandings of the participants. The following study provides an example of the use of ethnomethodology in nursing research.

Baker (1997) reported an ethnomethodological study titled "Rules Outside the Rules for Administration of Medication: A Study in New South Wales, Australia." The purpose of this study was to "improve understanding of how nurses define or redefine medication error." She used ethnomethodology as a research strategy "useful for making clearer the every-day, taken-for-granted understandings and practices of people as they make sense of their world" (p. 155). The researcher used participant observation over a period of 18 weeks, conducted formal interviews, and examined pertinent documents to gather data from nurses in an Australian hospital. She found that the nurses in the study defined medication errors in ways that were inconsistent with the institutional rules that required the reporting of medication errors; the nurses "adopted practices and embodied logic to accomplish tasks. They created criteria to decide when incidents were 'real errors' "(p. 155). These nurses did not believe that a medication error occurred if the hospital's rules or doctor's orders could not be followed as a result of what they perceived as extenuating circumstances, such as unavailability of prescribed medications, clerical errors, or intervals between doses that they perceived as not being time-critical (as opposed to those that were time-critical). Baker concluded that the findings of the study provided "a body of tacitly held knowledge about medication error that is shared among clinical nurses and redefines medication error" and that the study calls into question the way institutions seek to identify, document, and reduce medication errors by nurses (p. 155).

Ethnoscience.   Whereas ethnomethodologists analyze the tacitly held knowledge that people use in situations, ethnoscientists analyze the language used by the study's participants to determine how things are connected or recognized as belonging to the same categories. For example, an ethnoscientist might ask study participants to list various means of transportation. Categories of vehicles used for transportation, such as bicycles, automobiles, motorcycles, buses, and other transportation devices, might be listed. The researcher could then categorize these responses by the number of wheels they have, whether they are motorized, or in a number of other ways. In the simple taxonomy (classification system) of means of transportation displayed in Box 8-1, responses have been classified by whether or not the methods of transportation are propelled by engines and whether they are on the ground or in the air. Note that this simple taxonomy could have been expanded into a number of different categories, depending on the responses of the participants.

Ethnoscience could be a useful research strategy in areas related to health where there are many types of herbs and plants that are used in a variety of ways. An ethnoscientist might want to know how these are categorized in terms of their use and effects. For example, Barsh (1997) discussed various folk remedies and their effectiveness. He noted that many of the descriptions of plants that are described in traditional pharmacopoeias are based, in part, on ethnoscientific information elicited from various sources. However, "comparatively little attention has been devoted to the prescription of traditional remedies" (p. 28). Barsh pointed out that simply knowing which plants should be used for which diseases is not enough; it is also essential for the traditional healer to have learned, through experience, experimentation, and exchange of information, not only when these plants are to be used in prescribing remedies for individual patients, but also which parts and how much of the plant to use. Categorizing this information could be the task of the ethnoscientist.

Ethnonursing. **Ethnonursing**, a term unique to nursing, is used by Madeline Leininger (1991) in connection with her theory of culture care diversity and universality. Nurse researchers who propose to study phenomena uniquely related to culture care patterns can use the ethnonursing research method to contribute to an understanding of the caring patterns used in different cultures. Ethnonursing uses traditional ethnographic methods to gather data from informants; participant observation and interviews are an integral part of data collection. Data elicited from the participants are analyzed in a manner consistent with traditional ethnographic data-analysis methods.

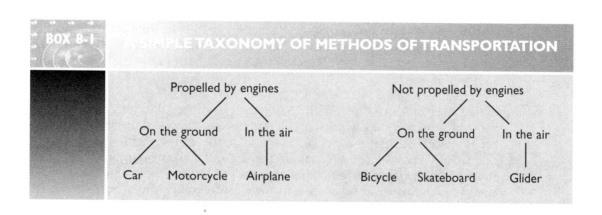

BOX 8-1   A SIMPLE TAXONOMY OF METHODS OF TRANSPORTATION

An example of the use of the ethnonursing research method is the study conducted by Wing, Thompson, and Heleshaya (1996). The authors used the theory of culture care diversity and universality as the theoretical base for their research: "The theory was appropriate because its goal is 'to discover inductively and explain, interpret, and predict culture care knowledge and its influences' " (p. 176). Because alcohol abuse is a major problem among Native Americans, the researchers sought information that would help to explain what alcohol means to traditional Muscogee Creek Indians in eastern Oklahoma. The researchers conducted in-depth interviews with 24 Muscogee Creek Indians who practiced traditional ways to elicit both the emic and etic meanings of alcohol. The interviews were conducted in English when possible, and in Muscogee Creek when necessary. Some of the conversations were tape-recorded; others, out of respect for the participant's beliefs, were recorded in the form of written notes. The Muscogee Creek speakers' comments were translated into English, using the English words that best fit the meaning of a word for which there was no direct translation. The researchers analyzed the data using both an etic (outsider's or non-traditional Muscogee Creek) perspective and an emic (insider's or traditional Muscogee Creek) perspective to determine the meaning of alcohol to traditional Muscogee Creek Indians. One major theme emerged from the study: "Alcohol represents a dichotomy of power to do both good and evil" (p. 177). The findings suggested culturally competent nursing implications for preserving, accommodating, and repatterning the meaning of alcohol to traditional Muscogee Creek Indians. The authors concluded: "Other culture-specific meanings of alcohol must be understood in order to plan culturally competent nursing care" (p. 180).

Historical Research

Nursing is both a very young profession and a very old one. Even before Greek and Roman soldiers were carried home on their shields, sometimes dead and sometimes wounded, someone has always been charged with the care of the ill or injured. **Historical research** deals with what has happened in the past and how these events affect the present. Historical research lends itself well to nursing; no professional group has been more in the forefront of world history than nursing. By its very nature, nursing is always "where the action is." Nurses have been active in all areas of the world both in times of conflict and in times of peace.

Historians piece together information from the past to get a picture of the actual lives and times of an era. They may use these data to determine the impact of history on the present and may even attempt to predict the future on the basis of this knowledge. Essentially, the historian follows the same research process as any other researcher. First, the problem to be investigated must be selected and formulated within the context of existing knowledge and theory. Like any researcher, the historical researcher must be particularly careful in gathering and interpreting data and in drawing conclusions based on these data. In some instances, the computer can be used to locate and reprint historical documents as well as to facilitate data analysis.

Historical research lends itself to the acceptance of evidence that is hard to verify. The careful researcher must do the utmost to corroborate data and to demonstrate their reliability and validity. Although the majority of data in historical research are qualitative, some historians have used computer programs to examine their numeric data statistically to draw conclusions about the conditions of individuals in a given historical period; this use of mathematics and statistics in historical research is called cliometrics.

SOURCES OF HISTORICAL DATA

Data sources available to the historical researcher fall into two categories: primary sources and secondary sources. Primary sources are those that provide firsthand information obtained from original materials, such as the originals of written documents, still pictures, paintings, and video and audio recordings. Secondary sources are those that provide secondhand interpretations of information, such as a document written by someone who has read all of the original source materials and then summarized them, or a newspaper article from the time of an event that is written by someone other than those who experienced the event.

Although primary sources have more credibility, historical researchers may choose to use a combination of both primary and secondary sources. In either case, the historical researcher must question the reliability and validity of sources by applying both external criticism and internal criticism to a written document. **External criticism** in historical research deals with the validity of the data sources: Are the data authentic—that is, are they what they purport to be? In determining the validity of a document, the researcher must ask such questions as, Where and when was this document written? By whom was it written? Why was it written? If the data source passes the test of external validity, the researcher can then apply internal criticism to the written document. **Internal criticism** deals with the reliability or accuracy of the information—that is, the authenticity and consistency of the information within the document itself. The historical researcher must become familiar with the milieu (the life and times) of the historical period to decide whether data sources are reliable. In applying internal criticism to a document, the researcher must ask such questions as, Is this document consistent with other documents written by this person? Does it have the same style? Does the style match the style of the time? Are the spelling and handwriting consistent with the time?

Locating Primary Data Sources.   Published materials can be an extremely valuable primary data source available to the historical researcher. Published sources may include the original documents: there is an increasing trend to store old newspapers, journals, magazines, and other published materials in microform. This may be advantageous to the historical researcher, who may not have to travel great distances to gain access to these materials. Rather, a microform copy can be ordered and reviewed by using a microform reader, which is readily available in most college and university libraries and in an increasing number of public libraries.

Original items of historical interest about nursing can often be found in popular literature, either in the form of articles about nurses and nursing or as fictional representations of nurses and their roles.

Government documents can also provide an excellent source of primary data for the historical researcher. In addition to the national government, state and local governments have compiled enormous quantities of official records and documents.

Official minutes of meetings and other written records of meetings can be an important primary source of data for the historical researcher. However, the researcher must bear in mind that more often than not, the minutes of a meeting reflect an abridged version of what actually transpired during that meeting. For example, acrimonious debate or issues that were not voted on may not be recorded in the minutes. It is also wise to remember that because each legislator has the privilege of editing what he or she has said on the floor of the U.S. House of Representatives or Senate before such information is finally placed in the *Congressional Record*, the information that is published may not necessarily be the verbatim report of what actually transpired.

Additional primary sources for written materials that may be available to the historical researcher include old telephone books, business directories, catalogues of local and national businesses, accounting books, and bank records.

Personal diaries can provide an invaluable source of documentation for the historical researcher. These diaries are often handed down from generation to generation in a family; the astute historical researcher must locate families who still have these documents in their possession and are willing to share their intimate contents. Diary research requires judicious questioning and the application of a substantial amount of external and internal criticism.

Historical societies are another source of primary data. These groups are justifiably proud of their community's history and may provide access not only to documents but also to key individuals within the community; these people may prove to be invaluable resources to an outside researcher.

An additional important primary source of material available to the historical researcher is physical evidence of change throughout the years. Many of the products of technical evolution have been added to the repertoire of nursing. The evolution of measurement of body temperature—from the mercury thermometer to the current, more technologically based methods—is a simple example of such change.

Oral history is another important source of primary data. Cameras and audio and video recordings can be used to assist the oral historian in recording the recollections of individuals or groups of people, thus providing records of what took place in specific places in past times. The remembrances of the older members of the professional community can be especially important for the oral historian. These older people are often invaluable resources, and as they die, their unique information is lost forever.

For example, Russell (1997) replicated an earlier oral history project in mental health nursing by interviewing 22 "trained nurses" working in a local mental health facility in greater London. The purpose of the study was three-fold:

1. To produce material that would support, or alternatively challenge, the content of a piece of historical writing, based largely on primary archival sources
2. To compare information with a previous study
3. To arrive at some opinions regarding the usefulness of such an investigation (p. 489).

The investigator was able to replicate as well as to expand on the original study. He taped each interview, using the same prepared interview schedule that had been used in the original oral history project and to which he added an additional unstructured interview. These enabled him to elicit information on topics regarding mental health nursing in the past as well as to include the contemporary concerns of "gender issues, ethnicity, management of violence, and nurses' roles in treatment" (p. 489). In discussing the results of his study, Russell made the following comments:

> Reminiscences taken at a distance, in this case up to 66 years ago, suffer distortion, favorable or unfavorable, and much may be simplified and exaggerated. However, it is possible by cross-checking to achieve some corroboration of the general thrust of accounts received, for example, by searching the hospital archives. *(pp. 494–495)*

He was able to determine that the responses of the study participants supported the information found in written records as well as providing data that enriched the description of the historical process. He concluded:

> In spite of the limitations of the oral method—the complexity of the testimony with its irrelevancies and obscurities—the anecdotes have an intrinsic value in giving some flavor of the basic day-to-day care in past times, through their provision of historically minute detail. *(p. 495)*

Life histories and career histories are an extension of the oral history technique. Researchers who gather data related to the life and/or career history of one individual or several individuals who are contemporaries can then go beyond the lives of these individuals and draw broader conclusions regarding the whole cultural milieu in which they lived and worked. For example, a life history approach was used by Barry and Boyle (1996) when they investigated the life and career history of a "granny midwife." For the purposes of their study, the researchers defined *granny* as "an African-American lay-midwife with specialized training who assisted women in childbirth and occasionally in other domestic duties" (p. 13). This focus on life history "facilitated the sharing of reflections and experiences about the informant's life as well as her

career as a granny midwife" (p. 14). The researchers interviewed Beatrice
Cody, a 75-year-old African-American woman who had practiced as a lay-midwife in rural Georgia most of her life. She had learned the required
lay-midwifery skills by reading about childbirth in texts and by assisting her
grandmother and another older woman in delivering babies. When she had
the opportunity to be trained and certified in midwifery by the county health
department staff, Mrs. Cody was the first to volunteer and to receive additional training. On her graduation in 1953 at the age of 32, "she was very
proud that she was the youngest midwife on the registry" (p. 16). Mrs. Cody
then became the primary caregiver to many patients who lived in small, rural
communities or on farms in four Georgia counties: "all of Mrs. Cody's clients
were African-American women who were poor and had no other access to
health care" (p. 16).

Data were collected by formal and informal interviews with Mrs. Cody at
her home and by a questionnaire designed to elicit her responses concerning
midwifery practices. The researchers used field notes from the informal interviews to expand and clarify the more formal interviews. After transcribing the
recordings of their interviews, all of which consisted of open-ended questions,
the researchers used the Ethnograph computer program to determine the categories and themes that emerged from her life history. Two major categories
emerged: "surviving hard times," especially in terms of being a member of a
minority group in rural Georgia during the Depression and World War II, as
well as during the turmoil of later times, and "serving God and others," a reflection of the deep religious convictions held by many who lived in the rural South.

This life history provided a picture of a vanishing segment of the American population: Mrs. Cody and "undoubtedly other African-American granny
midwives had a well-defined body of folk and professional knowledge that
guided their practices" (p. 17). In addition, the study provided a clearer historical picture of the life and times in rural Georgia during that era.

Secondary Data Sources.   There are two basic types of secondary data sources
available to historical researchers: interpretations of documented data and
hearsay evidence.

Historical researchers who use someone else's interpretation of documented data depend on another person's personal frame of reference for information. This means that these interpretations may or may not be accurate.
The farther a researcher is from the original source of historical data, the
greater the chance of misinterpretation. The historical researcher must go
back to the original sources whenever possible. The bibliography and footnotes of secondary documentary sources often lead to primary sources, which
can then be checked for the accuracy of interpretation and used for gathering
additional data. A secondary source, no matter how carefully evaluated, may
not provide a total interpretation of pertinent historical information. Historical researchers should select their information from a variety of secondary
sources and whenever possible should use primary sources.

The second, and a possibly naïve, secondary source is hearsay evidence.
Hearsay is simply what people think they heard or, even worse, the extension

of unproved rumors and gossip. Historical researchers must be extremely careful when dealing with hearsay data. These data may be old and valuable or may totally misrepresent the facts. The historical researcher must make every effort to corroborate any piece of hearsay data and to place it into proper historical perspective.

An example of historical research using extensive secondary sources is that reported by Nelson (1997). The purpose of her research was to reexamine "the role of the early nineteenth-century nurses, conventionally depicted in nursing histories as the well-meaning but untrained Catholic nursing nuns or, in post-Reformation Europe, servants and fellow patients" (p. 6). She used documentary sources to investigate the development of nursing before the mid-19th century, before the influence of Florence Nightingale and others of her time. Even though much of early nursing developed through the establishment of various religious orders that were first intended to minister to the poor by providing food, clothing, and shelter, Nelson argued that members of these religious orders (both Protestant and Catholic) became involved with poor people who were sick as a result of malnutrition as well as the lack of knowledge concerning bacterial infection and disease transmission at that time.

The early 19th century also saw many social reformers who felt morally obligated to aid in improving the moral character of the increasing population of the urban poor. These character-reformation schemes included the improvement of sanitation, housing, and health services through governmental agencies, with the cooperation of various nonreligious and religious bodies. When the Irish famine developed during the 1840s, many Irish emigrated to Great Britain, the United States, and Australia, bringing with them many of the religious orders that cared for the poor and sick. Nelson concluded that modern nursing started as the "extension of a religious form of life into the pastoral/government domain" (p. 13).

Action Research

Action research arose from social change theory and has become a valuable strategy in a variety of practice settings, including nursing. As its name implies, **action researchers** pursue action and research outcomes at the same time. "The purpose of action research is to solve practical problems through the application of the scientific method" (Gay, 1996, p. 10). Action research is concerned with a specific problem in a specific setting and is conducted in this setting, thus facilitating the development of knowledge or understanding as a part of practice. Action research has the advantage of allowing research to be done in situations where other research methods may be difficult or impractical to use: "To achieve action, action research is responsive, it has to be able to respond to the emerging needs of the situation. It must be flexible in a way that some research methods cannot be" (Dick, 1997, p. 3).

Proponents of action research find the strategy appropriate for nursing in the belief that traditional research may not allow practicing nurses to see the relevance of nursing research to their practice. Action research does not require expert researchers; the participants define the problem themselves, and the researchers and practitioners participate together in the process. Because it allows the participants to assume an active, collaborative role in the project, "action research is empowering for the participants and reflective of their practice . . ." (Brooker, 1997, p. 2).

CHARACTERISTICS OF ACTION RESEARCH

Action research is cyclic in that similar steps tend to recur in a similar sequence; it is participative because the clients and informants are involved as partners, or at least participants, in the research process; it is qualitative in that it deals more often with language than with numbers; and it is reflective because critical reflection upon the process and outcomes are important parts of each cycle (Dick, 1997). Action research is most effective

> when the end result emerges from the data. The conclusions drawn are data-based, preferably drawing data from multiple sources. The conclusions emerge slowly over the course of the study. At each cycle the researchers challenge the emerging conclusions by vigorously pursuing disconfirming evidence. *(Dick, 1997, p. 7)*

DATA COLLECTION AND ANALYSIS

After a problematic situation has been identified and the need for action research has been determined, individuals are identified to participate in the research; these individuals then become researchers. The aim is to improve the situation by proposing tentative changes, deliberately changing the situation (or parts of it), critically reflecting on the results through interactions with others in the project, and then determining whether the practice changes are effective. If the changes are effective, they continue to be implemented, and additional changes may be made. If the changes are ineffective, they may be discarded and other changes proposed, thus initiating the cycle once again.

The majority of action research is qualitative because developing quantitative measures may be too difficult and time-consuming, and it may prove to be more efficient to use qualitative data (that is, natural language rather than numbers): "Most action research is qualitative. Some is a mix of qualitative and quantitative" (Dick, 1997, p. 4).

ADVANTAGES AND LIMITATIONS OF ACTION RESEARCH

The flexibility and involvement of participants in action research makes it a useful method to use in practice settings, where it can be tailored to the specific setting: "I think that the major justification for action research methods is that they can be responsive to the situation in a way that many other research methods cannot be, at least in the short term" (Dick, 1997, p. 7). Because action research is site-specific in its processes and is not characterized by the same kinds of control as in other types of research, the results cannot be generalized to other settings:

> The primary goal of action research is the solution of a given problem, not contribution to science. . . The value of action research is confined primarily

to those conducting it. Despite its shortcomings, it does represent a scientific approach to problem solving that is considerably better than change based on the alleged effectiveness of untried procedures, and infinitely better than no change at all. *(Gay, 1996, p. 10)*

Because action research actively involves practitioners in the process, it can serve as a valuable strategy to facilitate the development of research-based nursing practice, as illustrated in the following study. Brooker (1997) described how an action research project was set up and implemented by nurses in a 16-bed surgical ward of a major pediatric teaching hospital in Australia. The aim of the project was "to improve and maintain the standard of wound care in a paediatric surgical ward" (p. 2). Two issues of concern had been raised by members of the nursing staff. The unit manager and clinical educator were concerned about the lack of observation and reflection on the part of nurses on their patients' wound care, and the nurses themselves were concerned about the many types of dressings and treatment used by the different surgeons. The nurse educator became the facilitator for the project and held in-service sessions to educate the nurses regarding action research. This helped "to solicit more participation and inform the nurses of their role in the process" (p. 3). The author described the first two cycles of the project, during which nurses were continuously involved in reviewing the literature related to wound care and implementing and evaluating a wound survey chart and a policy on wound care. Results indicated that the project helped the nurses to be more observant of their patients' wounds, increased their knowledge and skills on wound care, assisted them in acquiring more experience and skills in nursing research, and set up an ongoing framework for improvements in wound management.

> In the long term, by using this action research process, hopefully the nurses will acquire evidence-based knowledge and skills in wound management so that they will be able to challenge the hierarchical structures and participate in the decisions made in their patients' wound care. *(p. 6)*

Praxis Research.   Because you may occasionally see published studies using praxis as a research method, the following brief discussion is provided.

Praxis research has essentially the same goals as action research—that is, to change or improve a specific situation. The term praxis is a synonym for action. Praxis researchers are often deeply concerned with effecting social change to improve the human condition (thus returning to the roots of action research) and have goals beyond the simple changing of actions. Praxis researchers seeking changes in practice may opt to follow essentially the same process as action researchers. However, praxis research is usually reported with a philosophical framework as a part of the action. Lutz, Jones, and Kendall (1997) advocated the use of praxis in the field of nursing. They wrote that "praxis as an interpretive and critical methodology has been underutilized as an approach to clinical inquiry in nursing" (p. 23). They suggested that nurses need to use both the hermeneutic (descriptive) and eidetic (interpretive) systems in their practice to improve patient care and "to improve the human condition" (p. 30).

● USING COMPUTERS IN QUALITATIVE DATA ANALYSIS

Not unlike other researchers, qualitative researchers have turned to the computer for assistance in the analysis of qualitative data. Some have found that the use of a computerized word-processing program that displays word counts can aid in finding common themes or ideas. Qualitative researchers can choose from a number of programs mentioned in the literature, such as Ethnograph, Nud*ist, Martin, or Qualpro, which can facilitate the analysis of verbal data by finding themes or problem areas that are reported by subjects. However, although computers can assist in the management and analysis of data, they cannot fully analyze qualitative data. The focus of qualitative research is on the understanding that emerges; that understanding is a

> cocreation between the human researcher and the data . . . the focus on meaning is crucial to qualitative research, and meaning cannot be mechanically produced . . . while computers can assist in data analysis, they cannot do it; that requires contemplative work by the qualitative researcher. *(Pilkington, 1996, p. 6)*

● CRITIQUING THE DATA-COLLECTION AND DATA-ANALYSIS COMPONENTS OF A QUALITATIVE REPORT

The author should describe the specific qualitative method he or she used—phenomenology, grounded theory, ethnography, or another method. The research should focus on the human experience, and the method should be appropriate for the purpose of the study. For example, in the study in Appendix E the authors describe their research as an ethnographic study in the following statement: "The purpose of ethnography is to understand the lives of other individuals, in this case pregnant women on bed rest." The setting for the study should be described as to how and why it was selected.

Data-collection strategies, such as field notes, observation, interviews, and diaries, should be described and should be appropriate. Steps in the data-collection process should be described.

Data-analysis strategies should be discussed; a logical description should be provided of not only how the investigator moved from the raw data to the themes or hypotheses but also how these were related to the purpose of the study. If narrative data are cited, the themes or hypotheses should capture the essence of the narratives. An important consideration in evaluating the findings of qualitative research is the **confirmability** or trustworthiness of the finding; this serves as an indicator of the extent to which the researcher conducted the investigation in a rigorous manner. Three criteria should be used to evaluate confirmability or trustworthiness: credibility, auditability, and transferability. **Credibility** asks the question, "Are the reported findings true?" **Auditability** asks the question, "Can another individual follow the documentation of data collection and analysis that led to the conclusions of the researcher?" **Audit trail**, used in connection with auditability, refers to the systematic process by which an investigator records all activities related to the investigation so that an outside individual can examine the data and draw independent conclusions. **Transferability,** also termed fittingness, asks the questions, "Are the results applicable outside the research situation? Would the findings have meaning to others in a similar situation or situations?" For an example of how the researcher established auditability and credibility, refer to the discussion in the Methods section of the study in Appendix F.

Box 8-2 lists these points as evaluation guidelines.

BOX 8-2

GUIDELINES FOR EVALUATING THE DATA-COLLECTION AND DATA-ANALYSIS COMPONENTS FOR A QUALITATIVE REPORT

1. The research method is appropriate for the purpose of the study (ie, phenomenology, ethnography, grounded theory, or other).

2. Data collection

   a.. How/why was the study setting selected? Is the setting appropriate for the study?

   b. Data-collection strategies are described (such as personal diaries, observation, interviews).

   c. Data-collection strategies are appropriate for the research method and problem.

   d. Steps in the data-collection process are described.

3. Data Analysis

   a. Each data-analysis strategy is logically discussed and is appropriate for the purpose of the study.

   b. Data coding procedures are described.

   c. The themes and hypotheses are related to the purpose of the study.

   d. If narrative data are cited, do the themes capture the essence of the narrative?

4. Evaluating the Confirmability of the Findings

   a. Credibility: Did the participants validate that the reported findings truly reflect their own experiences?

   b. Auditability: Can another individual follow the documentation of data collection and analysis that led to the researcher's conclusions?

   c. Transferability (Fittingness): Are the findings transferable (that is, applicable outside the research situation)? Would the findings have meaning to others in a similar situation or situations?

SUMMARY

Validity and reliability are important considerations in conducting quantitative as well as qualitative research. Five of the major qualitative research methods were discussed in this chapter: phenomenology, which may employ one of two methods for describing lived experiences (hermeneutic [interpretive] or eidetic [descriptive]); grounded theory, which proposes to discover new theory based on "grounding" the theory in the data; ethnography, which is often used by cultural anthropologists and has many subfields that may be used by nurse researchers, including ethnomethodology, ethnoscience, and ethnonursing; historical research, which provides links to the past that may be used to increase our knowledge of how the field of nursing has evolved; and action research, in which researchers pursue action and research at the same time, with the potential to facilitate the development of research-based practice for nursing.

The following application activities will help you to apply this material and will assist you in developing your skills in evaluating published research.

REFERENCES

Addison, R. B. (1992). Grounded hermeneutic research. In B. Crabtree & W. Miller (Eds.), *Doing qualitative research* (pp. 110–124). Thousand Oaks, CA: Sage.

Baggs, J. G., & Schmitt, M. H. (1997). Nurses' and resident perceptions of the process of collaboration in an MICU. *Research in Nursing and Health, 20,* 71–80.

Baker, H. R. (1997). Outside the rules for the administration of medication: A study in New South Wales, Australia. *Image, 29*(2), 155–158.

Barry, D. G., & Boyle, J. S. (1996). An ethnohistory of a granny midwife. *Journal of Transcultural Nursing, 8*(1), 3–18.

Barsh, R. (1997). The epistemology of traditional healing systems. *Human Organization, 56*(1), 28–37.

Brooker, R. (1997). Improving wound care in a paediatric surgical ward. *Action Research Electronic Reader* [On-line]. Available: I.Hughes@cchs,usyd.edu.au

Davis, R. (1997). Community caring: An ethnographic study within an organizational culture. *Public Health Nursing, 14*(2), 92–100.

Dick, B. (1997). *A beginner's guide to action research.* Available FTP://www.scu.edu.au/www/arr/guide

Gay, L. R. (1996). *Educational research* (5th ed.). Upper Saddle River, NJ: Prentice-Hall, Inc.

Glaser, B., & Strauss, A. (1967). *The discovery of grounded theory: Strategies for qualitative research.* Chicago: Aldine.

Kavanaugh, K. (1997). Parents' experience surrounding the death of a newborn whose birth is at the margin of viability. *Journal of Obstetric, Gynecologic, and Neonatal Nursing, 26*(1), 43–51.

Leininger, M. (1991). *Culture care diversity and universality: A theory of nursing.* New York: National League for Nursing.

Lutz, K. L., Jones, K. D., & Kendall, J. (1997). Expanding the praxis debate: Contributions to clinical inquiry. *Advances in Nursing Science, 20*(2), 23–31.

Morse, J. M., & Field, P. A. (1995). *Qualitative research methods for health professionals* (2nd ed.). Thousand Oaks, CA: Sage.

Nelson, S. (1997). Pastoral care and moral government: Early nineteenth-century nursing and solutions to the Irish question. *Journal of Advanced Nursing, 26,* 6–14.

Pieranunzi, V. R. (1997). The lived experience of power and powerlessness in psychiatric nursing: A heideggerian hermeneutic analysis. *Archives of Psychiatric Nursing, 11*(3), 155–162.

Pilkington, F. B. (1996). The use of computers in qualitative research. *Nursing Science Quarterly, 9*(1), 5–7.

Powers, B. A., & Knapp, T. R. (1995). *A dictionary of nursing theory and research.* Thousand Oaks, CA: Sage.

Russell, D. (1997). An oral history project in mental health nursing. *Journal of Advanced Nursing, 26,* 489–495.

Strauss, A., & Corbin, J. (1990). *Basics of qualitative research.* Newbury Park, CA: Sage.

Wing, D. M., Thompson, T., Heleshaya [Medicine Man], (1996). The meaning of alcohol to traditional Muscogee Creek Indians. *Nursing Science Quarterly, 9*(4), 175–180.

BIBLIOGRAPHY AND SUGGESTED READINGS

Bogue, A. G. (1983). *Clio and the bitch goddess: Quantification in American political history.* Beverly Hills, CA: Sage.

Bowens, E. (1994). Ethnomethodology: An approach to nursing research. *International Journal of Nursing Studies, 29,* 59–67.

Coulon, A. (1995). *Ethnomethodology.* Thousand Oaks, CA: Sage.

Crabtree, B., & Miller, W. (Eds.). (1992). *Doing qualitative research.* Thousand Oaks, CA: Sage.

Denzin, N. K., & Lincoln, Y. S. (Eds.). (1994). *Handbook of qualitative research.* Thousand Oaks, CA: Sage.

Dick, B. (1997). *Frequently asked questions (FAQ file).* Available FTP://www.scu.edu.au/www/arr/arfaq

Dobbert, M. L. (1982). *Ethnographic research.* New York: Praeger.

Donahue, M. P. (1996). *Nursing, the finest art: An illustrated history* (2nd ed.). St. Louis: Mosby.

Doordan, A. M. (1998). *Research survival guide.* Philadelphia: Lippincott-Raven.

Fielding, N. G., & Lee, R. M. (Eds.). (1991). *Using computers in qualitative research.* Newbury Park, CA: Sage.

Fairman, J., & Lynaugh, J. D. (1998). *Critical care nursing: A history.* Philadelphia: University of Pennsylvania Press.

Fessler, D. B. (1997). *No time for fear.* East Lansing: Michigan State University Press.

Guba, E. (Ed.). (1990). *The paradigm dialog.* Newbury Park, CA: Sage.

Kalisch, P., & Kalisch, B. J. (1995). *The advance of American nursing* (3rd ed.). Philadelphia: Lippincott-Raven.

Lincoln, Y. S., & Guba, E. G. (1985). *Naturalistic inquiry.* Beverly Hills: Sage.

Morse, J., & Field, P. A. (1985). *Nursing research: The application of qualitative approaches.* Rockville, MD: Aspen.

Morse, J. M. (Ed.). (1989). *Qualitative nursing research: A contemporary dialogue.* Rockville, MD: Aspen.

Munhall, P. L., & Boyd, C. O. (1993). *Nursing research: A qualitative perspective* (2nd ed.). New York: National League for Nursing Press.

Streubert, H. J., & Carpenter, D. R. (1995). *Qualitative research in nursing: Advancing the humanistic imperative.* Philadelphia: Lippincott.

Thorne, S. E., & Hayes, V. E. (Eds.). (1997). *Nursing praxis.* Thousand Oaks, CA: Sage.

Werner, O., & Schoepfle, G. M. (Eds.). (1987). *Systematic fieldwork.* Beverly Hills: Sage.

APPLICATION ACTIVITIES

1. Distinguish between validity and reliability in qualitative research.

2. List the four levels of participant observation and discuss the major differences between them.

3. Discuss primary and secondary sources in historical research in terms of their meaning and potential sources of information.

4. Select two of the five qualitative methods presented in this chapter and discuss each in terms of definition, purpose, data-collection process, and data-analysis process.

5. Compare internal and external criticism as they relate to historical research.

6. If any or all of the three research studies you selected to critically evaluate are qualitative, use the guidelines in Box 8-2 or in Appendix H to evaluate the data collection and data analysis sections. If none of the three research reports you selected to critique are qualitative, use the guidelines in Box 8-2 or in Appendix H to evaluate the data collection and data analysis of the reports in Appendices E and F.

7. Explain the importance of evaluating the confirmability or trustworthiness of the findings of qualitative research. Discuss the meaning of the following terms: credibility, auditability, and transferability.

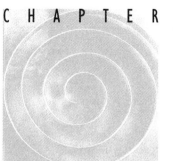

C H A P T E R

9

Quantitative Research Methods

TRUE EXPERIMENTAL DESIGNS
TYPES OF EXPERIMENTAL RESEARCH DESIGNS
QUASI-EXPERIMENTAL RESEARCH DESIGNS
NONEXPERIMENTAL QUANTITATIVE
    RESEARCH DESIGNS

CRITIQUING THE RESEARCH DESIGN IN A
    QUANTITATIVE REPORT
SUMMARY

OBJECTIVES   *On completing this chapter, the student will be able to:*

1. Identify three major categories of quantitative research design.
2. Discuss the essential characteristics of experimental research.
3. Discuss considerations related to internal and external validity in experimental design.
4. Compare five types of experimental research designs.
5. Discuss the differences between quasi-experimental and true experimental designs.
6. Identify five types of quasi-experimental designs.
7. Discuss the nature of nonexperimental quantitative research design.
8. Identify and discuss eight types of nonexperimental designs.
9. Define key terms.
10. Use evaluation guidelines to critique the research design of quantitative research reports.

KEY TERMS   Attrition   Hawthorne effect
Case study   Historical factors
Cohort   Longitudinal research design
Content analysis   Meta-analysis
Control group   Mortality threat
Correlational research design   Prospective research design
Cross-sectional research design   Quasi-experimental research design
Demographic variable   Randomization
Descriptive research   Regression toward the mean
Double-blind study   Retrospective research design
Ex post facto research design   Secondary data analysis
Experimental group   Self-report
Experimental research design   Single-blind study
Experimenter effect   Subject sensitization
Fatigue   Survey research
Focus group research design

*T*his chapter presents basic principles and methods related to quantitative research design. A research design is the overall plan for gathering the data to answer the research question that has been proposed for the study. Quantitative research designs can be divided into three major categories: true experimental designs, quasi-experimental designs, and nonexperimental designs. Each of these categories is discussed in this chapter. Critical evaluation of this component of a published research report is also discussed.

● TRUE EXPERIMENTAL DESIGNS

The Nature of Experimental Research

Experimental research design is a quantitative research design in which the independent variable(s) is manipulated by the researcher, subjects are randomly assigned to groups, and the experiment is conducted under controlled conditions. The primary purpose of experimental research is to investigate the effect of the independent variable(s) on the dependent variable(s) to determine the existence of a cause-and-effect relationship between the variables.

It is important to note the three major characteristics of experimental design: manipulation of a variable or variables by the researcher; random assignment of subjects to groups; and controlled conditions.

Manipulation of a variable or variables occurs when the researcher controls the movement of these variables—that is, the actual treatment or intervention for the experiment is done to only part of the study subjects.

Second, random selection of subjects from the target population and random assignment of subjects to the groups in an experimental study (also termed **randomization**) ensure that every subject has an equal chance of being assigned to either an experimental group or a control group on a random basis. Random assignment of subjects to groups on the basis of chance alone is used to avoid the possibility of systematic bias in assigning the subjects to the groups. Subjects in the **experimental group** (also termed the treatment group) receive the experimental treatment or intervention; subjects in the **control group** (comparison group) do not receive the experimental treatment or intervention and serve to provide a comparison with subjects in the experimental group.

Third, control of the setting in experimental research is crucial. In Chapter 1, the term "control" was defined as the process of holding constant—that is, eliminating or reducing the influence of variables that may interfere with the direct causal relationship between the primary variables of a research investigation. To achieve control in the experimental setting, the researcher must take measures to identify and isolate potential factors that could affect the variables under investigation and thereby affect the outcome of the research.

The primary purpose for conducting experiments is to determine the existence of cause-and-effect relationships between the independent variable(s) and the dependent variable(s) under investigation when a hypothesis is being tested. Observed instances of an activity may or may not be the cause of an observed effect or consequence. The experimenter wants to determine whether the activity was really the cause of the effect observed. For example, children are often admonished not to get their feet wet lest they catch a cold. Although this may seem to be a reasonable admonition, in fact we know that colds are caused by viruses that are transmitted from one person to another. Wet feet in and of themselves will not cause a person to catch a cold; they may make the person uncomfortable, disturb his or her physiologic balance, and lower resistance to infection. However, wet feet are not the causal factor in colds. Many so-called "common-sense ideas" are rooted in the folklore of cause and effect; the careful researcher designs experiments to verify whether, indeed, the cause does bring about the observed effect.

For example, to test the statement that getting one's feet wet will cause one to catch a cold, a researcher might compare two groups, one of which is exposed to foot wetting over a period of time and the other (control group) that is not exposed to foot wetting during the same period of time. Then the researcher could compare the frequency of colds in each group.

Conducting research with human beings as subjects puts the experimental researcher under many constraints. Controls are difficult to apply, and many experimental techniques used on plants and animals are certainly not open to experimenters who work with human subjects. Because of problems with randomization and control, few nursing studies, with the exception of physiologic research, use true experimental research designs. You may want to re-examine the discussion of the protection of human subjects in Chapter 7 to gain a fuller appreciation of the researcher's responsibilities for the protection of human rights.

Blind Studies

One of the ways to achieve control in experimental research is to use a design technique called a blind study. A blind study can be designed to be either single-blind or double-blind. A **single-blind study** may be carried out in one of two ways. In one method, the subjects know whether they are in the experimental group or the control group, but the experimenter does not know which group each subject is in. In the other single-blind method, the experimenter knows which group the subjects are in, but the subjects do not know which group they are in. The preferred method of designing blind studies is the **double-blind study**, in which an outside, neutral party has assigned subjects to both the experimental and the control groups, and neither the subjects nor the experimenter know which subjects are in which group.

Considerations in Experimental Research Design

In all experimental studies, the researcher must keep in mind certain major considerations concerning both internal validity and external validity. Internal validity in experimental research design refers to whether or not manipulating the independent variable(s) really does make a significant difference on the dependent variable(s). External validity refers to the ability to generalize the findings of the study. Following are major considerations regarding internal validity.

HISTORICAL FACTORS

If an experiment is carried out over a period of time, **historical factors** that are extraneous to the experiment, such as maturation or increased knowledge on the part of the subjects, may affect responses. Also, the occurrence of an event in the environment that is related to the topic of the study, such as a new breakthrough in the treatment of a disease, may affect the outcome of the study. These become confounding variables and must be accounted for.

FATIGUE

Not only the subjects of a study but also the researchers can become fatigued, bored, or inattentive during the course of an experiment. This means that either the treatment or the response measurement, or both, may not be consistent during the course of the experiment. There may come a time when both subjects and researchers have the feeling of "let's get this thing over with and get out of here." This natural **fatigue** must be recognized and guarded against to ensure accurate and consistent measurement.

ATTRITION

In research conducted over a period of time, there may be **attrition** or loss of study subjects. Subjects move, become ill, withdraw because they are tired of the research, or are lost to the experiment for any number of other reasons. An experimenter who starts with too small a sample or samples at the beginning of the experiment may obtain insufficient data for valid analysis. The term **mortality threat** refers to a threat to the internal validity of an experimental study when the dropout rate is different between the experimental and the control groups.

EXPERIMENTER EFFECT

Experimenters can unconsciously bias subjects merely by the tone of their voice, facial expressions, or other behavioral mannerisms. Such characteristics as gender, clothing, and age of the researcher can also influence the results. Unfortunately, some experimenters who have a vested interest in the outcome of their experiments may attempt to influence the results, either consciously or unconsciously. A truly scientific researcher remains objective and attempts to control these **experimenter effects** as much as possible.

REGRESSION TOWARD THE MEAN

When a group of individuals is given the same test several times, there is a tendency for their scores to change even if the test is extremely reliable. This universal statistical phenomena, known as **regression toward the mean**, occurs even in the best-designed studies. In most cases, the changes in scores tend to come closer to the mean scores of the group. Thus, experimenters who misinterpret this normal change as an experimental effect may draw incorrect conclusions.

External validity problems in some research studies, such as experimental conditions and/or the number and types of subjects selected for the study, do not allow for generalization of the findings. For example, if the experimenter administers a pretest to establish a baseline before introducing an experimental variable or variables, **subject sensitization** may occur. This means that the subjects have become sensitized to or knowledgeable about the procedures used for the research. This is especially true where a psychological rather than a physiologic response is measured. By its very nature, a pretest gives information about what the experimenter wants to discover. Even if the pretest questions are masked, subjects will often learn something about the research. Physiologic measurements can also be affected; as knowledge of biofeedback has increased, it has been demonstrated that subjects may be able to control many of their physiologic responses, even if they are doing it subconsciously. Subjects may also respond to being studied.

The **Hawthorne effect** is the term used to describe the psychological reactions to the presence of the investigator or to special treatment during the study, which may alter the responses of the subjects. The Hawthorne studies were a series of classic studies conducted in the late 1920s and early 1930s at the Hawthorne plant of the Western Electric Company in Chicago in which investigators observed that subjects may change their behavior in an effort to please the experimenter. Over the years there have been many studies of the Hawthorne effect and its influence on research.

SUBJECT SELECTION

When the researcher cannot randomly select subjects, there may be differences between the experimental and control groups of which the researcher is unaware. These differences may have an unintended impact on the results of a study.

● TYPES OF EXPERIMENTAL RESEARCH DESIGNS

There are a number of ways to design true experimental research; the designs range from simple to extremely complex. In incorporating the characteristics of a true experiment, each of these designs is characterized by manipulation of the independent variable by the investigator and by some form of control and randomization. Of the many designs that have been developed to meet the requirements of a true experiment, the following five are discussed here:

1. Pretest/posttest control group design
2. Solomon four-group design
3. Two-group random sample design
4. Matching samples design
5. Factorial designs.

The *pretest/posttest control group design* uses a control group to determine whether a treatment (or other experimental intervention) makes a difference. For example, an experimenter may design a study to measure the effect of reducing cholesterol in subjects with mild angina pain. The subjects would be randomly assigned to two groups: an experimental group and a control group. The subjects in the experimental group would then alter their diets, while the control group subjects would change nothing. At the conclusion of the experiment, the researcher would determine whether there was a statistically significant difference in the cholesterol levels of both groups. If this difference was indeed significant, and if there was a significant difference in the reported incidence of mild angina pain between the experimental and the control group, the experimenter could then conclude that the reduction of blood cholesterol did have an effect on the occurrence of angina. It is important to note there was no attempt to match or otherwise compare the members of either group; the only common element of control the control group shares with the experimental group is mild angina pain. Note also the term "mild." Pain perception varies greatly from individual to individual, and response to pain varies between cultures as well as between the sexes within a culture. None of these factors were taken into consideration in this example, only the common diagnosis of mild angina pain.

The *Solomon four-group design* is a frequently used and highly valid experimental design. In this experiment, the investigator would randomly divide the sample into four separate groups, effectively constructing two experimental groups and two control groups. The first experimental group would receive the same procedures as in the pretest/posttest design; that is, subjects would be randomly assigned, pretested, given the appropriate treatment, and then given the posttest. The first of the control groups is given the pretest, no treatment, and then the posttest. Up to this point, the Solomon design is precisely the same as the pretest/posttest control group design. However, group 3 is also defined as an experimental group. In the cholesterol example, it would consist of subjects diagnosed as having mild angina. They would not be given the pretest; that is, their cholesterol level would not be measured at all. However, they would receive the treatment; that is, their intake of cholesterol would be reduced and they would be given the appropriate blood tests at the end of the experimental period. Subjects in the fourth group in the Solomon design would have nothing done until the posttest. They would not be pretested for cholesterol levels at the beginning of the experiment and would not receive any treatment. Only at the end of the experiment would their blood cholesterol levels be measured (posttested) and then compared to the incidence of anginal pain in the other groups. Because two of the groups (groups 1 and 3) received the experimental treatment, any differences noted by the experimenter can be more confidently attributed to the treatment, rather than to subject sensitization due to the pretest, if both experimental groups show similar results at the end of the treatment and there is a significant difference between the experimental and the control groups. Similarly, a lack of statistically significant differences between the four groups enables the investigator to accept the null hypothesis that there was no significant difference in the blood cholesterol levels of the subjects in any of the four groups.

In the *two-group random sample design*, the experimenter may choose to use only the last two groups of the Solomon four-group design; that is, one group is given the treatment and then posttested with no pretesting, and the control group is given only the posttest. The theory behind this design is that the experimenter, adhering rigorously to the random assignment of subjects to the groups, can say that the two groups were essentially the same because random assignment should avoid any systematic bias in the two groups. This design not only simplifies the experiment but also eliminates the effect of a pretest on the subjects; in effect, it maintains the subjects' naïveté. It is also noteworthy that there are some things that cannot be pretested or accurately predicted. Patients who already have mild angina pain may or may not have elevated cholesterol levels. The angina pain already exists. If treatment or lack of treatment (cholesterol in the diet) is a factor, there should be a difference between the two groups at the end of the treatment. The researchers whose study is reprinted in Appendix C used this type of design to determine the impact of social support boosting interventions on caregivers of children with HIV/AIDS.

The *matching samples design* is more rigorous than those previously discussed. In this design, the researcher attempts to match (or to pair) the subjects in the control and the experimental group. For example, in the cholesterol study, the experimenter might match the subjects in each of the groups on such characteristics as height, weight, gender, age, smoking or nonsmoking, the results of psychological stress tests, and so on. A major problem with this type of experimental design is that unless the subject pool is infinitely large, the experimenter reduces the available sample with each matching or pairing situation. Males can be matched only with other males. Age further reduces the sample size. Eventually, it is entirely possible to reduce the sample down to two very well-matched people! The problem then becomes one of maintaining a sample size large enough to be generalizable.

In the experimental designs discussed so far, the experimenter identifies one independent variable and one dependent variable. Through the use of various forms of control, the effect of the independent variable on the dependent variable is then measured. However, there may be a situation when there are two or more independent variables that are manipulated simultaneously and, through interaction, may cause the dependent variable or variables to appear in the way that they did. Each of the independent variables is considered a factor influencing the dependent variable, either alone or in interaction with the other independent variables. Using the cholesterol example, suppose the subjects were overweight when placed on the low-cholesterol diet. In some cases, weight might be maintained because, although saturated fat intake was reduced, nonsaturated fats could be substituted for the saturated fats. The experimenter, however, might want to reduce both the weight and the intake of saturated fats of the subjects simultaneously. At the end of the experiment, it might be found that angina pain had been reduced in both intensity and frequency. It would then become very difficult to ascribe the causal effects to either of the two independent variables. Experimenters can more easily control experiments in which one and only one independent variable is introduced, as in the case of cholesterol intake reduction alone or a weight-loss diet alone. Often the interaction of two or more variables produces more significant results than a single variable does. The experimenter must then use what is called a *factorial design*. In this type of design, groups of subjects are assigned into all possible combinations of treatments to determine the effect of the independent variables alone and the effect of the interaction of the independent variables. Such factorial designs can grow to enormous complexity very quickly, but such is the work of researchers. Human beings are enormously complex; even the simplest and most tightly designed and tightly controlled experiment has results that are probably influenced by interaction effects. Factorial designs attempt to get at these interactive effects and determine their impact on the experiment.

Table 9-1 summarizes the experimental designs using the diagrammatic explanation of each.

TABLE 9-1   Summary of Experimental Research Designs

DESIGN	NUMBER OF GROUPS USED	PRETEST?	TREATMENT?	POSTTEST?
Pretest/postest	2	X Yes	X Yes	X Yes
		C Yes	C No	C Yes
Solomon four-group	4	X_1 Yes	X_1 Yes	X_1 Yes
		C_1 Yes	C_1 No	C_1 Yes
		X_2 No	X_2 Yes	X_2 Yes
		C_2 No	C_2 No	C_2 Yes
Two-group random sample	2	X No	X Yes	X Yes
		C No	C No	C Yes
Matching samples	2	X Yes	X Yes	X Yes
	Matched	C Yes	C No	C Yes
Factorial	Varies	X Yes	X Yes	X Yes
		C Yes	C No	C Yes

X: experimental group(s)
C: control group(s)

● QUASI-EXPERIMENTAL RESEARCH DESIGNS

The Nature of Quasi-Experimental Designs

When a researcher cannot design a true experimental study because of constraints imposed by subject selection or the study setting, he or she may use a **quasi-experimental design**, a design that is similar to a true experimental design (*quasi* means similar to or resembling). A quasi-experimental design may be defined as a quantitative research design in which there is always manipulation of the independent variable(s) and control measures are employed, but the other element of a true experiment, random assignment of subjects, is absent. For example, a researcher may want to investigate the differences between patients who may or may not receive a certain protocol that is routinely ordered by three different physicians. Physician A never orders the protocol, Physician B always orders the protocol at a set time, and physician C always orders the protocol at a set time that is different from physician B's time. In this case, the researcher cannot randomly assign the study subjects to the treatment groups, even though the impact of the time of the protocol or the lack of it can be measured. This is in contrast to a true experimental design, in which a researcher would be able to randomly assign the study subjects to either the experimental or the control group.

Five types of quasi-experimental designs will be presented here:

1. One-group pretest/posttest design
2. Nonrandomized control group design
3. Counterbalanced design
4. Time series design
5. Control group time series design.

The *one-group pretest/posttest design* is the simplest type of quasi-experimental design. Although this design leaves many things to chance, it is often the only available way to determine the effectiveness of a treatment. Essentially, this design measures what has happened to the experimental group based on the way it was before the beginning of the experiment (pretest state), and the differences achieved at the end of the experiment (posttest state). For example, using the study of a group of subjects with mild angina pain, the experimenter could measure the subjects' cholesterol level and then ask them to restrict their intake of cholesterol through changes in their diets. After a given period of time, the experimenter would determine whether the mild angina pain had been reduced and whether the blood cholesterol levels had dropped. If the blood cholesterol levels had dropped and angina pain had been reduced, the experimenter might then conclude that lowering cholesterol levels in the blood reduces angina pain. Note that no comparison in cholesterol levels is made in a control group or in a group of subjects who do not make changes in their diets. Minimal control is placed on other variables that might affect the evidence in the study subjects: changes in stress patterns, weight, exercise patterns, or many other factors might have contributed to the change.

The *nonrandomized control group design*, also termed the nonequivalent control group design, is often used in nursing research studies. When circumstances preclude random assignment of subjects to an experimental and control group at the beginning of an experiment, a nontreatment group may be established for the purpose of comparing outcomes. However, there is no way to guarantee that the groups are equivalent as to other characteristics. For example, the experimenter may wish to compare a sample of angina patients from a local Veterans Administration hospital with a sample of angina patients from a privately funded hospital. One of the hospitals may insist on a standardized routine of treatment for angina patients, whereas the other hospital may be available for the experimental treatment. In this case, the subjects in both samples would be given the pretest and one group would be given the experimental treatment. However, the researcher would not be able to control various interaction effects from the confounding variables at the beginning of the experiment. In this instance, where it is impossible to develop controls by assigning subjects randomly to control and experimental groups, alternative methods of statistical analysis are required. The method commonly used is the analysis of covariance, a statistical technique that allows the experimenter to statistically control for varying potential interaction effects after the experiment has been performed.

The *counterbalanced design* is a more effective design than the nonrandomized control group design, or at least one that attempts to remove some of the previously described problems. This design can be used when more than one treatment method is attempted. Each group of subjects is given a different treatment at the same point in time during the course of the experiment. This means that each group of subjects becomes both the experimental group and also control groups for themselves and for another group. Because of the nonrandom nature of group assignments, the experimenter cannot control for differences between groups. In many instances, the researcher may not be able to give a pretest. However, the testing does allow for greater flexibility in the interpretation of results; differences are noted both between groups and within groups. Using the statistical test of analysis of variance, the experimenter may be able to determine that the effects were caused by the treatment.

For example, two groups of psychiatric patients might be subjected to a computer program designed to interact with individuals and give the illusion of eliciting feelings at different times during their treatment. At the time of the first treatment session, group A would be given the computerized intervention and group B would receive a standard psychotherapeutic intervention. Both groups would then be given the same test to determine the subjects' responses to the treatments. At a later time, the treatments would be reversed: group A would receive the standard psychotherapeutic intervention and group B would be given the computerized intervention, and the same test would be given to determine the subjects' responses to the treatments. The differences in test scores, if any, between the two treatments could be recorded.

A number of variations to this design should be noted. More experimental variables could be introduced, such as another type of treatment in addition to computer and standard psychotherapeutic intervention. There would then have to be three groups of subjects, each receiving the treatments in a different order.

The *time series design* is useful when an experimenter wants to measure the effects of a treatment over a long period of time. In this design, the experimenter would continue to administer the treatment and measure the effects a number of times during the course of the experiment.

In the cholesterol example, instead of testing patients with mild angina pain only once (at the end of the diet restriction), the design would call for testing them at stated intervals. Chemical or behavioral changes in a human being can be very subtle and difficult to measure. Responses can vary daily, and some unrecognized confounding variables may lead to incorrect conclusions. Testing over a long period of time helps to reduce such pitfalls and improves the experiment. With a time series experiment, however, variables occurring during and after treatment may go unnoticed by the experimenter and can lead to a false or inappropriate conclusion.

A special case of the time series design is known as single-subject research, in which the researcher carries out an experiment on one individual or on a small number of individuals by alternating between administering a treatment and then withdrawing the treatment, with the purpose of determining the effectiveness of the intervention. Single-subject research has proven to be especially suited for psychiatric and other behavioral settings.

The *control group time series design* can be used to diminish the problems inherent in a time series design, such as subject sensitization or the Hawthorne effect. This design requires that a control group be tested simultaneously with the experimental group without being given the treatment. In our cholesterol example, two groups of randomly selected angina patients would receive a sequential series of blood tests over a period of time. The experimenter would then determine whether blood cholesterol levels had diminished significantly between the experimental treatment group and the control group, as well as the frequency and intensity of angina pain. This technique, obviously, provides far greater control than a single time series design and is preferable to the single time series design.

Table 9-2 summarizes the quasi-experimental designs using the diagrammatic explanation of each.

● NONEXPERIMENTAL QUANTITATIVE RESEARCH DESIGNS

The Nature of Nonexperimental Design

In nonexperimental research, the researcher collects data and describes phenomena as they exist. Unlike experimental research, variables are not manipulated because no interventions take place, there are no control measures, and there is no random assignment of subjects to groups. Much of the research that has been conducted in nursing has been nonexperimental due to difficulty in controlling variables in humans and with random assignment to groups, as well as ethical constraints incumbent on researchers who design experimental research involving human subjects. This type of research often relies on convenience samples. Although descriptive researchers often use simple statistics to analyze their data, they may also test hypotheses and use more complex statistics.

The following nonexperimental designs will be discussed:

1. Correlational designs
2. Descriptive designs
3. Time perspective designs
4. Retrospective designs
5. Prospective designs
6. Designs that use existing data
7. Focus group research
8. Content analysis

DESIGN	NUMBER OF GROUPS USED	PRETEST?	TREATMENT?	POSTTEST?
One-group pretest/posttest	1	Yes	Yes	Yes
Nonrandomized Control Group	2	X Yes C Yes	X Yes C No	X Yes C Yes
Counter balanced	Varies		Treatment A* X Yes*	X Yes
			Treatment B* Y Yes	Y Yes
			Later Time Treatment A* X Yes	Y Yes
			Treatment B* Y Yes*	X Yes
Time series (one group only)	1	Yes	Yes over time	Yes over time
Control group time series	2	X Yes C Yes	X Yes over time C No over time	X Yes over time C Yes over time

TABLE 9-2 *Summary of Quasi-Experimental Research Designs*

X: experimental group(s)
C: control group(s)
*Both groups receive treatment at the same time.

Correlational Designs

Correlational designs are nonexperimental designs that allow the researcher to infer relationships among two or more variables, rather than to draw conclusions about cause and effect. In these designs, the relationship between two or more variables is measured by correlation statistics, often called measures of association. Correlations range from -1.0 to +1.0 and are expressed numerically as correlation coefficients. A negative correlation means that as one variable increases, the other decreases. A positive correlation means that as one variable increases, the other increases, or as one variable decreases, the other decreases. A correlation of -1 is just as strong as a correlation of +1. The closer a correlation coefficient is to either -1 or +1, the stronger the relationship is between the variables being studied. The closer a correlation coefficient is to 0, the weaker the relationship between the variables. Correlations, however, do not imply cause-and-effect relationships. For example, the correlation between houses with roofs and houses with kitchens probably approaches +1.0, but this does not mean that the presence of roofs causes kitchens to be present.

A research study using a correlational design was conducted by Kennedy and Farrand (1996). The investigators examined the relationship between emergency nurses' attitudes toward organ and tissue donation and their intention to ask potential donor families to donate family members' organs and tissues. The results of the study indicated that emergency room nurses' willingness to approach a family regarding organ and tissue donation was positively correlated with the nurses' personal attitudes toward organ and tissue donation, with their confidence in asking families about donation, and with the frequency with which they approached a family. Although this study reported a positive correlation between nurses' attitudes toward organ and tissue donation and their willingness to approach a family, the researchers could not assign causality—that is, they could not conclude that nurses' willingness to approach a family was caused by their positive attitudes toward organ and tissue donation. Data-analysis techniques used in correlational designs will be discussed in Chapter 11.

Descriptive Designs

Descriptive research is often a preliminary to correlational research or to experimental studies. Descriptive research studies (not to be confused with qualitative research) can serve to discover new meaning and to provide new knowledge when there is very little known about a topic of interest. They also provide a knowledge base

> when a research problem needs to be refined, when hypotheses need to be formulated or data collection and analysis procedures need to be designed. . . Descriptive research is not the same as qualitative research. Qualitative research, although descriptive or narrative in nature, is a cover term for a number of research traditions that are distinct in purpose, orientation, and design. *(Powers & Knapp, 1995, p. 42)*

Survey research and case studies are two types of descriptive research.

Survey research is the term used to refer to the collection of data directly from the study subjects, usually by questionnaire or interview. When subjects respond to a survey, their responses are known as **self-reports** because it is the subjects themselves who are providing the information. Survey data are most often collected by questionnaires and interviews, both of which will be discussed in detail in the next chapter. Most survey researchers also collect demographic data to describe the characteristics of their subjects as part of their surveys. A **demographic variable** is a characteristic or attribute of a subject, such as age, gender, marital status, ethnicity, educational level, employment status, and family income. Although surveys can be conducted on an entire population of interest to the researcher, they are most often conducted on a sample of the population. Survey researchers use either probability or nonprobability sampling, depending on the purpose of the study. Also, surveys can either be **longitudinal**, in which case data are collected from the same subjects at different points in time, or **cross-sectional**, in which data are collected at one point in time. An example of a very extensive survey familiar to all of us is the United States census survey that is conducted every 10 years by the Census Bureau.

Schoenberg (1997) used various structured questionnaires and unstructured interviews in her survey to assess the influence of health beliefs on prescribed dietary behaviors in chronic hypertension management among 41 older (65+), hypertensive, rural African-Americans. Adherence was evaluated through a 24-hour dietary recall, food frequency, and physicians' consultation. The results of her study indicated that "the influence of health beliefs on the decision to follow treatment recommendation is complex, as study members tend to maintain both 'traditional' and biomedical health orientations and practices" (p. 174).

A **case study** is an intensive and in-depth investigation of a single unit of study. The single unit may be a single subject or it may be a family, a community, or an institution, such as a hospital or a university. Although case study data may be both quantitative and qualitative, "case study research should not be confused with qualitative research. Not every case study incorporates a qualitative perspective, and qualitative investigations can but do not always produce case studies" (Powers & Knapp, 1995, p. 19). In the case study method, either a single subject or a general population sharing a common background is identified, thus permitting the researcher to work with a limited number of individuals ranging from one to a large number of persons. Social anthropologists have a long tradition of using the case study method to study both small and large groups, especially those sharing a common culture or background. Multiple techniques may be used to collect the data, depending on the purpose of the study. Data-collection techniques may include interviews, questionnaires, records and documents, observations, and artifacts, such as cultural art and pottery.

Miller and Miller (1997) used the case study methodology in a freestanding rehabilitation hospital to determine the impact of the program-management model of administration on the quality of nursing care and changes in patient outcomes. They found that even though the discipline model of management was eliminated (each discipline, such as nursing and occupational therapy, had a separate administrator), most patient outcomes improved. Also, nursing employees had a mixed reaction to the change: equal percentages of staff reported greater satisfaction and less satisfaction, and 26% reported the same level of satisfaction with their work.

Time Perspective Designs

In *time perspective designs* (also called time dimensional designs), time is an important factor. Time perspective designs are concerned with examining trends or changes across time. Two major types of time perspective designs are longitudinal designs and cross-sectional designs.

In longitudinal designs, data are collected from the same subjects over a period of time. Typically, these subjects are members of a single **cohort**—that is, a group of persons who share a common characteristic, such as age, occupation, or a delineated area of residence. (Although the term *cohort* was originally used to refer to age as the common phenomenon, the meaning has now expanded to include additional characteristics of the subjects.) In a longitudinal study, the cohort is followed over a designated period of time with the purpose of describing changes that occur during that time. The time intervals may range from months to years. One of the most preeminent longitudinal studies in the health field is the Nurses' Health Study, which has been ongoing for more than 20 years. Initiated in 1976 by the Harvard Medical School, the purpose of the study was to investigate health risks that pose a special threat to women. The original cohort consisted of more than 100,000 married women born between 1921 and 1946 who lived in the 11 states with the largest total populations. (The senior author of this textbook has served as a subject for this study and has faithfully responded to a yearly questionnaire from the inception of this study to the present.) A similar, but younger, cohort has been added to the study with the purpose of examining the long-term effects of contraceptive use.

In 1998, Dr. Frank Speizer, Principal Investigator, reported the following:

> When the Nurse's Health Study began back in 1976 few of us had any idea that this research would continue for over 22 years and become one of the preeminent investigations of women's health . . . In the past year, we have published articles which reported that adult weight gain is strongly related to risk of hypertension, ischemic stroke and post-menopausal breast cancer. Physical activity, including brisk walking or more strenuous activity, reduces the risk of colon cancer. Saturated fat and transunsaturated fats are associated with increased risk of coronary heart disease, while high intakes of folate and vitamin B_6 (from diet and supplements) almost halved the risk. *(Speizer, 1998)*

In contrast to longitudinal studies, in which data are collected from the same subjects over a period of time, in cross-sectional designs data are collected from each subject at only one point in time, with the purpose of investigating differences in a specific variable or variables. For example, a cross-sectional study could be designed to study developmental issues, such as age-related phenomena, by taking a cross-sectional sample of different age groups and then comparing the data for each age group. The assumption would be made that each age group sampled is representative of that particular age group. A cross-sectional study has the advantages of being less expensive and easier to conduct than a longitudinal study. The obvious disadvantage of this design is that developmental trends over time cannot be established with the credibility of longitudinal research.

Armstrong and Murphy (1997) conducted a cross-sectional study to query 2,101 adolescents from eight junior and senior high schools across the United States regarding their interest in tattooing. Subjects responded to a 72-item self-reporting, anonymous survey tool that was distributed in their classrooms. The results indicated that permanent markings and blood-borne diseases were reasons subjects refrain from tattooing, but 55% (n = 1,159) expressed an interest in tattooing. The 10% of adolescents with tattoos described their experiences; tattooing was most frequently done "around the 9th grade and as early as 8 years of age; . . . over half report academic grades of As and Bs" (p. 181). Findings of the study indicate that adolescents who want a tattoo will obtain one, regardless of money, regulations, or risks. Adolescents view tattoos as objects of self-identity and body art, whereas adults perceive them as deviant behavior. The investigators recommended that informed decision-making be promoted through health education about "the possibility of blood-borne diseases, permanent markings, and themselves as growing and changing people" (p. 181).

Retrospective Designs

In **retrospective designs** (retrospective means "looking backward"), changes in the independent variable have already occurred before the research due to the natural course of events. The dependent variable (Y) is identified in the present, and then the researcher looks to the previous event that has already occurred to identify the possible independent variable (X). For example, a group of people attending a family reunion experience gastrointestinal symptoms serious enough to seek medical care. The purpose of a retrospective investigation would be to attempt to determine the possible cause for the current gastrointestinal symptoms. The investigator would "look backward" to determine the possible cause (X) of the present symptoms (Y). Retrospective studies have the same purpose as **ex post facto** studies (literally, "after the fact" studies).

Brown and Heermann (1997) conducted a retrospective comparative study in which they compared the charts of 25 preterm infants cared for in an NICU before 10% of the NICU nurses receiving training in the Neonatal Individualized Developmental Care and Assessment Program (NIDCAP) with 25 preterm infants cared for in the NICU after the training. They found that even with only a small percentage of nurses receiving the training, and with professional support from experts in developmentally supportive care, the preterm infants required less ventilation and less time in the NICU. These findings indicated that such training could reduce the costs of care for both consumers and hospitals.

The case-control study is frequently designed as retrospective research in epidemiologic investigations when investigators are attempting to determine possible causes of observed symptoms. In the case-control design, "a subject (case) with the condition of interest is compared with a subject (control) without the condition" (Doordan, 1998, p. 40). For example, a subject who had contracted hepatitis B would be compared with a similar subject who had not contracted hepatitis B.

Prospective Designs

In contrast to retrospective studies, which identify the dependent variable in the present and look to the past to identify the independent variable, **prospective designs** identify the independent variable (X) in the present and look to the future to identify potential effects (Y). The Nurses' Health Study, previously discussed as an example of a longitudinal study, is also an example of a prospective study. At one point in the study during the 1980s, the investigators identified intake of milk and dietary calcium as the specific independent variables (X) they planned to investigate into the future. They then continued to analyze the data over the next 12 years to determine the relationship of these variables to hip fractures (Y), the dependent variable. The results of the study were published in 1997:

> Among Nurses' Health Study participants, we found no evidence that high consumption of milk or other food sources of calcium protects against hip or forearm fracture. . . . Further follow-up will help us address this issue in more detail and thus inform future dietary guidelines. *(Speizer, 1998)*

Designs That Use Existing Data

Meta-analysis is a technique in which the investigator examines research findings across a number of research investigations relating to the same general phenomenon. The investigator then pools the results of these studies and synthesizes the findings—that is, brings together the findings of the many separate investigations relating to the same general phenomenon. "The original investigators have done the analyzing; the meta-analyst synthesizes the results of these analyses" (Powers & Knapp, 1995, p. 101). Meta-analyses may be performed either quantitatively or qualitatively. The basic procedure for both types of analyses is essentially the same: defining the research problem and identifying the studies to be included; collecting the related data; classifying and coding the distinctive characteristics/variables of the studies; examining the variables; and finally compiling the meta-analysis results and comparing this compilation with the characteristics/variables of the studies that have been examined (Kylma & Vehviläinen-Julkunen, 1997).

Labyak and Metzger (1996) noted that back rubs using effleurage (long and gliding strokes) were a regular part of nurses' repertoire in the past but are seldom done today because of technological advances and time demands. The investigators performed a quantitative meta-analysis on patients' responses—heart rate, blood pressure, and respiratory rate—before and after effleurage back rubs. Nine studies met the criteria of (a) back rub length of at least 3 minutes; (b) pre- and post-back rub vital signs being reported; and (c) statistical data reported in such a way that mean and standard deviation could be determined. The investigators, using statistical techniques to integrate the results of the nine studies, found that declines in heart rate, blood pressure, and respiratory rate were associated with back rubs lasting 3 minutes or more. Female subjects' blood pressure rose during the massage and declined during a 10-minute rest period after the back rub. Both males and females had immediate declines in heart and respiratory rates. The investigators concluded that effleurage back rubs are a "non-pharmacological form of nursing therapy that promotes biological and subjective relaxation" (p. 62) and suggested that this type of activity might well be reintroduced as a part of nursing activity.

Kylma and Vehviläinen-Julkunen (1997) used qualitative meta-analysis to analyze and synthesize 46 research studies published between 1975 and 1993 that examined the concept of hope, focusing on "the essence and distinctive characteristics of hope" (p. 364). Although hope is not easily quantifiable, many of the studies used questionnaires as the method of data collection on the concept of human hope. The researchers chose to do a qualitative meta-analysis of the articles based on the grounded theory techniques of Strauss and Corbin. They found that there are several dimensions to the concept of hope, including: (a) an affective dimension (hope and despair); (b) a functional dimension (activities both mental and physical); (c) a relational dimension (relation to self, others, and a higher power); (d) a temporal dimension (past and present experiences as well as a future orientation); and (e) a contextual dimension (environmental conditions). The authors concluded that more research must be done on hope as it relates to both sick and well individuals.

Secondary data analysis is a technique in which the investigator uses existing data that were collected for another purpose, either to design research studies to answer new questions and/or to test new hypotheses, or to reinterpret the existing data. Sources of data for secondary analysis include the results of research studies as well as other sources, such as information collected by state and federal governments. Census Bureau data often are a valuable source. Secondary researchers can usually gain access to these data and use them to answer their questions and to test a variety of hypotheses. However, investigators need to proceed with caution when using existing data for secondary analysis research, considering such issues as who collected the data, how rigorous the data-gathering techniques were, whether data are missing, the validity of the data, and whether the quality of the data is consistent or variable.

Secondary analysis as a research technique is sometimes confused with meta-analysis. Although both use existing data, secondary analysis is the analysis of a set of data from a research study or other source of existing data that is used by an investigator to design another study. Meta-analysis is a Psynthesis of the findings of many separate investigations relating to the same general phenomenon.

In the following example of a secondary analysis, a multisite survey provided the data for the secondary analysis research design. The original study by White and colleagues (1997) was conducted in Montreal over a 6-month period with the purpose of describing the prevalence and severity of pain in hospitalized patients. Secondary analysis of the original data led the researchers to develop a prospective study to explore the role of potential risk factors in predicting the development of chronic pain. In their study, "Predictors of the Development of Chronic Pain," the investigators re-examined data from the original study that were related to demographic, medical, psychological, cognitive, and pain-related variables measured during the acute phase of the pain experienced by the 2,415 patients in the original multisite study. They then analyzed data on the 371 patients who met all of the criteria for inclusion in their study. By performing a number of statistical tests, the researchers attempted to determine which set of variables measured in the acute-pain phase best predicted the development of chronic pain. The investigators found that no single variable predicted the development of chronic pain: chronic pain was best predicted by the interaction of medical, psychological, cognitive, and pain-related variables. Because the predictors of chronic pain are multidimensional, the researchers suggested that a team approach, rather than a single-discipline approach, is the best solution to the problem of pain and its resolution.

Focus Group Research

Focus group research design is a method that allows the researcher to examine the points of view of a number of individuals as they share their opinions/concerns about a topic. Essentially, a focus group consists of a small number of individuals who share a common bond. This bond might be any number of things such as age, number of children, wealth or lack of it, a specific disease, or any other commonality defined by the researcher. Focus groups have been a popular strategy for various commercial enterprises, who use them to determine whether a new product or idea would be accepted by the general public. Focus groups can also be used to evaluate changes in health care delivery systems, educational systems, or health care products. This type of research can provide a great deal of information at a relatively low cost. The focus group usually gathers in an informal setting, where the researcher or the researcher's designee serves as a moderator to collect data on a specific topic. It is the task of the moderator to keep the group focused on the topic to be discussed by using a series of questions designed to elicit pertinent information. Because of the shifting discussion pattern, audio and/or video recordings may be made of the session, with the permission of the participants. A researcher may use more than one focus group to gather data on a topic to gain more confidence in the responses.

Because the purpose of a focus group is to provide data about a topic, it is not important that the group reach a consensus. In analyzing the participants' responses, the researcher identifies common themes and patterns that reflect the responses of the group (or groups).

Butterfoss and colleagues (1997) reported the results of using focus groups for strategic planning by a community-based immunization coalition. A work group identified and selected 41 mothers for six focus groups representing private, military, and public sectors, as well as those who might not otherwise have been represented (such as the homeless). The focus groups were conducted to identify barriers that mothers of young children face when trying to obtain immunizations from public health, military, and private providers. The interview framework included questions to encourage discussion of "mothers' knowledge and attitudes about immunizations, as well as positive and negative experiences during their child's last immunization visit" (p. 51). The researchers found that although the mothers were deeply concerned about getting immunizations for their children, the clinic staff and facilities were not inviting to parents and children. Also, mothers lacked information concerning where immunizations were available, when to return for additional immunizations, and the availability of free immunizations. As a result of this research, a public awareness campaign was mounted to increase speakers' bureaus and to distribute informational packets, and media campaigns were developed to increase awareness in the community about the availability of immunizations:

> Coalition work groups used the data to develop strategies to improve access and delivery of immunizations including a public awareness campaign, increased clinic hours and sites, free transportation, parent incentives, and staff training. *(p. 49)*

Clinic facilities were also upgraded to provide a more positive environment for mothers and children.

Content Analysis

Content analysis is a data-analysis method that is used not only in quantitative research but also in qualitative research.

In quantitative research, content analysis can be used as "a method to make inferences based on systematic, objective, and statistical analyses of written text or oral communication and documentation" (Doordan, 1998, p. 47). In conducting a research study using content analysis, the investigator first formulates a research question, then selects an appropriate communication medium to be analyzed, establishes categories of information to be included in the analysis, then codes the content of the medium according to pre-established rules. Once the content has been coded, the categories are scored and scaled (usually statistically) and comparisons are made. Researchers use content analysis to analyze information from such sources as documentation found in written materials, videotaped and audiotaped materials, and still photographs and pictures. Essentially, any medium of communication can be analyzed for content, depending on the purpose of the research.

In qualitative research, content analysis is a process to analyze the content of qualitative information gathered from the study participants by "categorizing observations into themes and concepts emerging from the data" (Doordan, 1998, p. 47). For example, in the qualitative study reprinted in Appendix F, the researcher used content analysis as a process for categorizing the data relating to students' experience with bathing an adult patient for the first time.

The following examples describe two research studies. One study used content analysis as a quantitative data-analysis process; the other used content analysis as a qualitative research method.

"Tobacco and Alcohol Use Behaviors Portrayed in Music Videos: A Content Analysis" was published by Durant and colleagues in 1997. The purpose of the study was to analyze music videos from five genres of music (adult contemporary, country, rock, rap, and rhythm and blues) for portrayals of tobacco and alcohol use and for portrayals of these behaviors in conjunction with sexuality. Five hundred eighteen music videos were recorded during randomly selected days and times from MTV, VH1, Country Music Television, and Black Entertainment Television. The four networks were randomly assigned to morning, afternoon, and evening time slots and to days of the week by means of a random numbers table. The videos were recorded during the times when adolescents would have the most opportunity to view them.

Four teams of college students (four men and four women) were trained in the content analysis technique. The eight students were then randomly assigned to rotating two-person, male–female teams to analyze the content of the videos. In using the content analysis techniques, both members of the team had to agree that a targeted behavior occurred before it could be recorded on the data-collection instrument; when the team members could not agree, the principal investigator observed the video scene and made the final decision regarding the targeted behavior. Data were analyzed using both descriptive and inferential statistics. Network and music genre differences in alcohol and smoking behavior and in sexuality were tested with chi-square techniques.

The results indicated that when compared to the other networks, a higher percentage (25%) of MTV videos portrayed tobacco use; the percentage of videos showing alcohol use was similar on all four networks. In videos that portrayed both tobacco and alcohol use, the lead performer was most often the one smoking or drinking. The use of alcohol was associated with a high degree of sexuality on all videos. The researchers concluded that "even modest levels of viewing may result in substantial exposure to glamorized depictions of alcohol and tobacco use and alcohol use coupled with sexuality" (p. 1131).

Riesch and colleagues (1997) used content analysis as a qualitative data-analysis process in their study designed to determine what mothers of young adolescents perceive as important about themselves and parenting. The researchers collected data by requesting brief written statements from a sample of 538 mothers of young adolescents in which they reported their perceptions about themselves and parenting. After coding the responses within

BOX 9-1

GUIDELINES FOR EVALUATING A QUANTITATIVE RESEARCH DESIGN

1. The design is clearly identified.
2. The design is appropriate for the purpose of the study.
3. If a pilot study was conducted, the results are discussed.

themes, the researchers determined the categories within each theme. Six themes emerged: differences between ideals and practice; guiding principles (that is, the abstract and philosophical beliefs held by the participants); self-doubt (feeling ineffective, unique, or isolated despite their best efforts); parenting styles; stressors (events or situations that resulted in worry and that required the use of coping strategies); and communications (being an approachable parent, using communication to solve problems, to show affection, and to express opinions). The researchers recommended that professionals use the themes as a framework for anticipatory guidance not only when working with mothers about to embark on parenting an adolescent but also with families during adolescence.

CRITIQUING THE RESEARCH DESIGN IN A QUANTITATIVE REPORT

The research design is usually specified in the methodology section of the research report. The design should be clearly identified by the author and should be appropriate for the purpose of the study. The study in Appendix D was designed as a nonexperimental study, and a correlational design was used. In the true experimental study reported in Appendix C, the authors originally planned to use a four-group design that was collapsed into a two-group design. If a pilot study was conducted before the study, the results should be discussed. Box 9-1 lists these points as evaluation guidelines.

SUMMARY

Quantitative research designs can be divided into three major categories: experimental research designs, quasi-experimental research designs, and nonexperimental research designs. True experimental research design is characterized by manipulation of the independent variable by the investigator, who exercises some form of control over the experimental situation, including random assignment of subjects to groups (randomization). Researchers who carry out quasi-experiments cannot randomly assign their study subjects to either an experimental or a control group.

In nonexperimental investigations, researchers collect data to describe phenomena as they exist. Although often using simple descriptive statistics to analyze their data, they also test hypotheses and use more complex statistics. Much of the research that has been conducted in nursing has been nonexperimental due in large measure to the ethical constraints incumbent on researchers who design experimental research involving human subjects. Correlational designs examine the relationship between variables without assigning cause and effect. Descriptive research studies, such as surveys or case studies, can serve to discover new meaning and to provide new knowledge when there is very little known about a topic of interest. Descriptive research is often a preliminary to correlational research or to experimental studies.

A case study is an intensive and in-depth investigation of a single unit of study. The single unit may be a single subject or it may be a family, a community, or an institution. Although case study data may be both quantitative and qualitative, case studies are not necessarily qualitative.

In time perspective designs (also called time dimensional designs), time is an important factor. Longitudinal studies are designed to collect data from the same individuals over a period of time, whereas cross-sectional studies collect data from individuals one time only. In a retrospective study, changes in the independent variable have already occurred before the research due to the natural course of events. In contrast to retrospective studies, which identify the dependent variable in the present and look to the past to identify the independent variable, prospective studies identify the independent variable in the present and look to the future to identify potential effects.

Designs that use existing data include meta-analysis and secondary data analysis. Although both use existing data, meta-analysis is a synthesis of the findings of many separate investigations, either quantitative or qualitative, relating to the same general phenomenon, whereas secondary analysis is the analysis of a set of data from a research study or other source of existing data that is used by an investigator to design another study.

Focus group research design is a quantitative method that allows the researcher to examine the feelings, beliefs, and needs of a number of individuals as they share their viewpoints/concerns about a topic.

Content analysis is a technique that is used in both quantitative and qualitative research. In quantitative research, content analysis is used as a method to analyze written text or oral communication; in qualitative research, content analysis is a process used to categorize the data into themes and concepts emerging from the data.

The following application activities will help you to apply this material and assist you in developing your skills in evaluating published research.

REFERENCES

Armstrong, M., & Murphy, K. (1997). Tattooing: Another adolescent risk behavior warranting health education. *Applied Nursing Research, 10,* 181–189.

Brown, L. D., & Heermann, J. A. (1997). The effect of developmental care on preterm infant outcome. *Applied Nursing Research, 10*(4), 190–197.

Butterfoss, F. D., Houseman, C., Morrow, A. L., & Rosenthal, J. (1997). Use of focus group data for strategic planning by a community-based immunization coalition. *Family Community Health, 20*(3), 49–59.

Doordan, A. M. (1998). *Research survival guide.* Philadelphia: Lippincott-Raven.

Durant, R. H., Rome, E. S., Rich, M., Allred, E., Emans, S. J., & Woods, E. R. (1997). Tobacco and alcohol use behaviors portrayed in music videos. *American Journal of Public Health, 87*(7), 1131–1135 and *87*(9), 1514.

Kennedy, H. B., & Farrand, L. F. (1996). Attitudes of emergency nurses toward organ and tissue donation. *Journal of Emergency Nursing, 22*(5), 393–397.

Kylma, J., & Vehviläinen-Julkunen, K. (1997). Hope in nursing research: A meta-analysis of the ontological and epistemological foundations of research on hope. *Journal of Advanced Nursing, 25*, 364–371.

Labyak, S. E., & Metzger, B. L. (1996). The effects of effleurage back rub on the physiological components of relaxation: A meta-analysis. *Nursing Research, 46*(1), 59–62.

Miller, M. A., & Miller, L. D., (1997). Effects of the program-management model: A case study on professional rehabilitation nursing. *Nursing Administration Quarterly, 21*(2), 47–54.

Powers, B. A., & Knapp, T. R. (1995). *A dictionary of nursing theory and research* (2nd ed.). Thousand Oaks, CA: Sage.

Riesch, S. K., Coleman, R., Glowacki, J. S., & Konings, K. (1997). Understanding mothers' perceptions of what is important about themselves and parenting. *Journal of Community Health Nursing, 14*(1), 49–66.

Speizer, F. E. (1998). Cover letter. *Nurses' Health Study.* Boston: Harvard Medical School.

Schoenberg, N. E. (1997). A convergence of health beliefs: An "ethnography of adherence" of African-American rural elders with hypertension. *Human Organization, 56*(2), 174–181.

White, C. L., LeFort, S. M., Amsel, R., & Jeans, M. E. (1997). Predictors of the development of chronic pain. *Research in Nursing and Health, 20*, 309–318.

BIBLIOGRAPHY AND SUGGESTED READINGS

Campbell, D. T., & Stanley, J. (1963). *Experimental and quasi-experimental designs for research.* Chicago: Rand McNally.

Gray, D., Amos, A., & Curry, C. (1997). Decoding the image—consumption, young people, magazines and smoking. An exploration of theoretical and methodological issues. *Heath Education Research, 12*(4), 505–517.

Krueger, R. A. (1994). *Focus groups* (2nd ed.). Thousand Oaks, CA: Sage.

Solomon, R. C. (1949). An extension of control group design. *Psychological Bulletin, 46*, 137–150.

APPLICATION ACTIVITIES

1. Explain the differences between a true experimental design and a quasi-experimental design.

2. Discuss the purpose of blind studies.

3. List three considerations in establishing internal validity in a true experimental study, and discuss each of these.

4. Explain how the experimental study in Appendix C fulfills the following requirements for experimental research:

   a. Manipulation of the independent variable

   b. Random assignment of subjects to experimental and control groups

   c. Control measures

5. How does a nonexperimental design differ from an experimental design?

6. Distinguish between longitudinal designs and cross-sectional designs.

7. Distinguish between retrospective design and prospective design.

8. Discuss two purposes for conducting a meta-analysis.

9. Describe a situation in which a focus group research design might be used.

10. Use the guideline in Box 9-1 (or the guidelines in Appendix G) to critique the design for any of the quantitative studies you have selected to evaluate.

11. Locate one published true experimental research study and determine what type of experimental design was used. Record the title of the study, the author, and the journal source.

12. Locate one published research study using a quasi-experimental design and explain why the study has a quasi-experimental rather than a true experimental design. Record the title of the study, the author, and the journal source.

13. Locate two published research studies that use any of the following nonexperimental designs as a research technique: correlational design, descriptive design, time perspective design, focus groups, or content analysis. For each study you select, discuss the type of design that was used. Record the title of the study, the author, and the journal source for each.

10

Quantitative Data Collection

OBJECTIVES *On completion of this chapter, the student will be able to:*

1. Describe three approaches for establishing the validity of a quantitative measurement instrument.
2. Discuss four approaches for estimating the reliability of a quantitative measuring instrument.
3. Explain the importance of evaluating the usability of a quantitative measuring instrument.
4. Explain why validity and reliability are critical attributes in evaluating a quantitative research report.
5. Describe the characteristics of major quantitative data-collection instruments and techniques.
6. Define key terms.
7. Use evaluation guidelines to critique the data-collection components of published research reports.

KEY TERMS   Alternate forms reliability   Opinionnaire
                 Concurrent validity   Predictive validity
                 Construct validity   Projective test
                 Content validity   Proxemics
                 Criterion-related validity   Questionnaire
                 Delphi technique   Rating scale
                 Ethology   Semantic differential scale
                 Face validity   Sociometric techniques
                 Interrater reliability   Split-half reliability
                 Interview   Test-retest reliability
                 Kinesics   Unobtrusive measures
                 Likert scale   Visual analog scale (VAS)
                 Observation

As discussed in previous chapters, relevant data for a research study may be collected in either quantitative (numeric) form or in qualitative (verbal/descriptive) form. In either case, it is the task of the investigator to plan for appropriate data-collection techniques that will ensure that the data gathered are not only accurate but are also amenable to appropriate analysis. The purpose of this chapter is to present principles and techniques of quantitative data collection. Critical evaluation of the data-collection component of a published research report is also discussed.

● SELECTING A DATA-GATHERING INSTRUMENT

When talking about quantitative data-collection techniques, we are referring to the research instruments or the tools (such as devices or equipment) that are used to collect the relevant research data. The quantitative researcher's decision as to which data-collection technique to use depends on the nature of the research approach, the need for precision, and the availability of appropriate data-collection instruments. Quantitative researchers may use only one or two techniques to gather data, or they may choose to triangulate their data collection (that is, use three or more techniques to collect data). For example, in a study designed to describe the learning achieved by student nurses when caring for terminally ill patients, learning could be measured in the cognitive, affective, and psychomotor domains. A paper-and-pencil test could be used to gather data measuring cognitive learning (knowledge); an interview schedule could be used to ascertain attitudes on the affective domain; and an observational checklist might be used to gather data on the student's technical proficiency in performing psychomotor skills (procedures).

CHARACTERISTICS OF QUANTITATIVE DATA-GATHERING INSTRUMENTS

Because the outcome of a research study depends largely on the quality of the instruments used to collect the data, quantitative data-gathering instruments or tools must possess certain basic attributes to ensure that they will provide accurate and dependable measurement of the variables under investigation. The most important of these attributes are validity, reliability, and usability.

In quantitative research, the validity of an instrument refers to the extent to which a data-gathering instrument measures what it is supposed to measure—that is, the extent to which the instrument obtains data that are relevant to what is being measured. The more evidence of validity that is provided concerning a measuring instrument, the more confident a researcher can be that the instrument does indeed measure what it purports to measure. In establishing the validity of a measuring instrument, the questions "Valid for what?" and "Valid for whom?" must be answered.

In addition to validity, reliability is an important characteristic of a quantitative data-gathering instrument. Reliability in quantitative research refers to the ability of a measuring instrument to do consistently whatever it is designed to do in the same way each time it is administered. The ability to obtain consistent results when it is reused enables the researcher to be more confident that the scores will not fluctuate too greatly with repeated administration of the instrument. Reliability asks the question, "Does the instrument consistently measure whatever it is supposed to measure in the same way each time?"

Usability of a quantitative data-collection instrument refers to the practical aspects that the researcher must consider in selecting a data-gathering instrument, such as ease of administration and time constraints.

Approaches to Establishing Validity

There are three main approaches for establishing the validity of a quantitative measuring instrument: content validity, construct validity, and criterion-related validity.

The **content validity** of a measuring instrument is the extent to which the instrument represents the phenomena under study. Each content area must be defined, and representative items are then identified. Typically, a judge panel of experts is then requested to determine content validity. This means that a number of experts in the field of the specific study topic are asked to examine each item and to judge how well each of the items and the entire instrument reflect the previously defined content area(s). There are no statistical procedures involved in determining the content validity of a measuring instrument.

This type of validity is especially useful when developing instruments that measure specific areas of knowledge. For example, in a study designed to elicit the knowledge that teenage subjects have about teenage pregnancy, the researcher would formulate items related to the topic of teenage pregnancy, would then request that experts in the field of teenage pregnancy examine each item to determine whether it accurately reflects knowledge that teens would/should have regarding teenage pregnancy, and then would incorporate the valid items into the measuring instrument.

A subtype of content validity is **face validity**, in which validity is determined by inspecting the items to determine whether "on the face of it" the instrument contains important items that measure the phenomena under study. Face validity is the least time-consuming and least rigorous method for determining validity because it is based entirely on the subjective judgment of the investigator. Although estimating the face validity of an instrument is better than establishing no validity at all, face validity is seldom used due to its lack of true confirmability.

Construct validity is the degree to which a measuring instrument measures a specific hypothetical trait or construct, such as intelligence, grief, or prejudice. Establishing construct validity is a complicated and time-consuming process because it requires that the measuring instrument be used in a succession of different studies, each of which uses various methods for evaluating construct validity. A basic approach to establishing construct validity is the known-groups technique, in which the instrument is administered to several groups known to differ on a certain construct. If the results obtained demonstrate statistically significant differences as expected, then the instrument is said to have a degree of construct validity. For example, in establishing the construct validity of an instrument for measuring preoperative anxiety, it would be expected that the preoperative anxiety reported by a group of patients having minor surgery in an ambulatory care unit would differ significantly from the preoperative anxiety reported by patients admitted to the hospital for major surgery. Other procedures for demonstrating construct validity (such as factor analysis) are discussed in more advanced research and statistics textbooks. Although construct validity is considerably more difficult to establish than content validity, it is important to establish construct validity when complex concepts are being measured.

Criterion-related validity refers to the relationship of the measuring instrument to some already known external criterion or other valid instrument. Criterion-related validity is the general term that includes both predictive and concurrent validity. **Predictive validity** is the ability of the instrument to predict an individual's behavior in the future. For example, the scores received on the Graduate Record Examination (GRE) are supposed to predict a student's potential for success in graduate work in a college or university. **Concurrent validity** is a measure of how well an instrument correlates with another instrument that is known to be valid. For example, an individual's score on the Stanford-Binet IQ test should be very similar to that individual's score on the Wechsler Intelligence Test.

Approaches to Estimating Reliability

As noted above, the reliability of a measuring instrument refers to the ability of the measuring instrument to do consistently whatever it is designed to do in the same way each time it is administered. Reliability is usually expressed as a number, called a coefficient. A high coefficient indicates a high reliability. A measuring instrument that has a perfect reliability would have a coefficient of +1.00. Rarely, however, is a measuring instrument perfectly reliable. Reliability is more often reported as less than 1.00—that is, 0.80, 0.75, or 0.50. Less-than-perfect reliability of an instrument can be due to errors in measurement, such as the conditions under which the instrument was administered (for instance, improper directions); problems with the instrument itself (for instance, poorly constructed items); or characteristics of the individuals responding to the instrument (for instance, illness or fatigue).

There are several types of reliability that may be determined through various correlations: test-retest reliability, alternate forms reliability, split-half reliability, and interrater reliability.

Test-retest reliability indicates variation in scores from one administration of the instrument to the next, resulting from measurement errors. The procedure for determining test-retest reliability is to administer the instrument to individuals similar to the ones the researcher plans to study, let some period of time elapse (say a week) to allow for some loss of memory of the items, then give the instrument to the same individuals again. The scores on the two instruments are then correlated statistically to yield a coefficient referred to as the coefficient of stability. If the results are the same or similar, the coefficient will be high—say, 0.90—and the instrument is said to have high test-retest reliability. One of the major problems with this method of estimating reliability is that of deciding realistically how long the time interval between the test and the retest should be. If the interval is too short, the individuals tend to remember their responses to the items on the first administration. This results in an artificially high coefficient of reliability. If the time interval is too long, some individuals may do better on a retest because of their own learning and maturation during the interval between the test and the retest.

Alternate forms reliability is also called equivalent forms reliability. To establish this type of reliability, at least two different forms of the instrument are constructed. Although the actual items on the instruments are not the same, each form has the same number of total test items, is designed to measure the same variable or variables, and has the same level of difficulty. Both use the same procedures for administration, scoring, and interpreting results. At least two different forms of the instrument must be available. The procedure for determining alternate forms reliability is to administer one form of the test to a group of individuals and then, at the same session or very shortly thereafter, administer a second form to the same individuals. The two sets of scores are then statistically correlated, and the instrument is said to have good alternate forms reliability if the correlation coefficient is high. There are two major problems with this method. One is the difficulty involved in constructing two forms that are equivalent; this can result in measurement errors. The second is the difficulty in administering two different instruments to the same individuals within a relatively short time period.

Split-half reliability, also called odd-even reliability, yields the coefficient of internal consistency. Historically, this estimate of reliability has been used because it requires only one administration of an instrument. The entire instrument is administered to a group of individuals, and then the responses for each individual are divided into two comparable halves: all the responses to even items in one half and all the responses to odd items in the other. The response score for each individual is then computed separately for the two halves, resulting in a response score for the even items and a response score for the odd items. The two sets of scores are then correlated statistically to yield a correlation coefficient. If this is high, the instrument is said to have good split-half reliability. This method is more effective for longer instruments. For an instrument consisting of a limited number of items, a correlation formula such as the Spearman-Brown prophecy formula must be applied. The split-half method of estimating reliability has the advantage of requiring only one administration and one form of the instrument; it also eliminates the problems associated with more than one administration of the instrument to the same individuals. Cronbach's alpha is a statistical procedure to measure internal consistency. This technique allows the researcher to compare the results of each item on a questionnaire with every other item and average the results to achieve a correlation coefficient. This correlation coefficient is the average of all of the possible split-half reliabilities of an instrument when the responses to the questions on the instrument can be scored as having several possible responses (that is, 1, 2, 2, 4, and so forth). The Kuder-Richardson formula (K-R 20) is a special case of Cronbach's alpha and is used when the items measured are scored in a dichotomous fashion (yes or no; right or wrong).

Interrater reliability is also called interobserver reliability. When a researcher uses observational techniques and two or more different observers independently observe the same activities and record their observations using the same recording format, the strength of the agreement between the two sets of observations may be computed as a correlation.

Evaluating Usability

The usability of a measuring instrument refers to the practical aspects of using it. Among usability considerations in selecting an instrument are ease of administration, scoring, and interpretation of the results. Energy expenditure for both the administrator and subjects as well as cost and time requirements are also important. These and other practical aspects must be considered when selecting a measuring instrument.

● SELECTING APPROPRIATE MEASURING INSTRUMENTS

In selecting a measuring instrument, first, as with any research study, an appropriate research question or problem must be formulated. The problem statement and the purpose of the study should guide the selection of an appropriate research design as well as the choice of data-collection instruments that meet the criteria of validity, reliability, and usability. Given that it takes a great deal of time and skill to develop a measuring instrument, researchers may be well advised to consider selecting an appropriate already-developed instrument that has good validity and reliability as well as usability. If it is necessary to use a self-developed instrument, the researcher may be able to take parts from one or more instruments to develop the new instrument. To test the new instrument's effectiveness for gathering appropriate data, the researcher must then administer the new instrument to a group of subjects who meet the same criteria as the subjects to be used in the study. The researcher then uses these data to evaluate the instrument's strengths and weaknesses, making any necessary revisions in the instrument before using it in the study.

● QUANTITATIVE DATA-COLLECTION INSTRUMENTS AND TECHNIQUES

Although your primary purpose as an undergraduate research student is to develop skills in critically evaluating published research for its application to practice, it is also important for you to understand not only the purpose and characteristics of the various data-gathering instruments but also the process by which researchers develop them. Ten of the data-collection instruments and techniques most often used by quantitative researchers are questionnaires, interviews, self-report scales, observation, Delphi technique, unobtrusive measures, sociometric techniques, ethology (including proxemics and kinesics), biological and physiologic instruments, and psychological and projective tests.

Questionnaires

A **questionnaire** is a paper-and-pencil data-collection instrument that is completed by the study subjects themselves. The questionnaire is often mailed to the respondents; it can also be administered face to face. If the researcher finds it necessary to construct a questionnaire to collect the study data, great care must be exercised so that the items will allow the respondents to provide the information that directly relates to the design of the study. If the study is designed within a theoretical or conceptual framework, this framework should provide the rationale for the development of the questionnaire. Researchers should probably spend more time formulating their questionnaires than they do analyzing their research data. Well-constructed questionnaires allow for relatively easy interpretation and analysis. Poorly developed questionnaires may cost more in time and effort and prevent the investigator from achieving the purpose of the study.

Questionnaires are constructed to be either open-ended or closed. Open-ended questionnaires allow the respondents a variety of ways to answer questions and permit the researcher to make inferences from the responses to the questions. Closed questionnaires allow for certain structured answers (yes or no) or a limited selection of choices. Researchers who want to eliminate ambiguity and expedite the coding of data often opt for a closed questionnaire.

Every questionnaire item must be clear and unambiguous. We tend to assume that people understand what we are talking about, but the naïve respondent may not have the same frame of reference as the researcher. The question, "Are the chickens ready to eat?" is an example of the ambiguous use of the English language. Questions that could have multiple interpretations should also be avoided. Also, respondents not familiar with the vocabulary will not give accurate or valid answers; at the same time, the researcher must respect the respondent's intelligence. The wording of questions should also be concise. Any amount of confusion, or even mistrust, that the instrument causes reduces the chance that the respondent will return the questionnaire.

The questionnaire should be as simple and short as possible. There is something very threatening about an instrument with many pages and a multiplicity of choices. The shorter the instrument (within reason), the more likely it will be completed and returned. The researcher should place relatively simple items at the beginning of the instrument, thus allowing the respondent to succeed and be reinforced to continue. Researchers should provide cross-check questions to be sure that the respondent is answering consistently. Rewording the same question and asking it again, either positively or negatively, is a good way to provide this insurance, but questions should be sufficiently separated so that the subject will not see through this technique. Finally, careful development of the instructions for the respondent involves a clear statement of what the researcher wants the respondent to do. Validity and reliability must be determined by using the appropriate techniques described in the previous section of this chapter. A pretest of the questionnaire should be conducted to correct any problem with the questionnaire before it is administered to the study subjects.

Mailed questionnaires are answered in much larger numbers if a self-addressed, stamped envelope is included with each questionnaire. Most people are willing to respond but may be unwilling to subsidize the researcher. If a follow-up letter is sent, it may be wise to send yet another self-addressed, stamped envelope and questionnaire. Granted, this may add to the researcher's expenditures, but all research should be planned to include the total cost of all items.

It is important to include a cover letter with the questionnaire. This letter not only informs the respondents about the study but also serves as informed consent. The study subjects who choose to return the completed questionnaire have provided their implicit consent by returning it to the investigator.

A cover letter should include the following items:

1. Name of the researcher
2. Address of the researcher
3. Purpose of the study
4. The approximate length of time required to fill out the questionnaire
5. A statement safeguarding the confidentiality of the responses
6. Any additional information the researcher thinks is important.

When using a mailed questionnaire, the investigator should determine an acceptable percentage of responses to be obtained and should then allow a specific amount of time to elapse after the instrument has been mailed. There are many reasons for nonresponse, especially if the questionnaire is mailed. Although lower response rates are common, a response rate of 55% or more is usually considered to be acceptable. Thus, an investigator who expects a 100% response will probably never draw any conclusions from the study!

An **opinionnaire** is a questionnaire designed to elicit data about subjects' opinions. For example:

People have strong opinions and attitudes about a national health care program. Which of the following statements best represents your opinion about national health care? Place a circle around the letter of the response that most accurately reflects your point of view about the following items:
  a. National health care will cost too much to be practical and should be avoided.
  b. National health care is the only way to provide adequate health care for all people.
  c. National health care should be limited to catastrophic illnesses.
  d. National health care would subvert our free enterprise system.

Note that in this instance respondents may not agree with any of the choices. Care must be exercised in developing this kind of instrument so that any bias on the part of the investigator does not creep in through the use of slanted questions.

An opinionnaire may also be designed to request respondents to rank their responses from the most important to the least important. If the list is too long, however, the subjects may have difficulty in keeping the whole list in mind. For example:

Nurses should be capable of participating in research. The following is a list of settings in which nursing research can be carried out. Please rank each in order of importance as a setting for nursing research by placing a 6 by the most important, a 5 by the second most important, and so on down to number 1 (least important):
  ( ) hospital
  ( ) community health center
  ( ) visiting nurse association
  ( ) hospice
  ( ) day-care center
  ( ) home health agency.

Interviews

The term **interview** refers to verbal questioning of respondents by the investigator to collect data; interviewing requires interaction between people. There are two basic kinds of interviewing techniques: structured and unstructured. In the structured interview, the interviewer has a list of prepared questions that the researcher believes will provide a format for the respondent's answers. For example:

1. How competent do the nurses in ZZZ Hospital seem to be?
2. Why do you answer as you do?

The interviewer thus guides the respondent to determine what information is to be elicited and then records the answers.

An unstructured interview is more like a conversation and takes more time than a structured interview. Here the researcher has a general framework of questions to elicit answers concerning the information sought but uses the respondent's answers to enlarge on the topic and to ask additional questions. The topics flow from the conversation's progress; there is no set pattern or ordering of the categories that the researcher is exploring.

If the researcher is not the sole interviewer for the study, it is the researcher's responsibility to provide adequate training for the interviewers who may be assisting in the collection of the study data to ensure interrater reliability. A pilot or preliminary study is extremely valuable as a part of the training process. Debriefing after a few interviews allows the interviewers to point out flaws not initially discovered in the interview schedules and coding sheets. It also provides for a check on interviewing techniques. Face-to-face interviewers should be nonthreatening to the respondent, and the interviewer must establish rapport with each respondent. Interviewers should be trained to remain neutral when eliciting answers to the survey instrument. Some people will give the answer they think the interviewer wants to hear rather than what they really believe. Interviewers who encourage such responses, whether overtly or unconsciously, cannot gather valid data. Certain styles of dress and manners may be appropriate in one setting but not in another.

As in all research involving human subjects, informed consent must be secured. In the case of a face-to-face interview, the informed consent should be completed before the beginning of the interview so that the subjects are fully aware of the nature of the study and are free to make an informed decision as to whether or not to participate. If the interview is to be recorded either by audio or visual means, the informed consent must include this information.

Telephone interviewers should also be selected with care because respondents usually visualize the individual on the other end of the line. The interviewer should have a pleasing telephone voice and should have practiced using the data-collection instrument a number of times before actually talking to potential respondents. People seem increasingly resistant to responding to telephone surveys. This is probably due to a number of factors. First, with the increasing popularity of telephone surveys, individuals find that their time is being demanded more frequently, and they resent the intrusion on their privacy. Secondly, there have been frequent misrepresentations by telephone solicitors who claim to be conducting research but are actually selling a product.

The following is an additional principle of face-to-face interviewing that the senior author of this text learned through first-hand experience while conducting research designed to study community satisfaction and psychological well-being in a very small rural community in northeast Texas. On the first day of interviewing, one of the two interviewers who were assisting me with the interviews in the homes of the subjects happened to interview the wife of the town mayor, who eagerly signed the written consent form to participate in the interview. She was so excited about being interviewed that, after completing the interview, she phoned her husband to share the experience. Her husband immediately reported the interviewer to the police, who proceeded to pick up both interviewers. I then found myself at the police station explaining the situation. Fortunately, a full explanation sufficed. After providing the mayor with an official letter from the university explaining the study, we were each given written permission from the mayor to continue with the interviews and were able to complete the other 98 interviews with no further problem. The lessons learned: When planning to interview members of a community, it is wise for the researcher first to contact local city officials for permission. They may be willing to provide a letter, badge, or other symbol of official recognition that will give interviewers easier access to study subjects. It is also helpful to remember that in a small community, news travels fast. In the event that interviewing techniques should prove to be displeasing, potential respondents may reject the interviewers on the basis of what they have heard from others in the community.

Self-Report Scales

In relation to data collection, a scale is a self-report measure that consists of a series of items designed to measure the attributes being investigated. The subject is presented with the items and responds to each item on the scale provided. Self-report scales are usually designed to be summated—that is, each response can be given a value and the responses for the entire scale can then be totaled to obtain a single score. Four types of self-report scales will be discussed: rating scales, Likert scales, semantic differential scales, and visual analog scales.

A **rating scale** is a type of data-collection instrument that allows the respondents to place their responses, such as feelings or attitudes, on a scale that has a range of potential responses. For example:

How would you rate the nursing care in this hospital?
Very Good __: __: __: __: __ Very Poor
Please check the appropriate blank.

The number of response options on rating scales may vary considerably. Although five options occur most frequently, and this appears to be the minimum acceptable number, six, seven, or even eight options can also be presented.

The **Likert scale** is a commonly used self-report measure that is designed primarily to measure attitudes. A Likert scale consists of a series of statements, each of which has a number of possible responses, such as strongly agree, agree, uncertain, disagree, strongly disagree. Although five responses is typical, up to seven responses may be provided.

There is a definite advantage in using scales that have an even number of responses; these are called forced-choice scales. When given an odd number of choices, subjects may respond to the middle choice and thus appear to be neutral, choosing neither high nor low ratings. If a scale has an even number of options, however, the subject must respond with a high or low ranking or rating. Given the previous question, the even-numbered forced-choice rating scale compels the respondent to either like or dislike the nursing care:

The nursing care in this hospital is:
Very Good __: __: __: __: __: __ Very Poor

The scale might similarly have been written as a Likert scale:

The nursing care in this hospital is very good.
Very strongly agree; strongly agree; agree; disagree; strongly disagree; very strongly disagree.

In this instance, the respondent would probably be asked to circle the appropriate response.

Often, adequate statistical analysis cannot be done if the sample size is small. Forced-choice scales allow for the collapsing of cells (categories of data), for dichotomization, or for bringing cells together in statistically valid groups. Neutral responses might otherwise have to be discarded or divided, giving an unclear picture of the respondents' feelings or attitudes.

The **semantic differential scale** is used most often to elicit the attitudes and beliefs of respondents. The scale consists of a listing of bipolar adjectives with a five- to seven-point scale between them that may describe a setting, object, profession, or any other variable of interest. For example, a researcher who wanted to determine how people from different cultural and ethnic backgrounds perceive hospitals might construct the following scale:

Below is a checklist of words that describe a hospital. Please place a check mark in the space that best shows how you feel about hospitals. Be sure to place a check mark on each line.

Good __:__:__:__:__:__ Bad
Busy __:__:__:__:__:__ Quiet
Warm __:__:__:__:__:__ Cold
Clean __:__:__:__:__:__ Dirty

Analytical techniques specifically designed for semantic differential scales would then be applied to the data to determine whether different subjects perceive the hospital setting in different ways. Walker and Sofaer (1998) developed a 12-item, 5-point semantic differential scale in their study of psychological distress in patients attending pain clinics. The scale was validated by factor analysis and its reliability was obtained by the test-retest method. They asked subjects to mark the box that "represents how you feel MOST OFTEN these days." For example:

Calm __:__:__:__:__ Irritable
Happy __:__:__:__:__ Sad

The results of this study are discussed in greater detail in Chapter 11.

The **visual analog scale** (VAS) is a self-report paper-and-pencil scale that consists of a straight line that has the extreme limits of the variable being measured at each end of the line. The straight line may be either vertical or horizontal. The scale is designed to have the respondent indicate a point on the line that indicates where his or her pain is most like (analogous to) the intensity of the specific attribute being measured. The VAS has proven to be a useful research tool to measure such subjective experiences as pain and anxiety reported by subjects in a clinical setting.

Following is an example of a horizontal VAS that could be used to measure fatigue:

No Fatigue ├────────────┤ Fatigue As Bad
                              As It could Possibly
                              Become

The subject would be asked to select a point along the line that best expresses the intensity of his or her fatigue and to place a mark through the line at that point.

Observation

When the researcher is concerned with attributes other than attitudes and beliefs, **observation** permits the researcher to watch and note actions and reactions. Observational data-collection techniques may lend themselves to description and analysis of behavior. The structured checklist is often used to collect observation data. The researcher records what happens and how frequently it happens to determine the nature and frequency of events or activities of interest. For example, a study's purpose might be to determine whether laryngectomy patients behave differently as a result of structured preoperative teaching about their surgery, as opposed to a different kind of instruction. The researcher creates a checklist of significant behaviors of the patients being observed in the study. The researcher then determines the frequencies of occurrence and tallies the results. This provides a foundation for interpretations and conclusions about the effect of structured preoperative teaching on the postoperative behavior of laryngectomy patients.

Observation research often requires that several observers be used. This means that there is a potential for differences of observations among the observers. Consequently, the researcher must be extremely careful to train observers by providing common experiences so that observer reliability can be established. Given the example of the laryngectomy patient study, observers could be shown films or videotapes of patients performing a range of behaviors. The observers would then mark the designated activities on their observation checklist, and their perceptions could be checked by the researcher. After a number of training sessions, interrater reliability could be determined by correlational techniques.

Delphi Technique

A data-gathering technique that has become popular with researchers is known as the **Delphi technique**. Named after the famous Oracle of Apollo at Delphi in ancient Greece, the process attempts to predict what will be important to the surveyed group in the future. The Delphi technique consists of identifying a group of experts or persons concerned with a certain area or program. Their concerns about their area or program are elicited and ranked. Once a total list of concerns has been acquired, it is given to the experts, who are asked to rank the items on the list in order of importance. The responses are again tallied by the researcher and sent back to the same panel, with response totals given. The panel members are then asked to rerank their responses on the basis of the total responses and their peers' evaluations. The researcher can then focus on those items considered the most important by the experts.

For example, a researcher could use the Delphi technique to examine nurses' concerns in a community health agency by sending the following questions to all, or a sample, of the staff nurses:

> We are attempting to determine the future goals for patient care in a community setting. Please list at least five of your major concerns about nursing service as it is currently practiced in a community setting.

Each of the respondents then has an opportunity to express concerns and predictions about the future of nursing care in the community. After the first round of responses is returned, the researcher lists each comment—with similar comments organized into a single topic—and a questionnaire is developed. The same respondents are used in all rounds of questioning, so a letter like the following might be sent to the initial respondents:

> Several weeks ago you were asked to list your major concerns about the patient care in your community. As a result of your responses and those of your peers, we have been able to develop the following list of concerns. We would now like you to rate these concerns on a scale of 1 to 5, with 1 being of little importance and 5 being of great importance.
>   1. Patient loads are too large for adequate care to be given. 1 2 3 4 5
>   2. Patients are unable to get additional care from other community agencies. 1 2 3 4 5

After the subjects respond to this questionnaire, the researcher then calculates how each response was evaluated by determining the percentages of the total responses in each category. For instance, the group sampled on the question concerning patient loads might have responded 60% 5's, 20% 4's, and 20% 3's. Another survey is then sent to the respondents with a letter that might read like this:

> You and your colleagues have responded to a series of questions concerning nursing care in your community. Each of you was asked to rank a list of questions as to their importance. Based on your responses, the questions were rated by the percentages in the categories which you see below. Please rate the questions as to their importance again, based on your own beliefs and your knowledge of your peers' responses.

At this point, the subjects may also be supplied with their own previous responses. The subjects then respond and rate the questions as to their relative importance. The researcher re-evaluates the scale and determines which items are now considered the most important by the respondents. The researcher then identifies the main areas of concern and makes recommendations.

The Delphi technique has the advantage of identifying the major concerns and recommendations of a specific group and may provide the potential for alleviating these concerns. It can also help an organization to focus on and take direction toward the future.

Goossen and associates (1997) contacted an international panel of 36 experts and used a three-round Delphi process to gain consensus on criteria that would be useful in the application of information policy and information systems in nursing.

Unobtrusive Measures

In using **unobtrusive measures** to collect data, the researcher decides what needs to be measured and then determines how to measure it without direct intervention. A time-honored way to measure the most popular exhibits in a museum would be to determine the dirtiest display cases at the end of the day; this is done on the assumption that the more people who touch or press their noses against a display case, the dirtier it will be. Over a period of time, certain exhibits would show the most consistent usage. Unobtrusive measures might be used in a study designed to measure anxiety levels of patients by observing the wear and tear on magazines placed in waiting rooms—perhaps more anxiety is exhibited in the office of a dentist than in the office of a dermatologist?

Unobtrusive measures can also be used to collect data when people are unaware that they are being studied, such as installing hidden hardware for bedroom "bugging" to study sexual behavior (Powers & Knapp, 1995). Such research raises serious ethical concerns regarding informed consent and the right to privacy.

Sociometric Techniques

Sociometric techniques can provide valuable data when a researcher is interested in determining the social interaction and leadership patterns within a group, such as the group's informal structure, who the informal leaders are, and where the power really lies. Essentially, the researcher structures a questionnaire to determine the most desirable or the most favorably perceived individuals in a group. Questions used in sociometrics might include the following:

1. Who is the best nurse on the unit?
2. Which nurses are the most effective? Name three.
3. Which three nurses do you like working with the best?

The researcher may then want to develop a sociogram to diagram the responses (Fig. 10-1), as well as a social matrix showing the responses in tabular form (Table 10-1).

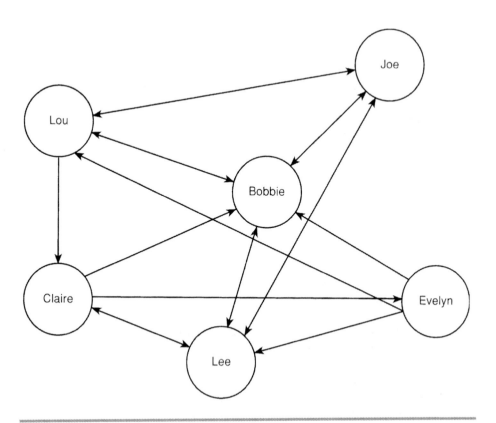

FIGURE 10-1. Sociogram.

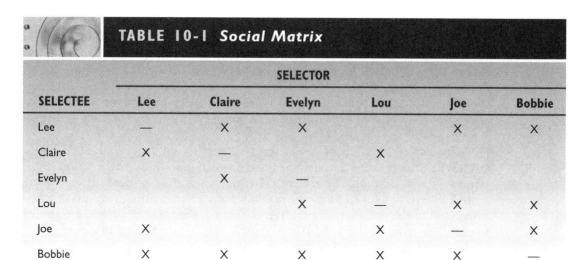

TABLE 10-1 *Social Matrix*

SELECTEE	SELECTOR					
	Lee	**Claire**	**Evelyn**	**Lou**	**Joe**	**Bobbie**
Lee	—	X	X		X	X
Claire	X	—		X		
Evelyn		X	—			
Lou			X	—	X	X
Joe	X			X	—	X
Bobbie	X	X	X	X	X	—

Ethology

Ethology is the observation and measurement of behaviors in animals. A number of researchers have used ethologic techniques to study human behaviors and interactions, often using films or videotapes to record interactions between individuals and groups of individuals. **Proxemics** is the study of body language, such as facial expressions, proximity to one another, touch, and gestures, all of which can be analyzed to determine patterns of behavior accompanying various tasks. When individuals from different cultures meet, they may have difficulty in communicating because of their backgrounds. For example, Americans often become uncomfortable when people from other countries or cultures approach and engage them in conversation. The person may be felt to be standing too close, and this makes the American nervous because his or her "body space" is being invaded. The other person is also uncomfortable and feels that the American is being standoffish. Both individuals are right.

Data collection in proxemics requires that the researcher observe and/or film or videotape situations to collect instances of the activities being analyzed. The researcher uses a pre-established data-gathering instrument, often a structured checklist, to determine the type and frequency of the activities being measured. For example, if the researcher is interested in facial expression during a conversation, data related to smiles, frowns, grimaces, or other expressions associated with the conversations would be recorded. The data are analyzed by counting the occurrences of the behaviors that the researcher is interested in.

Routasalo (1996) used proxemics to investigate "non-necessary" touching by nurses working with elderly patients in a ward in a facility in Finland. The results of the study indicated that non-necessary touching was used by the nurses in many situations in communicating with patients, but patients seldom touched the nurses unless it was necessary. The study raises cross-cultural questions for researchers: are there differences in non-necessary touching strategies used by nurses and patients from different cultural backgrounds?

Kinesics is the study of physical activity exhibited by individuals. Kinesic studies can range from the activities of the neonate to those of the wheelchair-bound elderly. Data can be collected by questionnaires or observation of the actual activities, as well as by film or videotape. For example, an investigator interested in the activities of children might ask them what games they prefer to play. The investigator could then observe the same children in informal situations to determine whether they actually did play these games. Data could be analyzed by determining what kinds and how much of various physical activities took place. (The investigator might also choose to analyze rule-determining behavior in this situation: what rules are broken? how are conflicts over rules resolved?)

Biddle and Goudas (1996) used kinesics in their study designed to determine whether schoolchildren aged 13 to 14 were influenced by encouragement from teachers and parents to participate in strenuous physical activities. Responses to their questionnaire indicated that "adult encouragement was a significant predictor of children's self-reported strenuous physical activity, as well as their intentions to be active" (p. 79).

Measuring Biological and Physiologic Responses

By its very nature, nursing research lends itself to the measurement of numerous biological and physiologic responses of research subjects. Measuring devices, ranging from the fever thermometer and sphygmomanometer to the electroencephalogram, the electrocardiogram, and magnetic resonance imaging can all be used to collect useful research data. Blood chemistries, microbiological samples, and tissue samples may also provide valuable sources of data. Clark (1997) obtained a portion of the data for her study by measuring bone-mineral density of the femoral neck and lumbar spine in a small sample of alcoholic women who were identified as either having multiple eating disorders or not having an eating disorder. She collected information by using a Lunar DPXL dual-energy densitometer that was operated by a licensed nuclear medicine technician. The results of her study indicated that women with eating disorders had a significantly greater median bone-mineral density than those without eating disorders. As in all research dealing with human subjects, researchers have the ethical responsibility to explain the purpose of any measurement device that is used and to obtain the informed consent of the subjects.

Psychological and Projective Tests

Psychological and projective tests may be used when a researcher is conducting an investigation to determine more than the subject's surface attitudes. Perhaps the intent is to understand why a subject feels the way he or she does. Because it is obviously not possible to read a person's mind, inferential instruments must be used to collect this type of data. Consistency of responses can indicate a frame of reference, a mindset, or a set of ideas. There are a number of psychological pencil-and-paper tests that require the subjects to agree or disagree at varying levels with a statement. Instruments such as the Minnesota Multiphasic Personality Inventory (MMPI) are quite long and lend themselves to numeric analysis and interpretation.

Other techniques, termed **projective tests**, require that the subject project a meaning into materials that are essentially ambiguous or meaningless. For example, in the Rorschach (ink blot) test, the individual is asked to look at a standard series of abstract forms (ink blots) and tell what he or she sees. Because the forms are random in shape, the subject must project—that is, put meaning into them from his or her own beliefs or ideas. By presenting a series of these items, the researcher can draw conclusions about the subject's state of mind. Another projective test, the Thematic Apperception Test (TAT), may also be used to determine feelings and ideas. In this test, subjects are shown pictures of people in ambiguous situations and are asked to describe what is happening. The subject must project his or her own feelings into the situation, allowing the researcher to draw conclusions about the individual. The self-portrait method is a projective technique in which subjects are asked to draw a self-portrait. This self-portrait gives the researcher important data as to how the subjects feel about themselves and what their self-image is like. Glaister (1996) used the self-portrait method to monitor the impact of therapy on adult survivors of childhood sexual abuse. She found that as therapy progressed, the self-portraits demonstrated a growth in self-confidence. She concluded that this technique gives nurses a way to practice therapeutic interventions in a holistic and caring way.

Although psychological and projective tests can be very useful in collecting research data, their results must be interpreted extremely cautiously because the very nature of these tests can lead to misinterpretation of the results. It is critical that a researcher either have special training to use these tests or rely on those who do have this specialized training.

● *CRITIQUING THE DATA-COLLECTION COMPONENT OF A QUANTITATIVE REPORT*

Data-collection instruments should be appropriate for the design of the study. The rationale for selecting each instrument should be discussed. Each instrument should be described as to purpose, content, and strengths and weak-

---

BOX 10-1

GUIDELINES FOR EVALUATING THE DATA-COLLECTION SECTION OF A QUANTITATIVE REPORT

Data-Collection Instruments
1. Instruments are appropriate for the study design.
2. The rationale for selecting each instrument is discussed.
3. Each instrument is described as to purpose, content, strengths, and weaknesses.
4. Instrument validity is described in terms of type and coefficients (if appropriate).
5. Instrument reliability is described in terms of type and size of reliability coefficients (if appropriate).
6. If the instrument was developed for the study:
   a. Rationale for development is discussed.
   b. Procedures in development are described.
   c. Validity and reliability are addressed.
   d. A pretest is discussed, if appropriate.

Data-Collection Procedures
1. Steps in the data-collection procedure(s) are clearly described.
2. The data-collection procedure(s) is appropriate for the study.

---

nesses. Validity should be discussed in terms of type and coefficients, if appropriate. Reliability should be discussed in terms of type and size of reliability coefficients, if appropriate. If instruments were developed for the study, the rationale for development, procedures used in development, and validity and reliability should be described. If a pretest was conducted, the process should be discussed. Steps in the data-collection procedure should be clearly described and should be appropriate for the study. The order in which data-collection instruments and data-collection procedures are reported varies with the author. Note that in the experimental study in Appendix C, the data-collection procedures are described before the data-collection instruments; in the study in Appendix D, the author describes the instruments and then describes the procedures. Box 10-1 lists these points as evaluation guidelines.

● SUMMARY

The essential characteristics of quantitative data-gathering instruments that must be examined by researchers and critical reviewers alike are validity, reliability, and usability. Validity is the ability of an instrument to measure what it is supposed to measure. Validity may be established in a variety of ways, including content validity, construct validity, and criterion-related validity, depending on the nature of the instrument. The reliability of a measuring instrument is the ability of the instrument to obtain consistent results when reused. Reliability is established numerically as a coefficient of reliability by using either alternate forms reliability, split-half reliability, test-retest reliability, or interrater reliability. The usability of a data-gathering instrument means that it is practical in terms of time, energy, financial, and other such considerations. Quantitative data-gathering instruments and methods include, but are not limited to, surveys or self-reports, such as questionnaires, interviews, and rating scales; unobtrusive measures; sociometrics; the Delphi technique; observation; ethologic studies, including proxemics and kinesics; and psychological and projective tests. Evaluating the data-collection component of a research report was also discussed.

The following application activities will help you to apply this material and will assist you in developing your skills in evaluating the data-collection component of published research reports.

REFERENCES

Biddle, S., & Goudas, M. (1996). Analysis of children's physical activity and its association with adult encouragement and social cognitive variables. *Journal of School Health, 66*(2), 75–79.

Clark, K. (1997). Disordered eating behaviors and bone-mineral density in women who misuse alcohol. *Western Journal of Nursing Research, 19*(1), 32–35.

Glaister, J. A. (1996). Serial self-portraits: A technique to monitor changes in self concept. *Archives of Psychiatric Nursing, 10*(5), 311–318.

Goossen, W. T. F., Epping, P. J. M. M., & Dassen, T. (1997). Criteria for nursing information systems as a component of the electronic patient record: An international Delphi study. *Computers in Nursing, 15*(6), 307–315.

Powers, B. A., & Knapp, T. R. (1995). *A dictionary of nursing theory and research* (2nd ed.). Thousand Oaks, CA: Sage.

Routasalo, P. (1996). Non-necessary touch in the nursing care of elderly people. *Journal of Advanced Nursing, 23*(5), 904–911.

Walker, J., & Sofaer, B. (1998). Predictors of psychological distress in chronic pain patients. *Journal of Advanced Nursing, 27*, 320–326.

BIBLIOGRAPHY AND SUGGESTED READINGS

Crisp, J., Pelletier, D., Duffield, C., Adams, A., & Nagy, S. (1997). The Delphi method? *Nursing Research, 46*(2), 116–118.

Osgood, C. E., Succi, G., & Tannenbaum, P. H. (1957). *The structure of inquiry*. Urbana: University of Illinois Press.

Poyatos, F. (Ed.). (1988). *Cross cultural perspectives in nonverbal communication*. Toronto: Hogrefe.

Webb, E., Campbell, D. T., Schwartz, R. D., Sechrest, L., & Grove, R. (1981). *Unobtrusive measures: Nonreactive research in the social sciences* (2nd ed.). Boston: Houghton Mifflin.

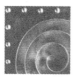

APPLICATION ACTIVITIES

1. Distinguish between the meaning of validity and reliability as attributes of quantitative data-collection instruments.

2. Look at the research report in Appendix D and note that the author used various approaches for establishing the validity of the instruments used to collect the data for the study. List each of these approaches and define the meaning of each.

3. Discuss the approaches for estimating reliability used by the author in the same study (Appendix D).

4. Why it is important for the researcher to evaluate the usability of a quantitative measuring instrument? List three considerations for evaluating usability.

5. Select a nursing journal that publishes research studies. List the techniques for gathering data used by the researchers in at least three issues of the same journal. Be sure to record the title of the article, the author, and the journal. Was any one technique used more frequently than others?

6. Complete one of the following options:

   a. Use the guidelines for evaluating quantitative data collection in Box 10-1 or the guidelines in Appendix G to evaluate the data-collection component of each of the quantitative studies you have chosen to critique.

   b. Use the above guidelines to evaluate the data-collection component for each of the reports in Appendices C and D.

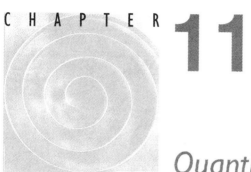

CHAPTER 11

Quantitative Data Analysis

OBJECTIVES *On completion of this chapter, the student will be able to:*

1. Describe four levels of measurement.
2. Distinguish between descriptive and inferential statistics.
3. Distinguish between parametric and nonparametric statistics.
4. Describe the function of correlations.
5. Define key terms.
6. Read and interpret statistical tables.
7. Use evaluation guidelines to critique the data-analysis component of published research reports.

KEY TERMS
Chi-squared
Descriptive statistics
Inferential statistics
Interval data
Mean
Median
Mode
Nominal data
Nonparametric statistics
Ordinal data
p

Parametric statistics
Pearson *r*
Percentile rank
Range
Ratio data
Standard score
Standard deviation
t test
type I error
type II error

*T*he purpose of this chapter is to present some very basic information about different methods of analyzing quantitative data and reporting these results in research studies. Critical evaluation of the data-analysis component of a published research report is also discussed.

QUANTITATIVE DATA ANALYSIS

It is highly significant that statistical analysis in nursing traces its roots to Florence Nightingale. Although Nightingale lacked the sophisticated techniques available to the nurse researcher today, she did use and publish descriptive statistical analyses using graphs and charts depicting the mortality rates of soldiers during the Crimean War. "Thanks to Nightingale's 1,000-page report, filled with horrifying detail, the Crimean War marked a turning point in military medicine. Nightingale's obsession with statistics started with botany" (Burke, 1997, p. 123).

THE USE OF STATISTICS IN DATA ANALYSIS

Statistics are ways of measuring things or groups of things. Any time opinions are measured, average miles per gallon are computed, or the odds in a card game are determined, statistics are being used. Basically, there are two kinds of statistics: descriptive and inferential. **Descriptive statistics** simply describe the population with which the researcher is concerned. **Inferential statistics** allow conclusions to be drawn about a population based on a sample or samples, and allow future happenings to be predicted. Although both quantitative and qualitative researchers may use a variety of statistical techniques to analyze their data, quantitative researchers tend to use more complex statistical analyses than qualitative researchers.

DESCRIPTIVE STATISTICS

Essentially, descriptive statistics describe. This type of statistical analysis is the simple reporting of facts and collective occurrences based on a number of samples. Sometimes the easiest way to describe a set of data is to draw a picture or pictures of the information. For example, suppose a researcher had the following set of scores on a test: 7, 6, 8, 9, 10, 9, 7, 11, 11, 9, 9, 9, 10, 8, 8. It is very hard to make any sense out of such data. But if the researcher organized the data by making a histogram (graph), the results are much clearer (Fig. 11-1). Another way to organize these data would be to make a bar graph (Fig. 11-2). This type of representation clearly shows the number of scores at each level of scoring. A third way to show these data would be by the use of a frequency polygon. In this instance, the midpoints on the bar graph are connected and the bars are eliminated (Fig. 11-3). The corners of a frequency polygon can be smoothed out so that a figure resembling a normal curve can be produced (Figure 11-4).

Descriptive statistics are concerned with several types of measures: centrality or central tendency; dispersion; and location or position within the

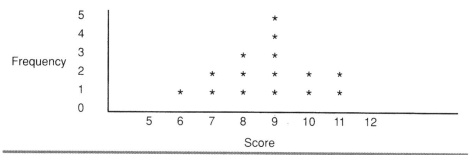

FIGURE 11-1. Histogram.

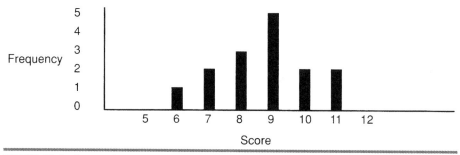

FIGURE 11-2. Bar graph.

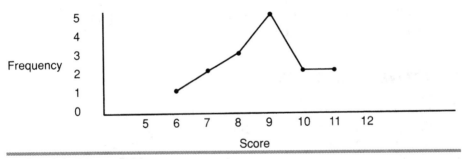

FIGURE 11-3. Frequency polygon.

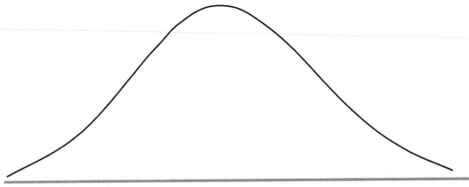

FIGURE 11-4. Normal curve.

sample or the population. In measuring any large population, the researcher finds that the characteristics of the members of the population distribute themselves across what is known as the normal curve.

Measures Of Central Tendency

THE MEAN

The **mean** may be thought of as the average. Most of the population clusters about the high point or the center of the curve. If the curve is perfectly symmetrical, the center of the normal curve is called the mean. Statistically, the mean of a population is shown by the symbol $\bar{X}$. The mean of a sample is shown by the symbol $\bar{x}$. For example, let us assume there are seven scores on a simple test: 5, 4, 3, 2, 6, 7, and 8. By adding these scores and then dividing the sum by the total number of tests, 5 is the mean, or average. Of course, means often describe essentially mythical characteristics. No one owns 1.3 cars or 2.2 television sets, or has 2.5 children. The mean gives some idea of what a total population may be like, but it is not a measure that can be completely trusted. For example, suppose there are seven more scores from a test: 6, 7, 8, 5, 4, 10, and 23. The mean of these seven scores is now

9, but only two scores are above 9. Thus, this average implies something that does not accurately reflect what happened with the test scores; the curve is distorted.

THE MEDIAN

The **median** is the number that divides the sample in half, so that 50% of the sample falls above the median and 50% falls below. In our first example of seven scores, the median is 5, the same as the mean. In the second example, however, the mean is 9, but the median is 7. In this particular instance, 7 is probably more descriptive of the data.

THE MODE

The **mode** is the most frequently occurring score. This statistic tells where scores tend to cluster. For example, consider these numbers: 4, 5, 6, 6, 6, 7, and 8. The most frequently occurring score or number is 6; consequently, the mode is 6. In this example the mean and the median also happen to be 6.

Figure 11-5 shows the mean, median, and mode graphically.

It is fairly unusual and inadvisable to use descriptive statistics exclusively with small samples because using such techniques distorts the data analysis.

Means, medians, and modes are used to describe central tendency. They give an idea of how alike members of a population are. Sometimes, however, the researcher wants to know how a population is actually distributed over the curve. This requires the use of measures of dispersion.

Measures of Dispersion

THE RANGE

The **range** is the difference between the lowest and the highest scores on an instrument. For example, in the following series of scores—4, 5, 6, 6, 6, 7, 8—the range is 4. However, ranges measure extremes, so the next set of scores—6, 7, 8, 5, 4, 10, 23—shows a range of 17.

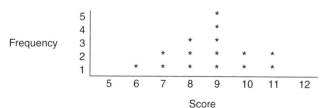

FIGURE 11-5. Mean, median, and mode shown graphically.

The mean equals 8.13
The mode is 9
The median is 9

PERCENTILE RANK

The **percentile rank** is the point below which a percentage of scores occurs. In percentile rank, the median is always the 50th percentile. A person scoring at the 60th percentile on a test is above 60% of the other test-takers and below the other 40%. Other percentage-based statistics commonly found in the literature are the decile (10%) and the quartile (25%).

STANDARD DEVIATION

The **standard deviation** is the general indicator of the dispersion or spread of scores from the mean. On all normal curves, certain proportions of the sample cluster around the mean. The standard deviation measures how widely distributed the scores are. When a curve is normal, about 68% of the population will be within one standard deviation, plus or minus, of the mean. The "average" characteristics of a population are discussed when the mean is reported, but usually this 68% (34% above the mean and 34% below the mean) is considered to be within the normal or average range. Ninety-five percent of the population will be within two standard deviations from the mean, and 99.7% will be within three standard deviations (Fig. 11-6).

The important idea is not the percentages of the population that are contained under any portion of a curve but, rather, the shape of the curve. There is one standard (imaginary) bell-shaped curve that has been used to illustrate the statistical curve. Curves can take many shapes, some with a narrow range and others with a wide range between standard deviations (Fig. 11-7).

If a test is given and the standard deviation is found to be 2 and the mean 16, this means that 68% of the population will fall between the scores of 14 and 18 on the normal curve. If the standard deviation of the same test is 4, the curve will assume a different shape; if the standard deviation is 8, still another shape will result. Consequently, a researcher can always describe the shape of

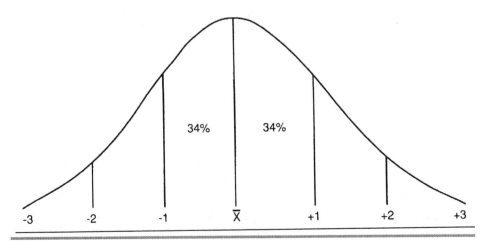

FIGURE 11-6. Normal curve showing standard deviation.

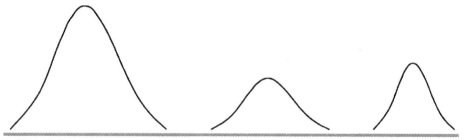

FIGURE 11-7. Three normal curves.

the curve on the basis of the standard deviation. This can also give some idea of the range of scores and a better feeling for an average individual. The most frequently used measure of dispersion is the standard deviation.

The standard deviation is sometimes described as the square root of the variance. The variance is used in analysis of variance techniques, which will be discussed in the next section.

STANDARD SCORES

A **standard score**, reported as a z, Z, or T, is used to indicate the distance a score is from the mean. Standard scores can be computed and compared to determine whether the differences between groups is significant. The researcher who carried out the study in Appendix D compared the standard scores of boys and girls on pain quality, general fears, medical fears, and temperamental intensity. She found that there was no significant difference in medical fears between boys and girls, but the other variables did differ significantly.

Reading Descriptive Tables

Many research reports include one or more tables to help the reader interpret the data presented. It is the author's task to present and interpret the basic information shown in a table in the text of the article. Frequently, not all of the information in a table is interpreted by the author, and it is up to the reader to interpret the rest of the information presented in a table. To that end, this section is designed to help you interpret descriptive statistical tables presented in the text of research reports.

Consider Table 11-1, which uses descriptive statistics. There are several bits of information contained in this table. First, it is labeled as Table 11-1. This means that the author will discuss the information it contains when referring to Table 11-1 (for example, "Table 11-1 contains . . ."). Second, this table has a heading or title, "Characteristics of Fictitious Group." This tells what the table is about. Third, there are a number of headings to read from left to right. These include the age range, which tells the ages of the individuals studied; number (n), which tells the number of individuals in each age

		TABLE 11-1 *Characteristics of Fictitious Group*	
AGE RANGE	**NUMBER (N)**	**MEAN ($\bar{X}$)**	**STANDARD DEVIATION (SD)** σ
20–29	47	25	1.8
30–39	43	36	2.1
40–49	41	44	2.5

range of the sample; mean (which may also be shown as $\bar{x}$); and standard deviation (which may be written as SD for a portion of the population or σ for the entire population).

In reading this table, we find that in the age group ranging from 30 to 39, the researcher had 43 individuals in the sample; their mean (average) age was 36; and most of this group (68%) fell between the ages of 33.9 and 38.1 (36 ± 2.1 [1 SD] = 33.9 − 38.1). This descriptive table might have included other information, such as median and modal ages for each age range. Additional tables could include percentages, percentile ranks, or other descriptive information that the author believes might be useful to the reader.

● INFERENTIAL STATISTICS

Descriptive statistics give us a quantitative way of viewing the world. They enable a researcher to describe certain factual aspects of a population. Most researchers, however, are concerned with other kinds of judgments as well. This leads to the use of inferential statistics. Inferential statistics do not examine a whole population. Rather, as described in Chapter 6, a sample (or samples) is drawn from the population, and the characteristics of the population are deduced or inferred from the responses of this sample or samples.

In addition to this type of inference, the quantitative researcher uses inferential statistics to test hypotheses and to determine whether certain experimental treatments or techniques are better, worse, or not significantly different from other types of treatments or techniques. Hypothesis testing is based on probability. When reading research, the statement "$H_0 = p < 0.05$" often occurs. (Remember that H_0 is called the null hypothesis, as discussed in Chap. 5.) Here, $p < 0.05$ is called the level of significance or level of confidence—that is, the researcher states that the results of the experimental treatment will probably not be significantly different from the standard or common treatment. Most researchers really want to reject the null hypothesis, but research convention has cast this as the most common type of research hypothesis. The symbol p stands for probability. The probability in the statement $p < 0.05$ means that there will be no conclusion of a significant difference between treatments unless 5 or fewer treatments out of 100 have the same result as the original or standard treatment. Probability is determined by computing the appropriate statistic and then reading the statistical table that gives the probability for that statistic.

When a level of significance is selected, the experimenter is telling the world that chance has little to do with the results of the experiment. Medically related experiments may set extremely high levels of significance; usually, one chance in a thousand or less ($p < 0.001$). In cases of life and death, the chance of error must be diminished as much as possible.

Levels of Measurement

When dealing with inferential statistics, a researcher must be concerned with what are called levels of measurement. Often, the researcher works with data represented by responses to questions that can be posed in various ways.

THE NOMINAL DATA SCALE

A **nominal data** scale deals only with data that can be separated into mutually exclusive categories. There are no qualifiers. For example, it is possible to classify all people in the world as having either light-colored eyes or dark-colored eyes. If this is done, anyone whose eyes are considered to be blue, green, brown, or black must be placed in the category light or dark. Nominal scales deal only with exclusive categories and do not attempt to find gradations between them. The categories are absolute, and the mode is the only measure of central tendency (Fig. 11-8).

In nursing research, the nominal scale might be used to determine whether pregnancies and abortions occur statistically more frequently in one of two socially different groups of women. This can be done by simply identifying members of one group or the other and asking each subject whether she has ever had an abortion. The responses of each group could then be tallied and analyzed statistically to determine whether there was a significant difference in the frequency of abortion between the two groups.

THE ORDINAL DATA SCALE

An **ordinal data** scale measures data that are ordered but for which there is no zero starting point, and the intervals between each individual datum are not equal. Subjects are asked to rank ideas, items, or other things. The subject can respond that item A is more or less than items B or C but cannot tell exactly how much more or less. For example, a patient may experience more or less discomfort, depending on certain postures or other physical phenom-

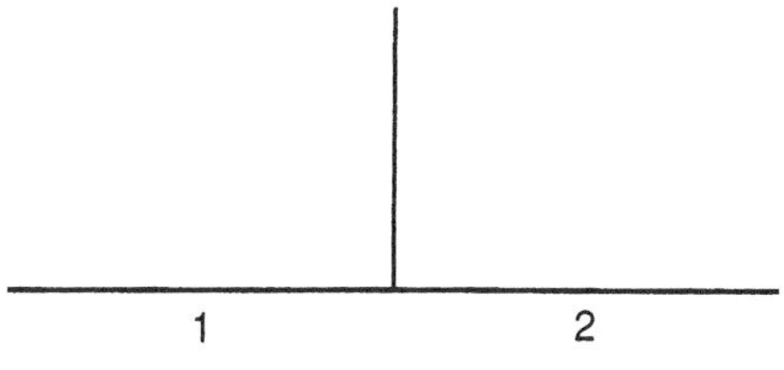

FIGURE 11-8. Nominal scale.

ena that can be adjusted. The amount cannot be quantified by saying, "I am twice as uncomfortable," but the feeling of more or less comfort can be experienced (Fig. 11-9).

THE INTERVAL DATA SCALE

An **interval data** scale has equal intervals, but there is no absolute zero starting point on an interval scale. Because temperatures can be measured in either Fahrenheit or Celsius, and neither of these scales has an absolute zero (that is, no temperature at all), a clinical thermometer is an example of an interval-measuring instrument. The interval scale is the most commonly used level of statistical measurement. Although many ordinal data are treated like interval data in the performance of statistical analysis, there is continuing philosophical debate in statistical circles as to whether this type of analysis provides valid conclusions (Fig. 11-10).

THE RATIO DATA SCALE

A **ratio data** scale has equal intervals and an absolute zero starting point (Fig. 11-11). All subjects start at zero and travel or respond in some manner along this same scale. Length, weight, and volume are examples of ratio measurements because they start with an absolute zero (no length, no weight, or no volume).

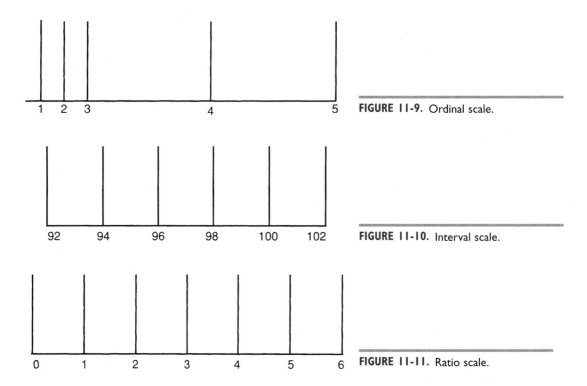

FIGURE 11-9. Ordinal scale.

FIGURE 11-10. Interval scale.

FIGURE 11-11. Ratio scale.

COMMONLY USED INFERENTIAL STATISTICAL TESTS

Regardless of the level of data used, the researcher must answer the question, "Are the differences I see caused by chance, or are other factors responsible, such as my treatment?" For example, when a researcher sees that two different groups have different means, the next task is to test the differences between the means to determine whether they are significantly different statistically. Based on the level of data, the researcher selects the statistical test that is the most appropriate to determine whether chance is the overriding factor.

The terms parametric statistics and nonparametric statistics are associated with level of measurement of the data to be analyzed. Each of these terms refers to a different group of inferential statistical techniques. Parametric statistical techniques are intended to be used with interval and ratio data; nonparametric statistical techniques are intended to be used with nominal and ordinal data.

Parametric Statistical Tests

The term **parametric statistics** is used to describe inferential statistics that assume a normal distribution of the variables and the use of interval or ratio measures. The most frequently used parametric tests include t tests, analysis of variance, and analysis of covariance.

t TESTS

To determine whether the differences between the means of two different sets of scores are statistically significant, the researcher can use the *t* **test**, a parametric statistical measure to determine the differences between the means of two groups. The researcher first determines whether the two samples are independent (such as in the case of an experimental and a control group) or dependent (using the same group of individuals and their responses before and after a treatment). This must be done because there are several ways to compute the t statistic. If an inappropriate method is used, the researcher might obtain incorrect results in either accepting or rejecting the hypothesis.

For example, consider Table 11-2 (this is for illustrative purposes only; there has been no attempt to calculate t scores). This table shows that on part A of a fictitious test, the probability of achieving this difference is less than 0.05, or $p < 0.05$. If the investigator sets a level of confidence at $p < 0.05$, then the differences in the scores between test 1 and test 2 are considered significant. The differences between the mean scores on part B of test 1 and part B of test 2 is -14. There are many reasons for negative numbers to occur in research design, and confidence levels can be assigned directionally—that is, the hypothesis indicates that there will be an increase or decrease in what is being tested, or the investigator may simply state that the difference is signif-

TABLE 11-2 *Paired t Test Results on Fictitious Test*					
VARIABLES	**N**	**TEST 1**	**TEST 2**	**MEAN DIFFERENCE**	**P VALUE**
part A	31	25	30	+5	0.04*
part B	31	41	27	−14	0.001*
part C	31	56	57	+1	0.37

*$p < 0.05$ level

icant regardless of whether the results show a positive or negative probability. An asterisk (*) shows that the result is significant. Part C shows that there is no significant difference between the two tests at the 0.05 level of confidence.

An example of the use of the *t* test statistic can be found in the study done by Sliwa (1997), in which the researcher used the paired *t* test to determine whether there was a significant difference between the mean hematocrit values of blood drawn through a saline lock device and blood drawn by traditional venipuncture. The investigator found that there was no significant difference in the hematocrit values of blood drawn by either method. This led to the conclusion that patients would be exposed to less pain and staff would have less difficulty in locating venipuncture sites if blood were drawn routinely through a saline lock. This study is also an example of establishing a probability level (in this case, $p < 0.05$) that the researcher hopes will not be met.

ANALYSIS OF VARIANCE

Sometimes the researcher has more than two means to test to determine whether there are significant differences between them. In this instance, using the *t* test statistic could be exceedingly tedious because of the number of possible permutations of the *t* test. Also, the more individual *t* tests conducted, the greater the possibility of what is called a **type I error** or a **type II error** (Table 11-3).

TABLE 11-3 *Type I and Type II Errors*		
DECISION	**IF STATEMENT OF THE H_0 IS REALLY TRUE**	**IF STATEMENT OF THE H_0 IS REALLY FALSE**
Accept H_0	Correct decision	Type II (Beta)
Reject H_0	Type I (Alpha)	Correct decision

TABLE 11-4 *Univariate Analysis of Three Dependent Variables by HIV Status Interaction Over Time*

VARIABLE	F	P
Stress	.197	.658
Coping	3.276	.075
Social support	10.391	.002*

Note: Univariate F test with (1, 66) df.
*$p < 0.05$

A type I error, also called the alpha error, means that the investigator has rejected the null hypothesis when it should be accepted. A **type II error**, also called the beta error, occurs when the investigator accepts the null hypothesis when it should be rejected.

Consequently, the statistical analysis of variance (ANOVA) is often used. With this technique, it is possible to determine whether there is a significant difference between several means simultaneously. The literature will report these differences as the F test, the F ratio, or the F statistic.

Also, when many means have been tested, the researcher will want to know exactly which means were significantly different from the other means. There are other methods, such as Sheffe's test or the Tukey HSD test, that can be applied to determine which means were significantly different from the other means.

Table 11-4 has been modified from the original table in the research report in Appendix C. When examining tables such as this, the critical reviewer needs to concentrate on the asterisks. These indicate footnotes that tell which findings are significant, and the level of significance (in this case, $p < 0.05$). The term *df* stands for degrees of freedom. Degrees of freedom are used when calculating many statistics and refer to the number of values in a set that are free to vary.

Sometimes additional information concerning sums of squares and mean squares is presented in an ANOVA table (Table 11-5) (this is a fictitious table;

TABLE 11-5 *Fictitious Table of Nursing Students' Test Scores Comparing Three Different Methods of Instruction*

SOURCE OF VARIATION	DEGREES OF FREEDOM	SUM OF SQUARES	MEAN SQUARE	F RATIO
Between groups	2	24.38	12.19	11.5*
Within groups	42	987.44		

*$p < 0.05$

no effort was made to calculate F ratios). Sometimes such tables also include other footnotes that contain additional explanations of the findings and the meanings of various abbreviations used in the table. The researcher should discuss the important parts of the findings in the text but probably would not include all of the detail shown in the table.

The use of ANOVA can be found in a study conducted by Gaffney and associates (1997) of pregnant Salvadoran women in the United States. The researchers compared stressful events occurring in the lives of women from three cultural groups, Salvadoran-Hispanic, non–Salvadoran-Hispanic, and non-Hispanic. By using ANOVA and the Tukey B test to identify specific group differences, the investigators found that Salvadoran women had significantly different kinds of life stress when compared to non-Salvadoran and non-Hispanic women.

ANOVA may be applied when there is more than one dependent variable to be examined. Statisticians call this multiple analysis of variance or multi-variate analysis of variance (MANOVA). MANOVA was used by the researchers whose report is found in Appendix C. This type of statistical analysis can become quite complex. The researcher reports the results of MANOVA using the F statistic, just like the researcher using ANOVA. The tables used by researchers reporting MANOVA are similar to those using ANOVA.

Gwele (1996) used MANOVA to examine how the imposition of curriculum reform on schools of nursing by legislative edict affected nurse educators in four institutions in South Africa. Using the Concerns-Based Adoption Model, the investigator examined the nurse educators' concerns about the new curriculum by testing six hypotheses that compared inexperienced users and "old hands" in determining differences in their levels of concern in reacting to the government's mandate for change. Gwele found that coercing staff to adopt change impedes the development of staff concerns, which may affect student learning. Gwele concluded that "legislated change is not the best means for facilitating adoption and implementation" (p. 614).

ANALYSIS OF COVARIANCE

Frequently, because of the nature of the research setting, it is impossible for a researcher to place subjects into truly randomly assigned groups. In this case, there may be variables that confound the variable under consideration. This means that the researcher's data may or may not show significant differences unless the confounding variable(s) is accounted for.

To account for the confounding variable(s), the researcher may use analysis of covariance (ANCOVA), which is also reported as an F statistic or F ratio. This procedure may also be used in place of the *t* statistic when two groups are involved and there is no way to achieve the requirements of randomness necessary for appropriate use of the *t* statistic. ANCOVA may also be used on more than two sets of subjects or when there is more than one dependent variable. The tables used by the researcher reporting ANCOVA are similar to those used to report ANOVA.

An example of the use of ANCOVA can be found in the 1997 study by Kerr and associates about the effect of short-duration hyperventilation during endotracheal suction on intracranial pressure in adults with severe head injury. The researchers compared the level of intracranial pressure resulting from severe head injuries in adults during endotracheal suctioning after providing short-term hyperventilation before the suctioning process. They found that there was a significant difference in the level of intracranial pressure and that short-duration hyperventilation helped to reduce intracranial pressure.

Examples of multiple analysis of covariance (MANCOVA) may also be found in the literature. For more information on this subject, discuss it with your instructor or find information in a statistics text.

Nonparametric Statistical Tests

The term **nonparametric statistics** is used to describe inferential statistics that do not require the same rigorous assumptions as parametric statistics. Nonparametric statistics are most often used when samples are small and/or when the data are measured on the nominal or ordinal scales.

Because there are literally dozens of nonparametric statistical tests available, only a few of the more commonly used will be discussed: chi-squared, Mann-Whitney U, Kruskal-Wallis one-way ANOVA, and Friedman two-way ANOVA.

CHI-SQUARED

Perhaps the most commonly used nonparametric statistic is the chi-squared (X^2; also called chi-square) measure. This statistic can be applied to nominal or higher levels of measurement and can be used in one or more samples. Essentially, the chi-squared test is used to determine whether the observed frequencies of events in certain categories fall within the range of frequencies expected to fall in these categories.

Chi-squared tables contain information similar to parametric statistics tables. Table 11-6 is a fictitious table meant to demonstrate the information commonly found in a chi-squared table (this table is for illustrative purposes only; there has been no attempt to calculate X^2 scores). This table shows the color preferences of a fictitious group of 84 nursing students. The numbers listed in the rows and columns shows the selection and the totals by groups. By comparing the actual numbers of color selection with the expected numbers of color selection (this is done mathematically), the chi-squared statistic is computed. Degrees of freedom (df) are also computed, and a chi-squared table is read to determine the level of significance. In this instance, $p > 0.05$ means that the differences between male and female nursing students' preference in colors is not statistically significant at the 0.05 level.

Brown (1997) used the chi-squared statistic to analyze differences between individuals complaining of chest pain and presenting in an emergency facility over a period of 6 months. The researcher found that there were statistically significant differences in the use of different kinds of licit and illicit drugs, including cocaine, and in complaints concerning cardiac and noncardiac chest pain.

TABLE 11-6 Fictitious Table of Preference of Colors Between Male and Female Nursing Students			
	YELLOW	BLUE	GREEN	TOTAL
Male	10	20	15	35
Female	12	24	13	49
Total	22	44	28	84

$X^2 = 1.98$; df = 4; $p > 0.05$

MANN-WHITNEY U

A very powerful nonparametric alternative to the t test is the Mann-Whitney U test. By using this statistic, a researcher can determine whether or not two groups are significantly different when the scores from two sets of data are ranked.

Lamond and Farnell (1998) compared the scores of seven novice nurses to the scores of seven expert nurses who sorted 16 cards, 8 with pictures of a variety of pressure sores and 8 others showing various dressings that might be used in dressing pressure sores. The subjects were asked to sort the cards into categories so that each category had something in common that was different from the other categories they developed. They were then asked to explain their reasons for placing the cards into the categories they had developed. The explanations were audiotaped and subjected to content analysis to determine the common categories used by the subjects. The subjects were also given a brief, fictitious case history using a photograph of a pressure sore and other data related to the factors thought to affect the healing of pressure sores for three imaginary patients. Subjects were then asked to recommend treatment on the basis of this information and were asked to explain their decisions. Their responses were also audiotaped for analysis. The investigators used a judge panel of experts in wound care to establish a "gold standard" for treatment against which the subjects' responses were measured.

The expert nurses made more accurate decisions than the novice nurses; when these data were analyzed using the Mann-Whitney U test, this was statistically significant at the level of $p < 0.05$. The researchers concluded that experts organize data in different ways than novices, and additional instruction on wound care and treatment decisions might result in benefits to patients.

KRUSKAL-WALLIS ONE-WAY ANOVA

The Kruskal-Wallis statistical test allows for a one-way ANOVA with ordinal data by establishing a rank order by examining the data. The Kruskal-Wallis statistic is reported as H.

Elnitsky and associates (1997) used the Kruskal-Wallis one-way ANOVA test to determine whether there were differences of opinions among nurses in their reporting of incidents in a hospital setting. They found there was a significant difference in incident-reporting behaviors based on educational background: "nurses with the lower educational levels were less likely to agree with appropriate incident *reporting* behaviors than were nurses with higher education levels" (p. 43).

FRIEDMAN TWO-WAY ANOVA BY RANKS

Occasionally there is a need to use a nonparametric ANOVA, such as the Friedman two-way ANOVA by ranks. The researcher ranks the scores on repeated measures of subjects and then compares the ranks of these repeated measures. Scores on the Friedman test are reported as χ_r^2, and tables that report this statistic are similar to the chi-squared statistic table.

CORRELATIONS

Correlational designs allow the researcher to determine relationships between variables rather than drawing cause-and-effect conclusions, which can lead to spurious (incorrect) conclusions. Researchers who conclude that a high positive or high negative correlation is necessarily a cause-and-effect relationship have failed to interpret correlations correctly.

Pearson r

The commonly used parametric statistic for correlation is the Pearson product-moment correlation coefficient, otherwise known as the **Pearson *r***, or more simply as *r*. The Pearson *r* can be either descriptive or inferential. As a descriptive statistic, the correlation coefficient demonstrates the size and the direction of a statistical relationship. As an inferential statistic, the Pearson *r* can be used to test hypotheses about relationships between data sets within and between populations. In this test, two different sets of interval or ratio data are compared to determine the degree of relationship between them. Because *r* values range from -1 through 0 to +1, pairs of items are related either positively or negatively. As the correlation coefficient approaches -1 or +1, the items become more highly related. If the correlation coefficient approaches 0, the items have little or no relationship. The researcher can then determine whether the correlation coefficient is statistically significant by referring to the appropriate statistical table.

Table 11-7 (based on information in Appendix D) shows the correlation between pain quality and pain intensity and behavioral responses. Pearson *r* values have been computed. The number in parenthesis shows the degrees of freedom. The asterisks refer to the level of significance.

The Pearson product-moment statistic was used by Clark (1997) "to determine associations between body composition and bone-mineral density . . . between women with and without evidence of disordered eating behaviors"

(p. 38). The investigator found a "moderate positive correlation between bone-mineral density of the femoral neck and body weight" ($r = 0.51, p = 0.01$) (p. 40).

Spearman's Rho Correlation

There are many nonparametric correlation techniques. One of the most common is the Spearman's rho correlation (r_s). Researchers using this statistic rank their observations of the two variables under consideration and then determine the level of relationship between them. For example, a researcher might want to test the relationship between patients' perceived level of comfort and their perception of the quality of care provided by the nursing staff in a hospital. In this instance, the patients would be given two attitude-evaluation scales (one to measure each variable), and then the two scores would be ranked and a Spearman's rho computed.

An example of the use of the Spearman's rho is the study conducted by Walker and Sofaer (1998) in their attempt to identify sources of psychological distress in patients attending pain clinics. Among other statistical measures, the investigators used the Spearman's rho to correlate ordinal scores between five measures of pain and six measures of psychological distress. The data analyses demonstrated that all the measures of psychological distress, except age, had statistically significant relationships with the measures of pain at the 0.01 level or below. The researchers concluded that the findings of this study might be used in developing an easily used nursing assessment instrument that might be used to improve the psychological well-being of patients with chronic pain.

Partial and Multiple Correlation

Occasionally, the researcher needs to analyze a number of variables that might be interrelated. In this instance, partial correlations can be computed. The intent of this method is to eliminate the confounding effects of one or more variables when measuring the relationships between a number of variables. This is shown as $r_{1,2:3}$ where variables 1 and 2 are correlated and variable 3 is eliminated mathematically. Conversely, if a researcher wants to combine the variables, this can be done by a technique called multiple correlation (symbolized by the letter R).

TABLE 11-7 *Pearson Product-Moment Correlation*		
	PAIN INTENSITY	**BEHAVIORAL RESPONSES**
Pain quality	$r(94) = 0.59^{**}$	$r(93) = 0.41^{**}$

$^{**}p < 0.001$

Correlations can be used for prediction by using a technique called regression analysis. This technique allows the researcher to predict the score an individual will make on a third assessment by correlating the scores obtained by that individual on two assessments.

The researcher whose study is reprinted in Appendix D used a multiple correlation technique known as canonical correlation that measured the relationship between a set of independent variables (age, medical fears, distractibility, threshold of pain) and a set of dependent variables (pain quality, behavioral responses, magnitude of heart rate change). Although canonical correlations can be used to determine regression scores, and thus can be used as predictors, the researcher chose not to do this.

Stein and colleagues (1998) used both partial and multiple correlations to determine whether self-reported risky behaviors (sexual intercourse, tobacco use, alcohol use, and poor school performance) by students in the eighth grade predicted risky behaviors by the same students in the ninth grade. They found that risky behaviors are intercorrelated and that adolescent self-concept, especially as being socially popular, was a predictor of engagement in risky behaviors, which then "contributed to the conceptualization of the self as currently deviant and expectation that one will be deviant in the future" (p. 103). The researchers concluded that interventions to limit risky behaviors may help prevent the development and continuation of risky patterns of behavior.

Table 11-8 summarizes selected statistical tests based on levels of data.

TABLE 11-8 *Summary of Selected Statistical Tests Based on Levels of Data*			
LEVEL OF DATA	**NUMBER OF SAMPLES**	**STATISTICAL TEST**	**CORRELATIONAL STATISTIC**
Nominal level	1 or more	Chi-squared	
Ordinal level	1 or more	Chi-squared	
	2	Mann-Whitney U	Spearman's rho
	3 or more	Kruskal-Wallace one-way analysis of variance by ranks	
		Friedman two-way analysis of variance by ranks	
Interval or ratio level	2	t test (must state if samples are independent or related)	Pearson's r
		Analysis of variance	
	3 or more	Analysis of variance	
		Analysis of covariance	
		Multiple analysis of variance	
		Multiple analysis of covariance	

CRITIQUING THE DATA-ANALYSIS COMPONENT OF A QUANTITATIVE RESEARCH REPORT

The section of a research report that discusses the data-analysis procedures and results or findings of a study is usually labeled "Results." Note the reports in Appendixes C and D. The choice of statistical procedures (descriptive or inferential statistics or both) should be appropriate. Each statistical test should be correctly applied for the level of measurement of the data. Data should be analyzed in relation to the purpose of the study; if hypotheses were tested, the author should report the results. Information in tables and figures should be clearly discussed in the text, and this information should be consistent with each table or figure that is displayed. Tables and figures should be clear and well labeled and should accurately reflect reported findings. Box 11-1 lists these points as evaluation guidelines.

SUMMARY

Quantitative researchers analyze data by using a variety of descriptive statistics, including measures of central tendency (mean, median, mode) and measures of dispersion (range, percentile rank, standard deviation, and standard scores). Quantitative instruments may be at different levels of measurement that range from the nominal (the lowest), to the ordinal, to the interval, to the ratio data scale (the highest). Researchers use inferential statistics when analyzing data to determine whether there are significant differences between or

BOX 11-1	GUIDELINES FOR EVALUATING THE DATA-ANALYSIS COMPONENT OF A QUANTITATIVE REPORT

1. The choice of statistical procedures is appropriate (descriptive or inferential, or both).
2. Statistical procedures are correctly applied for the level of measurement of the data.
3. Data are analyzed in relation to the purpose of the study.
4. Each hypothesis was tested, and the results are reported accurately.
5. Tables and figures:
   a. Information in the text is consistent with each.
   b. Reflect reported findings.
   c. Are clear and well labeled.

within groups. Parametric statistics are used when the data are at the interval or ratio level. Parametric statistical analysis may include *t* tests, ANOVA, ANCOVA, and MANOVA. Nonparametric statistical tests, including the chi-squared test, the Mann-Whitney U test, the Friedman test, and the Kruskal-Wallis two-way ANOVA test, are used to analyze data at the nominal and ordinal level. The Pearson product-moment (*r*), a parametric test, and the Spearman rho (r_s), a nonparametric test, are correlations or measures of association that are used to determine the degree or amount of relationship that exists between two variables. Multiple and partial correlations may also be used to describe relationships. Regression statistical analysis may be used to explain or predict causal relationships between variables.

The following application activities will help you to evaluate your understanding of this material and will assist you in developing your skills in evaluating published research.

REFERENCES

Brown, S. C. (1997). Chest pain and cocaine use in 18 to 40 year-old persons: A retrospective study. *Applied Nursing Research, 10*(3), 136–142.

Burke, J. (1997). Connections. *Scientific American, 277*(5), 122–123.

Clark, K. (1997). Disordered eating behaviors and bone-mineral density in women who misuse alcohol. *Western Journal of Nursing Research, 19*(1), 32–35.

Elnitsky, C., Nichols, B., & Palmer, K. (1997). Are hospital incidents being reported? *Journal of Nursing Administration, 27*(11), 40–46.

Gaffney, K. F., Choi, E., Yi, E., Jones, G. B., Bowman, C., & Tavangar, N. N. (1997). Stressful events among pregnant Salvadoran women: A cross-cultural comparison. *Journal of Gynecological and Neonatal Nursing, 26*(3), 303–310.

Gwele, N. S. (1996). Concerns of nurse educators regarding the implementation of a major curriculum reform. *Journal of Advanced Nursing, 24,* 607–614.

Kerr, M. E., Rudy, E. B., Weber, B. B., et al. (1997). Effect of short-duration hyperventilation during endotracheal suctioning on intracranial pressure in severe head-injured adults. *Nursing Research, 46*(4), 195–201.

Lamond, D., & Farnell, S. (1998). The treatment of pressure sores: A comparison of novice and expert nurses' knowledge, information use and decision accuracy. *Journal of Advanced Nursing, 27,* 280–286.

Sliwa, C. M. Jr. (1997). A comparative study of hematocrits drawn from a standard venipuncture and those drawn from a saline lock device. *Journal of Emergency Nursing, 23*(3), 228–231.

Stein, K. F., Roeser, R., & Markus, H. R. (1998). Self-schemas and possible selves as predictors and outcomes of risky behaviors in adolescents. *Nursing Research, 47*(2), 96–106.

Walker, J., & Sofaer, B. (1998). Predictors of psychological distress in chronic pain patients. *Journal of Advanced Nursing, 27,* 320–326.

BIBLIOGRAPHY AND SUGGESTED READINGS

Elmore, P. B., & Woehlke, P. L. (1997). *Basic statistics.* Reading, MA: Longman Publishing Group.

Pett, M. A. (1997). *Nonparametric statistics for health care research: Statistics for small samples and unusual distributions.* Thousand Oaks, CA: Sage.

Siegel, S., & Castellan, N. J. Jr. (1988). *Nonparametric statistics for the behavioral sciences* (2nd ed.). New York: McGraw Hill.

Sprinthall, R. C. (1996). *Basic statistical analysis* (5th ed.). Needham Heights, MA: Allyn & Bacon.

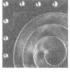

APPLICATION ACTIVITIES

1. Define the following terms:

   a. Nominal data

   b. Ordinal data

   c. Interval data

   d. Ratio data

   e. Mean

   f. Median

   g. Mode

   h. Percentile rank

2. How does standard deviation affect the shape of the bell curve?

3. Explain how inferential statistics differ from descriptive statistics.

4. Discuss when nonparametric statistics should be used to analyze data.

5. If the studies you have selected to critique are quantitative, examine the data-collection technique and determine the level of data used. If your studies are qualitative, locate two quantitative studies that use inferential statistics and determine the level of data used. Are they nominal, ordinal, interval, or ratio? If the data are ordinal, were they treated as interval?

6. Use the guidelines for evaluating the data-analysis component of a quantitative report (see Box 11-1) or the guidelines in Appendix G to critique the data-analysis section of the quantitative studies that you have selected to evaluate. If all of your studies are qualitative, find two quantitative studies that use inferential statistics and critique the data-analysis section for each of these studies.

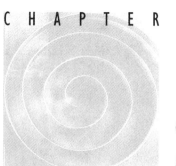

C H A P T E R 12

Communicating Research Findings

INTERPRETING THE FINDINGS,
    FORMULATING CONCLUSIONS,
    AND WRITING THE REPORT
A NOTE ON PUBLICATION
CRITIQUING THE DISCUSSION COMPONENT
    OF A RESEARCH REPORT

ADDITIONAL CONSIDERATIONS IN EVALUAT-
    ING A RESEARCH REPORT
RATING THE SCIENTIFIC MERIT OF A
    RESEARCH REPORT
SUMMARY

OBJECTIVES   *On completing this chapter, the student will be able to:*

1. Discuss the importance of careful interpretation of research findings.
2. Describe three ways of communicating research results.
3. Identify the components of a written research report.
4. Discuss the purposes for preparing an abstract of a research study.
5. Define key terms.
6. Use evaluation guidelines to critique the discussion component
    and additional features of published research reports.
7. Use guidelines to rate the scientific merit of published research reports.

KEY TERMS   Abstract   Scientific merit

Refereed journal   Serendipitous findings

*I*n previous chapters, material was presented related to the first two stages of the research process: the planning stage, during which the investigator develops a plan for the proposed research, and the implementation stage, during which the researcher puts the plan into action by collecting and analyzing the data. It is during the final stages of the research process that the investigator interprets the findings of the study, formulates conclusions, and writes the research report to communicate the findings so that others may have access to the new knowledge. The purpose of this chapter is to discuss these final steps in the research process and to present guidelines for evaluating these components and additional features of published research reports. Criteria for rating the scientific merit of published studies are also presented.

INTERPRETING THE FINDINGS, FORMULATING CONCLUSIONS, AND WRITING THE REPORT

Interpretation of data-based results is a subjective process on the part of the investigator, who must take great care not to interpret beyond what the data indicate. The findings of the study should be logically presented and interpreted in relation to the specific research question and purpose of the study. If the purpose of the study was to describe the interaction of certain variables, then meaningful descriptions are indicated. For example, if the purpose of the study was to describe the relationship between individualized breast-feeding instruction and successful breast-feeding by primiparas, the researcher should interpret the findings as a description of the nature of this relationship. If the study asked a question, the findings should be interpreted to answer this question. For example, if the purpose of the study was to answer the question, "Do primiparas who are provided with individualized breast-feeding instruction report a successful breast-feeding experience?" the researcher should relate the results of the study to this question. If a hypothesis was tested, the study findings should be interpreted as supporting (accepting) or not supporting (rejecting) the hypothesis.

For example, the investigator might have formulated a null (statistical) hypothesis (H_0) that stated: There is no significant difference at the $p < 0.05$ level in successful breast-feeding by primiparas who receive individualized breast-feeding instruction and primiparas who do not receive individualized breast-feeding instruction. If the researcher used a research hypothesis, he or she would then interpret the results of the study as either supporting or not supporting this hypothesis.

If the investigation was formulated within a specific theoretical or conceptual framework, the findings should be interpreted in relation to this framework. Note, for example, that the researcher who conducted the study that was guided by the Roy Adaptation Model (Appendix D) stated in the discussion section of her report that the results of the study provided limited support for this model.

To place the findings in the context of already existing knowledge, the researcher should discuss the study findings in relation to the review of the literature, discussing their agreement or disagreement with the findings of other relevant studies cited in the literature review.

Conclusions for the study must be supported by the data and must not go beyond the data. Any generalizations that are made must be consistent with the methodology and warranted by the findings. Conclusions must also be consistent with the analysis of the data and the interpretation of the findings of the study. The researcher should describe any limitations of the study, as well as the significance of the study for nursing practice.

Sometimes a study may have important and unexpected findings not related to the original purpose of the study. These are called **serendipitous findings.** The investigator needs to be aware of the possible existence of such findings and the importance of interpreting and reporting them.

As a final step in the research process, the investigator writes a research report to make the results available and known to others. A research report may communicate the research results to other investigators, in which case the report should communicate the purpose, procedures, findings, and recommendations in sufficient detail so that another investigator could replicate the study. In addition, consumers of nursing research need to become aware of reported research so that they may critically evaluate the findings and use them in practice. A research report should be objective, concise, and scholarly in spelling, grammar, and punctuation. A dictionary and a style manual should be used when writing the report. Authors such as Campbell and Turabian and associations such as the American Psychological Association and the Modern Language Association have developed style manuals.

Research Report Format

Researchers typically use the following format for preparing a detailed report of a research investigation. This detailed report provides the basis for writing an abridged report for publication in a journal, for oral presentations at conferences and seminars, or for participation in poster sessions.

A research report is divided into three major parts: preliminary materials, main body (text), and reference materials. Each major part consists of several sections:

    I. Preliminary materials
       A. Title page
       B. Table of contents

   C. List of illustrations (figures)
   D. List of tables
   E. Preface or acknowledgment (if any)
 II. Main body (text)
   A. Introduction
      1. Statement of the problem
      2. Review of related literature, including conceptual or theoretical framework (if appropriate)
      3. Research objectives, questions, or hypotheses
      4. Definition of terms
      5. Assumptions of the study
   B. Methodology
      1. Research approach
      2. Study subjects (participants)
      3. Techniques for data collection
      4. Procedures
   C. Findings
      1. Reporting of data and discussion of their meaning
      2. Tables and figures discussed in text, as appropriate
   D. Discussion
      1. Interpretation of findings
      2. Comparison of findings with those of other investigations
      3. Conclusions
      4. Limitations of the study
      5. Implications for nursing
      6. Recommendations for further study
   E. Summary of the study
      1. Brief restatement of problem
      2. Brief review of procedures, major conclusions, and recommendations
III. Reference materials
   A. Bibliography
   B. Appendix(es)—may include materials especially designed for the study, such as cover letters and questionnaires. Raw data from the study may also be included as an appendix.
   C. Glossary of terms (if appropriate).

Preparing an Abstract of the Study

An **abstract** is a concise summary of the study. Usually limited to 200 to 250 words, the abstract communicates the essential information about the study:

> A good abstract communicates the essential ideas in the work. It covers all the key points, is precise and accurate, logical and to the point. It is clearly and concisely written, and interesting. *(Brazier, 1997, p. 3)*

Researchers write abstracts for several purposes. When placed at the beginning of a research report published as a journal article, an abstract presents a concise overview of the research problem, the methodology for the study, an interpretation of the results, and the conclusions that were formulated for the study. This brief overview is helpful for the reader in deciding whether or not to read the complete article. Abstracts may also be written in response to a call for papers for professional meetings, primarily to determine whether the study topic is relevant to the sessions being planned for the meeting.

Because the abstract is the most permanent and public record of a research study, it is important that it provide an accurate and honest reflection of the content of the research report:

> A paper in a journal is likely to be read in its entirety by only a very small number of people, but many more will read the abstract. The abstract of a published paper may appear in a database such as CINAHL or MEDLINE and be accessible to thousands of people, very few of whom will ever see the journal. Conference abstracts are likely to be seen by many more people than attended the conference. *(Brazier, 1997, p. 3)*

A NOTE ON PUBLICATION

Researchers who plan to write an article for a professional journal usually find it advisable to look over current publications in the area of their study to see where it would have the best chances of being accepted. They may then write a query letter to the editor of the publication to which they would like to submit the article. The query letter usually includes a brief statement of the author's background relevant to the article and a brief description of the planned article; it may also include an outline of the article. Although it is permissible to submit query letters to several publication editors at the same time, journal stipulations and professional ethics dictate that the manuscript for the journal article be submitted to only one publication at a time (Brosnan & Kovalsky, 1980).

Some journals are known as **refereed journals** or peer-reviewed journals. The referee system is a process of having three or more experts independently review and judge the merits of the manuscript before a journal editor accepts the article for publication. Manuscripts are usually reviewed "blind"—that is, the referees do not know who wrote the article or who submitted it for publication. This review process is designed to provide objectivity in acceptance or rejection of an article:

> The implication is that refereed nursing journals are the source and repository of reliable, valid clinical papers through which the refinement of professional practice occurs—and hence, bring higher prestige to authors appearing in them than nonrefereed journals do. *(Clayton & Boyle, 1981, p. 531)*

● CRITIQUING THE DISCUSSION COMPONENT OF A RESEARCH REPORT

The Discussion section of both a quantitative and a qualitative report is that part of the report in which the researcher writes about the meaning of the results of the study. This section typically consists of the major findings of the study and their interpretation; conclusions; limitations of the study; implications for nursing; and recommendations for further research.

Points to Consider in a Quantitative Report

The researcher should discuss the data-based findings of the study in relation to the specific research question and the purpose of the study as well as the relevant findings of other studies. If a theoretical or conceptual framework was used to guide the study, the findings should be discussed within this context. Generalizations to a broader setting must be consistent with the methodology and the findings. It may be necessary for the researcher to distinguish between statistical significance and clinical relevance. A study can have statistically significant results that may not be of value when applied in a clinical setting. Conversely, findings from another study may not be statistically significant but may still be useful in a clinical setting.

Conclusions should be clearly stated, must be supported by the data, and must be consistent with the analysis and interpretation of the data. Because all research studies have limitations over which the investigator has no control, the researcher should cite these limitations, such as small samples or time constraints, and discuss the effect of any limitations on the outcome of the study. Implications of the study should be discussed and evaluated as being both plausible and relevant for nursing. Recommendations for further research should be appropriate as well as clearly formulated.

Box 12-1 presents these points as evaluation guidelines.

Points to Consider in a Qualitative Report

Interpretation of the data by the researcher should be appropriate to the phenomenon of interest and the qualitative design used for the study. The researcher should discuss the findings in relation to the specific research question or problem and place them within the context of relevant literature and the findings from other studies. Conceptual categories should be appropriately described and must be true to the data. A theory or conceptual model, if developed, must be supported by the data. Conclusions for the study must not only be clearly stated but must also be logically consistent with the phenomenon of interest and with the context in which the study was conducted. The researcher should discuss any limitations of the study. Implications for nursing should be plausible and relevant, and recommendations for further research should be clearly formulated and appropriate.

Box 12-2 presents these points as evaluation guidelines.

BOX 12-1

GUIDELINES FOR EVALUATING THE DISCUSSION COMPONENT OF A QUANTITATIVE REPORT

1. Interpretations are based on the data.
2. Findings are discussed in relation to the study's purpose.
3. Findings are discussed in relation to the theoretical or conceptual framework and/or previous studies.
4. Generalizations are warranted by the results.
5. A distinction is made between statistical significance and clinical relevance and discussed, if appropriate.
6. Conclusions are based on the data.
7. Conclusions are clearly stated.
8. Limitations of the study are appropriately discussed.
9. Implications for nursing are plausible and relevant.
10. Recommendations are clearly formulated and appropriate.

BOX 12-2

GUIDELINES FOR EVALUATING THE DISCUSSION COMPONENT OF A QUALITATIVE REPORT

1. Interpretations are appropriate for the phenomenon of interest.
2. Findings are discussed in relation to the research question or problem.
3. Findings are discussed in relation to relevant literature and the findings of other studies.
4. Conceptual categories are appropriately described and true to the data.
5. Theoretical formulations, if developed, are supported by the data.
6. Conclusions are logically consistent with the phenomenon of interest and with the context of the study.
7. Conclusions are clearly stated.
8. Limitations of the study are appropriately discussed.
9. Implications for nursing are plausible and relevant.
10. Recommendations are clearly formulated and appropriate.

● ADDITIONAL CONSIDERATIONS IN EVALUATING A RESEARCH REPORT

Although many authors rely on the abstract rather than providing a brief summary at the conclusion of the report, it is most helpful for the reader if the researcher does include a summary. If provided, the summary should present a brief restatement of the research problem, the purpose of the study, the methodology, and the major conclusions and recommendations of the study.

The final components of a research report that must be evaluated include the credentials of the investigator, the title of the study, the abstract, and the style and format of the article. The credentials of the investigator are typically listed as academic qualifications and institutional affiliation. Sources of external funding that may have been awarded to the investigator(s) are also included. Each of these has implications for the quality of the research. The title of the study should be concise and reflect the major ideas of the research. The abstract for the study, located at the beginning of the article, may be either in text format (see the abstracts in the studies reprinted in Appendixes D and F) or in topical format (Appendixes C and E). The abstract should present an accurate and concise summary of the content. The article should be well organized and should flow logically; the grammar, sentence structure, and punctuation should be correct. Finally, the reference section should list all sources used to write the report.

Box 12-3 presents these points as evaluation guidelines.

● *RATING THE SCIENTIFIC MERIT OF A RESEARCH REPORT*

After critically evaluating each of the components of a research report, the final step in evaluation is to determine the scientific merit of the entire study. The **scientific merit** of a study refers to the degree to which the study is both methodologically and conceptually sound. Scientific merit is a subjective decision that is based on the logic and judgment of the evaluator. It is a major criterion for determining the potential for using the study's findings in practice.

In determining scientific merit, some components of a report are more important than others. For example, an inadequate title is not as critical to the scientific merit of the study as inadequate interpretation of data. Likewise, if the whole data-collection section is unacceptable, the study's findings are not valid.

Box 12-4 presents evaluation criteria for scientific merit.

BOX 12-3 **GUIDELINES FOR EVALUATING THE ADDITIONAL COMPONENTS OF A RESEARCH REPORT**

1. The investigator(s) is qualified.
2. The title is appropriate, accurately reflecting the problem.
3. The abstract presents an accurate and concise summary of the content.
4. The report is well organized and flows logically.
5. Grammar, sentence structure, and punctuation are correct.
6. References are accurate and complete.

BOX 12-4   RATING THE SCIENTIFIC MERIT OF THE REPORT

4   Critique indicates that overall, the study satisfies the basic requirements of scientific research.

3   Critique indicates that overall, the study satisfies the basic requirements of scientific research, with the following exceptions: (state the exceptions)

2   Critique indicates that overall, the study does not satisfy the basic requirements of scientific research, with the following exceptions: (state the exceptions)

1   Critique indicates that overall, the study does not satisfy the basic requirements of scientific research.

RATING FOR SCIENTIFIC MERIT: _____ .

SUMMARY

Interpretation of data-based results is a subjective process on the part of the investigator, who must take great care not to interpret beyond what the data indicate. The findings of the study should be logically presented and interpreted in relation to the specific research question and purpose of the study. A research report should be objective, concise, and scholarly in spelling, grammar, and punctuation. Most research studies are accompanied by an abstract that presents a summary of the study. When researchers plan to write an article for a professional journal, they may find it advisable to look over current publications in the area of their study to see where it would have the best chances of being accepted. If a journal is refereed, the peer-review process is designed to provide objectivity in accepting or rejecting an article submitted for publication. Scientific merit refers to the degree to which a research study is conceptually and methodologically sound and is an important criterion for determining the potential for using the study's findings in practice.

The following application activities will help you to develop your skills in evaluating the remaining components of published reports and in rating research reports for scientific merit.

REFERENCES

Brazier, H. (1997). Writing a research abstract: Structure, style and content. *Nursing Standard Online, 11*(48).

Brosnan, J., & Kovalsky, A. (1980). Perishing while publishing. *Nursing Outlook, 28*, 688.

Clayton, B. C., & Boyle, K. (1981). The refereed journal: Prestige in professional publication, *Nursing Outlook, 29*, 531–534.

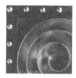

APPLICATION ACTIVITIES

1. Discuss the importance of careful interpretation of research findings, and cite three considerations in reporting these findings.

2. Describe the meaning of the term "serendipitous findings" in relation to a research study.

3. Discuss two major purposes for writing an abstract of a research report.

4. Explain the meaning of the term "refereed journal," and describe the refereeing purpose and process.

5. Discuss the meaning of the term "scientific merit" as you now understand it.

6. Use the following guidelines to evaluate the remainder of the reports you have selected to critique: Box 12-1 and/or 12-2 to evaluate the discussion component; Box 12-3 to evaluate additional components of the reports.

7. Use the guidelines in Box 12-4 to rate the scientific merit of each report, or use the above guidelines to evaluate two reports in the appendix.

USING THE RESULTS OF RESEARCH TO IMPROVE NURSING PRACTICE

Part III presents principles and techniques for using the results of research to improve nursing practice. Chapter 13 discusses current issues regarding the utilization of research-based knowledge and provides specific techniques and activities to prepare the baccalaureate graduate to begin to participate in research utilization in the clinical setting.

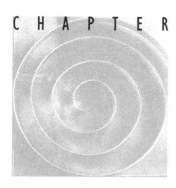

CHAPTER

13

Utilizing the Results of Research

*RELATIONSHIP OF RESEARCH CONDUCT AND
RESEARCH UTILIZATION*
THE RESEARCH–PRACTICE GAP IN NURSING
BRIDGING THE RESEARCH–PRACTICE GAP
MAJOR UTILIZATION PROJECTS
RESEARCH UTILIZATION MODELS
THE RESEARCH UTILIZATION PROCESS

*DEVELOPMENT OF A RESEARCH-BASED
PROTOCOL*
*DEVELOPMENT OF A RESEARCH-BASED
NURSING PROCEDURE*
*TOWARD EVIDENCE-BASED NURSING
PRACTICE*
SUMMARY

OBJECTIVES   *On completing this chapter, the student will be able to:*

1. Explain the relationship between the conduct of research and the utilization of research.
2. Define research utilization.
3. Discuss at least three potential facilitators for bridging the research–practice gap in nursing.
4. Identify three major federally funded research utilization projects.
5. Describe the purpose of research utilization models.
6. Discuss each of the steps in the research utilization process.
7. Identify the potential role of the baccalaureate-prepared nurse in the research utilization process.
8. Explain the relationship between research utilization and evidence-based nursing practice.
9. Define key terms.

The purpose of this final chapter is to discuss current issues related to using research in practice and to present the process for translating research-based findings into nursing practice. Techniques for the baccalaureate-prepared nurse to begin to participate in the research utilization process are presented, and the role of research utilization in furthering evidence-based nursing practice is also discussed.

● RELATIONSHIP OF RESEARCH CONDUCT AND RESEARCH UTILIZATION

Conducting research and utilizing research are distinct yet complementary and interdependent processes—that is, each is dependent on the other to further the development of a scientific basis for the practice of nursing. The purpose of conducting research is to identify valid scientific knowledge that can be used to guide nursing practice in the delivery of optimal patient care. The purpose of research utilization is to make use of this knowledge by transferring the research-based knowledge into the practice setting. The term **research utilization** has a simple, straightforward meaning: it is a systematic process by which the scientifically valid results of research are transferred for use in practice. Research utilization may mean changing a current practice by developing a new **research-based document**, such as a clinical protocol, a procedure, or a policy, that transforms research-based knowledge so that it can be used in practice. Research utilization may also mean updating already existing documents so that they are based on available scientific research.

Knowledge that has the potential to guide nursing practice is generated by using the research process. This knowledge is then evaluated and transformed for use in practice through research utilization, a process in which a nursing problem in need of a scientific basis is identified, the valid findings from scientific investigations in the research literature are located and critically evaluated for applicability to the clinical problem, research-based interventions for use in practice are formulated, and the outcome is evaluated. Each of these steps is detailed later in this chapter.

Grady (1998) aptly describes the relationship of research conduct and research utilization as we move into the 21st century—"to bring life to research and research to life"—and offers the following example that exemplifies the movement from knowledge generation to clinical research to translation at the bedside, thus making a difference in people's lives:

A routine clinical procedure—endotracheal suctioning—often is used to clear a patient's trachea. Although it is a necessary procedure to provide an open airway, it has risks, sometimes causing changes in central venous pressures that, in turn, can cause sudden high or increased intracranial pressure in the brain of head-injured patients. Because it may take more than 10 minutes for increased intracranial pressure to return to normal, this condition can pose serious problems for effective patient treatment and recovery. A National Institute of Nursing Research-supported researcher found that differences in intracranial pressure are most significant at the first and second suctioning. Additional evidence indicates that placing patients on pharmacological blocking agents in conjunction with mechanical ventilation protects them from the increased pressure in the brain induced by suctioning. Results from this study have been incorporated into practice guidelines endorsed by the American Association of Critical Care Nurses. The information also has been videotaped and disseminated around the country. *(p. 1)*

● THE RESEARCH–PRACTICE GAP IN NURSING

There is little disagreement that nursing should be a research-based profession in which nursing education, nursing practice, and nursing administration are based on the findings of scientific research. If the RU process can be used to transform the results of research for use in practice, why is there still a large gap between conducting research and utilizing the results in nursing practice? Why is the nursing profession still not making maximal use of the scientific findings of research, and why is much of nursing practice still based on tradition and ritual? "Even nurses who are aware of research and its implications for nursing practice often continue to base their practice on traditions, myths and rituals" (Tordoff, 1998, p. 2).

Tremendous volumes of research have been generated over the past 20 to 25 years, with much of it ready to be implemented in nursing practice. However, all too often there is a 10- to 15-year gap between the time the knowledge is generated and the time it is implemented in practice. Research finding are of little benefit if they do not find their way to practitioners and if practitioners do not integrate the findings into practice (Barnsteiner, 1996).

The current reality in the practice setting is that nurses have been mandated to base their practice decisions on up-to-date scientific information. Standard VII of the American Nurses Association (ANA) Standards of Clinical Nursing Practice states, "the nurse uses research findings in practice." Nurses use interventions substantiated by research and participate in research activities "as appropriate to the individual's position, education, and practice environment." The nurse participates in research through such activities as critiquing research for application to practice and "using research findings in the development of policies, procedures, and guidelines for client care" (ANA, 1991, p. 16).

Also, the Joint Commission of the Association of Health Care Organizations (JCAHO) accreditation guidelines specify that patient care must be based on information from up-to-date sources about the design and performance of the process (such as practice guidelines). The commission also specifies that the performance of this process must be compared to relevant scientific clinical and management literature. Not only are nurses being held increasingly accountable for current and scientifically based practice, but one writer asserts that "using research in practice represents a professional imperative. In fact, practice that does not incorporate up-to-date empirical findings may be unethical" (Mayhew, 1993a, p. 211).

In viewing RU from a historical perspective, it is interesting to note that using research in practice was not an issue for Florence Nightingale, who used data to change practices that were contributing to the high mortality rates in hospitals and communities. However, in the years that followed the Nightingale era, few nurses built on the solid foundation of RU that she exemplified:

> Separation of the conduct and use of research is rooted in the 1930s and 1940s—a period in nursing when there were few educationally qualified nurse researchers, most nursing research was being done by non-nurses, and hospitals were being used as the primary setting for nursing education. During the mid-1900s, nurses were being prepared as researchers in fields other than nursing and most research focused on nurses rather than on patients. *(Titler, 1997, p. 104)*

In a national Delphi survey conducted by Lindeman in 1975, 15 priorities were established that were considered to have the most significant potential for improving nursing care. One of the priorities emerging from this study was to determine strategies for greater utilization of research in practice; this priority continues to be discussed in the current literature. In the years since Lindeman's survey, the literature has consistently reflected widespread agreement among nursing professionals that nursing must establish itself as a research-based profession with a strong scientific basis for practice. However, numerous surveys conducted during these same years to determine not only nurses' use of research findings in their practice but also their knowledge and attitudes toward using research have shown that staff nurses are relatively unaware of research findings and that their use of research in practice has been limited.

For example, in one of the earliest surveys to be conducted (1975), Ketefian investigated the impact of nursing research on nursing practice to determine the extent to which a series of research findings on the mode of temperature determination were being used by nursing practitioners. Her conclusions demonstrated the major gap between knowledge and practice: "A clear picture emerged: The practitioner either was totally unaware of the research literature relative to her practice, or, if she was aware of it, was unable to relate to it or utilize it" (Ketefian, 1975, p. 91).

Kirchoff's 1982 report of a national survey of critical care nurses' coronary precautions revealed that the awareness of published studies had not significantly changed practice.

In a 1994 study, 212 medical-surgical nurses employed in six hospitals were asked to self-report their use of the methods and products of research and to identify their attitudes toward the use of research-based knowledge in clinical practice. Respondents rated research-based practice change as the most difficult, indicating their perception of the difficulty involved in changing practice based on research findings. Although they delegate the translation of research findings into usable formats to educators and researchers, most subjects reported they were interested in learning how to develop research-based patient protocols (Baessler et al., 1994, p. 120).

In another study, a group of 237 registered nurses described their perceptions of the barriers to and facilitators of RU at two hospitals in Sweden. These nurses perceived that the major barriers to RU were research that was not readily available, inadequate facilities for implementation of research findings, lack of competent colleagues with whom to discuss the research, lack of time for reading and implementing the research findings, and the lack of authority that nurses have in the organization. Nurses who had studied research methods in their basic nursing education seemed to perceive fewer barriers than those who had not (Kajermo et al., 1998).

● *BRIDGING THE RESEARCH–PRACTICE GAP*

Research utilization is a complex process. Experts in the field of RU have observed that in many ways RU presents more challenges to overcome than those faced in conducting research: "Influencing the behavior of multiple caregivers to let go of ritual-based practices is not an easy task" (Titler 1997, p. 106).

Nursing, however, is not alone in its concern with translating research findings into practice. Even though knowledge seems to be expanding at a rapid rate, every discipline has a research-practice gap—that is, a major time lag between the scientific knowledge generated by research and its implementation in practice. In many instances, this time lag is related to the obstacles encountered during the process of introducing **innovations** (changes perceived as new, such as new ideas or methods) within a social system. An innovation, such as introducing the valid results of a set of specific research studies into a social system, requires the changing of entrenched attitudes and practices on the part of the members of the social system as the innovation is spread through the system by **diffusion**.

A classical theory of innovation diffusion proposed by Rogers in 1983 serves to provide a clearer understanding of the complex process of introducing change within a social system. Rogers defines diffusion as "the process by which (1) an innovation (2) is communicated through certain channels (3) over time (4) among the members of a social system" (Rogers, 1983, p. 11). Diffusion of an innovation requires that the individual who is the adopter of the innovation must first gain the relevant knowledge, must then be persuaded of the value as well as the applicability of this knowledge, must decide to use this knowledge, must implement it, and then must evaluate or confirm it (Funk et al., 1995, p. 396).

Nurses' Perceived Barriers to Research Utilization

In 1995, Funk and colleagues published an integrative literature review in which they synthesized the specific literature generated over the years related to the barriers to and facilitators of research utilization. In reviewing 79 articles, they found that many authors reported potential barriers to research utilization, a few reported the results of data-based surveys of the perceptions of nurses in clinical, administrative, or academic positions, and others provided firsthand reports of informal or formal research utilization experiences. The authors concluded that "the numbers of barriers identified are great, and the consistency among the reports is striking . . . nurses see substantial barriers to the use of research findings in practice" (Funk et al., 1995, p. 396).

Although there were fluctuations in the numbers of nurses citing each barrier, the review showed results to be quite stable across time as well as among nurses serving in different roles. The reported barriers fell into four major categories: those related to nurses' research values and skills, those related to limitations in the setting, those related to how the research itself is communicated, and those related to the quality of the research itself.

In terms of their own research values and skills, over the years nurses have reported that they lacked awareness of the research that was being published and did not feel capable of evaluating the quality of the research that they were aware of. They reported feeling isolated from knowledgeable colleagues. Nurses also perceived that the benefits of changing practice would be minimal, saw little benefit in it for themselves, did not see the value of changing practice, and were unwilling to change or try new ideas.

Organizational limitations perceived by the nurses included insufficient authority to change patient-care procedures and insufficient time on the job to implement new ideas. They also perceived administrators as not allowing implementation of innovations and physicians as not cooperating with the implementation of innovations.

Nurses also reported that barriers related to the accessibility of research and how research is presented included statistical analyses that were not understandable, the fact that the relevant literature was not compiled in one place, that implications for practice were not made clear, and that the research itself was not reported clearly and readably.

In terms of the quality of the published research, nurses reported the lack of replication studies as a barrier. They also reported uncertainty about the believability of the results of the research, literature reports with conflicting results, methodologic inadequacies of the research, unjustified conclusions, and the fact that research reports and articles are not published fast enough.

Recommendations for Facilitating Research Utilization

One of the more prominent recommendations in the nursing literature for facilitating research utilization is related to the collaborative nature of activities required for research utilization—that is, the need for the entire nursing profession to work toward using research in practice: "if we are to improve practice through research utilization, it will take the commitment and collaboration of educators, researchers, clinicians, and administrators" (Funk et al., 1995, p. 404).

Nursing educators must socialize students into the research arena and must integrate research utilization knowledge and skills at both the baccalaureate and graduate levels. Crane (1995) recommended such specific educational strategies as requiring nursing students to develop one written research-based protocol at the baccalaureate level, completion of a research utilization practicum in a practice setting at the master's level, and dissertations dealing with the science of research utilization and with designing and conducting replication studies at the doctoral level.

In the organizational setting, facilitation strategies include a clear-cut commitment by administrators to the value that research and research utilization have within the organization; these values must be operationalized by incorporation into the governance documents and policies of the organization and by establishing a reward system within the organization that recognizes research activities. Organizations must allocate not only adequate financial resources but also human resources, such as the leadership provided by doctorally prepared nurse researchers.

To facilitate the communication of research findings, more practice journals need to include research columns, more journals need to emphasize the application of research findings to practice, and more journals need to publish research summaries. Titler (1997) recommended increased use of the electronic superhighway to show research utilization protocols and the establishment of a central clearinghouse for indexing, updating, and disseminating written research-based practice protocols. There is also a need for more local and national conferences that nurses can attend to increase their research utilization knowledge and skills.

Because research utilization must be based on the highest quality of research, a recurring theme in the nursing literature is the urgent need for more replication studies to build a stronger scientific basis for innovation. Also, compilation of research in the form of integrative reviews and more meta-analyses of existing research would assist researchers in their efforts to increase research utilization activities (Titler, 1997).

Research utilization can be viewed as a collaborative endeavor that requires the concerted efforts, knowledge, and skills of the members of the entire nursing profession:

- Researchers generate and disseminate the scientific knowledge base.
- Administrators facilitate organizational activities in numerous ways, ranging from providing open encouragement and leadership to securing the necessary organizational support and resources.
- Clinicians often begin the process by identifying clinical problems and by locating research findings relevant to practice and proposing ways to integrate these findings into clinical practice.
- Educators provide the knowledge and skills that graduates need to begin to participate in RU at the organizational level.

As a baccalaureate graduate, you will be prepared to participate in utilization activities by participating in journal clubs designed to review research articles for potential application to practice, taking part in RU discussion groups, and serving on RU committees.

● MAJOR UTILIZATION PROJECTS

Beginning in the 1970s, three large-scale research utilization projects received grant support from the Division of Nursing at the federal level:

- The Regional Program for Nursing Research and Development Project, carried out by staff members of the Western Interstate Commission for Higher Education (WICHE)
- The Nursing Child Assessment Satellite Training Projects (NCAST)
- The Conduct and Utilization of Research in Nursing (CURN) Project conducted under the auspices of the Michigan Nurses Association.

Each of these demonstration projects was designed to bridge the gap between the conduct of research and its utilization in clinical practice.

Regional Program for Nursing Research and Development (WICHE) Project

With the goal of increasing the quantity, quality, and use of nursing research in the western United States, WICHE, headquartered in Boulder, Colorado, was funded in 1971 by the Division of Nursing to establish a program to support collaborative research endeavors among prepared and potential nurse researchers in different settings. An additional grant, funded in 1974, enabled the project staff to begin the first large-scale structured approach to using valid clinical nursing research findings in the patient-care setting.

Three types of research groups for nurses were developed during the project: nontargeted groups, targeted groups, and utilization groups. The goal of the nontargeted groups was the generation of research hypotheses from care settings by nurses caring for patients. In contrast to the single-investigator/single-institution approach that characterized nursing research in the 1960s, the nontargeted, regional approach brought together groups of nurses with different skills and backgrounds. The long-term goal of the targeted research groups was to develop valid and reliable instruments for the purpose of assessing the quality of nursing care. The goal of the utilization groups was to help nurses to locate and evaluate research findings and to make plans for using research to change the care they provided to patients.

Nurses from the western region met in a series of workshops to develop plans for basing changes in nursing care in their own settings on research findings. Dracup and Breu's 1978 article "Using Nursing Research Findings to Meet the Needs of Grieving Spouses" is a report of their experiences with a utilization project in a coronary care setting developed at one of the regional workshops. In 1978, Krueger and associates provided the following recommendation regarding this pioneering large-scale RU project:

> On the basis of the experience gained in this project, it is apparent that it was ahead of its proper time. When and if nursing research is identified, evaluated, and collated systematically, this project should be repeated on local levels in such a way that it is available to all nurses. *(pp. 450–452)*

Nursing Child Assessment Satellite Training (NCAST) Projects

Three projects were carried out between 1976 and 1985 with the purpose of translating and disseminating research findings. These projects aimed at increasing the practicing nurse's awareness of new research and the value of using research in practice. The first project (1976–1978) tested the use of a communications satellite for rapid dissemination of new research results that focused on new assessment techniques in child health. The second NCAST project (1978–1983) provided learners with videotaped parent–child interactions with which to practice assessments. The objective of the third NCAST project (1983–1985) was to teach public health nurses to use a nursing protocol for the follow-up care of preterm infants and their families.

Conduct and Utilization of Research in Nursing (CURN) Project

CURN, a 5-year research development project, was funded by the Division of Nursing on the federal level from 1975 to 1980. The Michigan Nurses Association conducted the project with the assistance of faculty and graduate students at the University of Michigan School of Nursing, the Institute for Social Research, and the Michigan State University School of Nursing. The purpose of the project was to improve the practice of nursing through two types of activities: the use of existing research findings in the daily practice of registered nurses, and the design and conduct of research that was directly relevant and could be readily transferred to nursing practice. Thirty-four departments of nursing in hospitals throughout Michigan assisted the CURN project staff. The research utilization process developed and used by the project staff consisted of a systematic series of activities:

1. Identification and synthesis of multiple research studies in a common conceptual area (research base)

2. Transformation of the knowledge derived from a research base into a solution or clinical protocol
3. Transformation of the clinical protocol into specific nursing actions (innovations) that are administered to patients
4. Clinical evaluation of the new practice to ascertain whether it produced the predicted result (Horsley et al., 1983).

Ten research-based practice protocols, developed by CURN project personnel, were published by Grune & Stratton during 1981 and 1982:

1. Preventing decubitus ulcers
2. Structured preoperative teaching
3. Clean intermittent catheterization
4. Intravenous cannula change
5. Reducing diarrhea in tube-fed patients
6. Closed urinary drainage systems
7. Distress reduction through sensory preparation
8. Preoperative sensory preparation to promote recovery
9. Mutual goal-setting in patient care
10. Pain: Deliberative nursing interventions.

Published as separate books, each of the protocols in the series contains information regarding the need for the change (innovation), a description of the innovation, a summary of the research base provided by the conceptually related research studies that met specific criteria developed by CURN project personnel, a description of the research-based principles guiding the implementation of the innovation, and a description of the implementation and the systematic evaluation of its effects. Each protocol also includes a summary of the benefits to be anticipated from successful use of the innovation, as well as additional pertinent materials.

In 1987, Goode and colleagues described how they used the CURN protocols to utilize research-based knowledge in their hospital. The already active audit committee was charged by the nursing administrator with reviewing, discussing, and evaluating findings from current research and making recommendations regarding the use of research findings in the hospital. The intent was to substantiate practice procedures with findings from current research. They selected temperature-taking as their first project because they wanted to start with an aspect of patient care to which all of their nurses could relate and because there was concern about the basis for low temperature readings by the procedure currently in use. As a result of a review and evaluation of the related research literature, the committee found substantial support for making changes in procedures for temperature-taking. The group continued to use the CURN protocols to write additional policies and learned from this project that " 'Just because that is the way we've always done it' is not reason enough to explain our practice" (Goode et al., 1987, p. 13).

In an effort to determine the extent of use of the CURN models in the practice setting, Brett (1987) used research journals and CURN publications to identify 14 nursing research findings that met the CURN project criteria for clinical use. She then surveyed nurses practicing in small, medium, and large hospitals to determine the extent of their awareness of, persuasion about, and use of these research findings. All of the 216 respondents were full-time employees and were responsible for the direct care of patients; 86% were staff nurses and 14% were head nurses. Brett concluded, "The majority of nurses were aware of the average innovation, were persuaded about it, and used the average innovation at least sometimes" (p. 344).

In a 1990 report of a replication of Brett's study, Coyle and Sokop found that of the 113 nurses surveyed, the majority were aware of 9 of the 14 nursing practices and that 8 of the 14 practices were used regularly by more than half of the sample.

A major outcome of the CURN project was the development and refinement of an RU model for developing research-based protocols that represent a significant step in transferring research-based knowledge into clinical nursing practice.

Each of the three major large-scale demonstration projects—WICHE, NCAST, and the CURN project—has provided its own unique and significant contribution to the advancement of research utilization in the practice setting.

● RESEARCH UTILIZATION MODELS

During the past 25 to 30 years, a number of research utilization models have been developed with the purpose of providing a process for bridging the gap between nursing research and nursing practice. Each of these models can be viewed as a form of prescriptive information that specifies the process by which research utilization should occur. Examples of such models include the CURN project model, the Stetler model, the Iowa Model of Research in Practice, the Orange County Research Utilization in Nursing Project, the Horn model, and the Goode model.

The majority of models approach research utilization from an organizational perspective, as in the CURN model. When an organizationally focused model is used, research utilization is characterized by a process of planned change within the organizational setting. The organization must be committed to the utilization process, and the potential change must be very carefully evaluated before judiciously planned implementation. Also, "Visible, potent and enduring mechanisms" such as standing committees, policies and procedures, must be in place, and substantive resources must be provided, including personnel, equipment, time, and funds (White et al., 1995, p. 411).

While the CURN model and other organizational models were developed for organizational use, the Stetler model was developed for use by the individual practitioner. The Stetler model was unique in approaching research utilization from an individual practitioner's perspective. Unlike the organizational models, in which change in practice is the primary goal, the primary goal of the Stetler model is the incorporation of research findings into *individual* practice. This model was originally published in 1976 as the Stetler/Marram model of research utilization. "Its primary focus was to facilitate application of research findings at the practitioner rather than the organizational, level of practice" (Stetler, 1994, p. 15). The Stetler model, a refinement and expansion of the original Stetler/Marram model, is now being used as a framework to facilitate research utilization in the practice setting at both the practitioner and organizational levels. Stetler refers to this model as the practitioner model of research utilization in that it approaches research utilization as an integral part of the practitioner's routine activities, such as problem-solving and decision-making, with the purpose of integrating scientific knowledge to provide more scientifically based care. The formal organization may or may not be involved in the practitioner's use of research. One of the model's assumptions is that information from both experience and theory are more likely to be combined with research information than they are to be ignored. For effective as well as safe use of this model, the user must have sound knowledge of the research process, the research utilization process, and the area under review (Stetler, 1994).

Although different in their terminology, the Stetler model and the models for planned organizational change are similar in specifying that the utilization of research is an orderly process that should occur in a linear progression. Implicit in the process is that the proposed change must be based on the scientific merit of the research, must be relevant to the practice setting, and must have the potential for implementation in the practice setting.

THE RESEARCH UTILIZATION PROCESS

The research utilization process provides a step-by-step method that facilitates systematic movement from identifying a nursing problem in need of a scientific basis through formulation and evaluation of a research-based innovation in the practice setting. As a baccalaureate-prepared nurse, you need to become familiar with the basic steps in the research utilization process to enable you to begin participating in utilization activities at the organizational level.

The research utilization process includes the following steps:

1. Identify a nursing problem that has the potential to be addressed by the application of research findings.
2. Locate the relevant research literature.
3. Critically evaluate each research study for scientific merit and applicability to the problem being addressed.
4. Summarize the valid and relevant studies in a standardized format, such as the Research Utilization Worksheet in Table 13-1 and the examples in Tables 13-2 and 13-3.
5. Determine the consistency of findings across studies, and decide whether there is a sufficient research base that could guide practice.
6. If there is a sufficient research base, develop a research-based practice document (a protocol, procedure, or policy) to address the problem.
7. Identify the expected outcomes and formulate an evaluation plan.

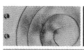

TABLE 13-1 *Research Utilization Worksheet*

Nursing problem being considered: _____

RESEARCH STUDIES	SUBJECT/ PARTICIPANTS: NUMBER AND DEMOGRAPHICS	VARIABLES: INDEPENDENT ANDDEPENDENT (QUANTITATIVE STUDIES)	PHENOMENON: DESCRIBE (QUALITAIYE STUDIES)	FINDINGS	IMPLICATIONS FOR NURSING
Study #1					
Quantitative or qualitative study? Author/ Journal/Date					
Clinical problem(s) addressed					
Critique rating:					
Study #2					

TABLE 13-2 *Sample Research Utilization Worksheet Using Fictitious Data*

Nursing problem being considered: <u>Effect of individualized vs. group instruction on successful breast-feeding in primiparas</u>

RESEARCH STUDIES	SUBJECT/ PARTICIPANTS: NUMBER AND DEMOGRAPHICS	VARIABLES: INDEPENDENT ANDDEPENDENT (QUANTITATIVE STUDIES)	PHENOMENON: DESCRIBE (QUALITAIYE STUDIES)	FINDINGS	IMPLICATIONS FOR NURSING
Study #1					
Quantitative or qualitative study? Author/Journal/ Date: Fictitious/ *Imaginary*/2002	N = 60 primiparas, 30 in each group; ages 18–25 55 married, 5 unmarried; 30 Caucasian, 15 African-American, 12 Hispanic, 3 Asian-American	IV = type of breast-feeding instruction (individualized vs. group) DV = successful breast-feeding experience for primiparas	NA	Primiparas who received individualized instruction were more successful in breast-feeding their infants.	Primiparas should receive individualized instruction in breast-feeding.
Clinical problem(s) addressed: Breast-feeding instruction for primiparas					
Critique rating: 4					
Study #2					

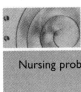

TABLE 13-3 *Sample Research Utilization Worksheet*

Nursing problem being considered: <u>Instruction of nursing students before bathing patients for the first time.</u>

RESEARCH STUDIES	SUBJECT/ PARTICIPANTS: NUMBER AND DEMOGRAPHICS	VARIABLES: INDEPENDENT ANDDEPENDENT (QUANTITATIVE STUDIES)	PHENOMENON: DESCRIBE (QUALITAIVE STUDIES)	FINDINGS	IMPLICATIONS FOR NURSING
Study #1 Quantitative or qualitative study? Author/Journal/ Date Wolf/ *Nurse Educator/* 1997	N = 16 nursing students X̄ age = 23.5 yrs.; 13 single, 3 married; 11 Caucasian, 4 African-American 1 Asian-American; genders not reported	NA	Nursing students' experience bathing patients for the first time	Students reported bathing first patient is stressful (fear of harming patient and touching private body parts); lack of skill bathing a stranger; were more confident when paired with another student and were surprised when patients helped them through the bath	Faculty should provide positive feedback; hold preclinical conferences to discuss students' fears; team students to bathe patients of the same sex.
Clinical problem(s) addressed: Nursing students' experience bathing adult patients for the first time Critique rating: 4 **Study #2**					

---

8. Conduct a trial run of the protocol or procedure on a pilot group, evaluate the process and outcomes, and make necessary modifications.
9. Educate all personnel who will be involved in implementation of the protocol or procedure.
10. Implement the protocol or procedure, evaluate, and revise as needed.

● DEVELOPMENT OF A RESEARCH-BASED PROTOCOL

The following description of the development of a research-based protocol for the management of asthma in elementary-school children illustrates the application of each of these steps of the research utilization process to the development of a research-based protocol to address a clinical nursing problem (Peugh et al., 1998).

In identifying a clinical nursing situation that could be improved if research findings were used, a group of elementary-school nurses decided to establish a research-based intervention protocol to help asthmatic students and their families to manage asthma better. In view of the fact that asthma is the number-one chronic illness of childhood, school nurses frequently encounter acute episodes and must be prepared to assess these students and refer them appropriately. Because it is unwise to change practice based on the results of a single study, each member of the group then worked to locate multiple published research studies related to interventions for increasing coping and management skills of school-age children with asthma. Because not all research reported in the literature is suitable for use in practice, the members critiqued each of their articles to determine its scientific merit and applicability to the clinical problem.

Using the worksheet in Table 13-1 to summarize the valid and relevant studies, the members then pooled their critiques to determine whether there was a sufficient research base that would be relevant to their clinical problem and that could guide the development of a research-based protocol that could be used by school nurses working with asthmatic children. The findings of their pooled critiques indicated that instruction and support for asthmatic children is basic to the development of coping and management skills, and that school nurses are in a position to provide this instruction and support by organizing support groups within the school setting. These support groups would address such problems as the proper use of inhalers, the use of peak flow meters as objective measures of lung function, the proper pacing of activities, attention to the control of environmental factors for prevention, and self-help breathing and relaxation techniques.

After evaluating their pooled research findings for applicability to the clinical problem, the group decided there was a sufficient research base to develop a research-based clinical protocol. They then wrote a protocol that incorporated what they determined to be the valid findings from their critical review of the research literature. Included in the protocol were management strategies during the acute phase of an asthmatic episode as well as long-term strategies that provided for student participation in an asthma-management support group. Their plan for implementing the asthma protocol in the school setting specified expected outcomes and proposed evaluation measures for both acute and long-term management. To educate the personnel who would be involved in using the protocol, they included plans for providing inservice education for all nurses who would be using the new protocol, as well as plans for the nurses to provide inservice sessions to school staff, counselors, and physical education teachers. The group planned to conduct a trial run of the protocol in one school, evaluate the process and outcomes, and then modify the protocol if indicated.

Text continues on page 268

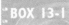

BOX 13-1   RESEARCH-BASED PROTOCOL FOR ASTHMA MANAGEMENT IN ELEMENTARY-SCHOOL CHILDREN

I. The purpose of the protocol is two fold:

   A. To provide school nurses with guidelines for management of asthmatic children during the acute phase of an asthmatic attack.

   B. To provide strategies for long-term management of asthmatic children.

II. Definition of asthma

   An allergic condition that causes edema, narrowing of the bronchial tubes, and excess secretions, resulting in the inability to breathe out. This reaction is caused by a response to a foreign substance (pollen, dust), virus or bacteria, physical factors (cold, sunlight, physical exertion), or any other agent to which the patient is allergic.

III. Use of peak flow meters

   A. Peak flow meter to be in every nurse's office.

   B. Establish a baseline reading before an acute episode.

   C. Obtain reading during acute episode.

IV. Coping/management during acute episode

   A. Children are capable of rating dyspnea and describing sensation.

   B. Determine peak flow; assess lung sounds, respirations, pulse, and color.

   C. NANDA Nursing Dx for Asthma: Ineffective airway clearance/impaired gas exchange/anxiety

   D. Assist child through acute episode:

      1. Rest

      2. Hydrate (sips of warm water)

      3. Relaxation techniques

      4. Metered dose inhaler with spacer

      5. Medication policy to be changed to allow elementary students to self-medicate if appropriate (determined by parent and physician).

(Continues)

BOX 13-1   *(Continued)*

V. Long-term management

   A. Refer children to the school-based asthma program called "Easy Breathers." This is a support group for students.

      1. This group will be generated from health problem lists, teacher/parent referral, and number of nurse office visits.

      2. Doctors caring for students will be informed of program so they can make referrals as well.

   B. Easy Breathers Support Group

      1. Facilitated by nurse/counselor/guest speakers, etc.

      2. Meetings will be conducted at school, once each week for 6 weeks initially, then each month thereafter for support and reinforcement of knowledge and skills.

      3. Nurses/counselors will teach the following:

         a. Basic information and feelings about asthma

         b. How to recognize and respond to symptoms of asthma, including use of peak flow meter

         c. Use of medications

         d. How to decide to seek help

         e. Exercise

         f. Identifying and controlling triggers of asthma symptoms

         g. Handling problems related to asthma in school

         Note: Treats for attendance as incentives to continue to come to meetings

   C. Inservice for teachers and parents

      1. Teachers will be taught about general asthma management in school, referral process to nurse's office, and availability of support groups for students.

      2. Parents will be taught general information on asthma and informed about information being taught to students.

Based on Peugh, S., Betts, M., Hamlin, P., & Krause, B. (1998). Development of a research-based protocol for asthma management in elementary-school children (unpublished manuscript). Las Cruces, NM.

The research-based protocol developed by this group is shown in Box 13-1. References for the protocol are listed at the end of this chapter.

These nurses addressed the management of elementary-school children with asthma from the perspective of their own practice setting by using relevant research findings to develop a research-based protocol unique to their identified need. This is but one example of a range of research-based practice protocols that could be developed to guide practice in a specific setting.

DEVELOPMENT OF A RESEARCH-BASED NURSING PROCEDURE

In the following example, the research utilization process was used to develop a research-based nursing procedure in response to a perceived need in the academic setting. Several years ago, a graduate nursing student who was helping nursing faculty to teach fundamental nursing skills to baccalaureate nursing students was also enrolled in a graduate-level nursing research course designed primarily to provide students with skills to use research in clinical settings. This student asked the following questions:

- Why do we teach our basic nursing skills procedures, such as bathing, hand washing, bed making, and others, in the way that we do?
- Are these procedures really based on valid scientific findings, or do we teach them in this way "because this is the way we have always taught them?"

With encouragement and assistance from the research course professor, she and her classmates used the research utilization process to write several research-based procedures. Graduate students enrolled in subsequent research classes, with the assistance of nursing faculty, have continued to use the RU process to develop additional research-based nursing procedures, such as hand washing, back rubs, indwelling urinary catheter, nasogastric tube placement, and a teaching plan for range of motion. All of these procedures have been incorporated into a research-based skills manual that nursing faculty now use to teach research-based procedures. To enable their students to understand the scientific knowledge base for each procedure, faculty require their students to read and discuss selected studies relevant to the research base for each procedure.

One procedure from the research-based skills manual—the procedure for wound care—is reprinted in Box 13-2. References for this procedure are listed at the end of this chapter.

In each of the above situations, the nurses identified a clinical nursing problem unique to their own setting. By using the research utilization process as a guide, they were able to transform research-based knowledge for use in clinical practice.

Although the research utilization process provides a valuable guide for transferring valid research into practice, it is not feasible to base all nursing

BOX 13-2   **RESEARCH-BASED CLINICAL PROCEDURE***

WOUNDS: Cleansing & Dressing

Wound healing is optimized and the potential for infection is decreased when all necrotic tissue, exudate and metabolic wastes are removed from the wound (USDHHS, 1994).

Cleansing the wound of necrotic tissue, excess wound exudate, dressing residue and metabolic wastes from the wound surface is essential for optimum healing. Wound cleansing involves using an appropriate solution and an adequate mechanical force. Every effort should be made to use biocompatible cleansing solution with the minimal mechanical force. The objective is to adequately cleanse the wound while preventing any unnecessary chemical or mechanical trauma to the wound surface (Barr, 1995)

Procedure	Rationale	Evaluation	Comments
Verify order and rationale for dressing change.		The student will: • check order and verbalize reasons for verification.	□ A pilot study of patients having elective gastrointestinal surgery found no difference in the rate of wound healing with clean versus sterile technique. In addition the clean technique was less expensive (Stotts, et al., 1995). These findings need to be confirmed with a larger sample.
Collect equipment/ materials: ➢ gloves ➢ tape ➢ scissors ➢ saline ➢ gauze ➢ disposable bag		• explain rationale: √ moist vs. dry dressings √ clean vs. sterile [differentiate aseptic at home vs. hospital]	
Wash hands.	RBSM - Handwashing*	• secure equipment/materials.	
Explain procedure to patient and encourage questions.		• wash hands. • explain procedure to patient.	Wound healing is optimized and the potential for infection is decreased when all necrotic tissue, exudate and metabolic wastes are removed from the wound.
Don gloves/protective clothing.		• provide for patient privacy.	
Remove dressing and dispose in plastic bag.		• evaluate wound healing and potential for infection.	Benefits of cleansing a wound must be weighed against the potential trauma to the wound bed as a result of such cleansing.
Assess wound site: ➢ color ➢ drainage ➢ bleeding ➢ swelling ➢ signs of infection/healing		• maintain aseptic technique. • cleans wound as appropriate • avoid cytotoxic agents • use lukewarm water • use sterile gauze • clean each side separately • dry skin	Some clinicians recommend no routine cleansing at all for wounds that have no exudate or necrotic tissue.

(Continues)

Procedure

If necessary, use sterile cleansing solution (preferably saline). Clean along wound edges using small circular motion from one end of the incision to the other. Clean each side of the incision line. Clean the drain site separately. Pat incision site and drain site dry with a sterile dressing sponge.

Apply sterile dressing.

Keep moist or per protocol.

Dispose of contaminated dressing and gloves in plastic bag.

Document procedure, wound status, and patient response.

Rationale

Cytotoxic agents like providone iodine, acetic acid, hydrogen peroxide, and sodium hypochloride (Dakins) should not be used for routine cleansing of wounds because they can inhibit healing by preventing re-epithelialization (Walker, 1996)

A wound with minimal surface debris can be cleansed using gauze saturated with normal saline and minimal mechanical force (Walker, 1996). Skin injury due to excessive thermal energy or accelerated metabolic activity induced by elevated temperatures should be minimized by only using wash water that is comfortable to the skin (USDHHS, 1992).

A moist wound environment dressing versus a wet to dry normal saline was more cost effective, faster and resulted in less pain (Gates, et al,, 1992).

Do not clean ulcer wounds with skin cleansers or antiseptic. Certain dilution levels are required to maintain white blood cell viability and phagocytic efficiency. Use normal saline for cleansing most pressure ulcers (USDHHS, 1994).

Evaluation

The student will:

- correctly apply sterile dressing—keep moist.
- dispose of contaminated materials properly.
- document patient respose, wound status, and nursing action.

Comments

Contamination by fecal or urinary incontinence should be removed ASAP to limit chemical irritation.

During the cleansing process care should be taken to minimize the force and friction applied to the skin.

A study to investigate patterns of temperature change in surgical wounds that are healing by primary intention found that during the first three days after surgery, temperatures rose in both the wounds themselves and their wider surroundings. From day 4 to day 8, temperatures in the wounds and surrounding tissue decreased gradually. After the stitches were removed on day 7, only the narrow zones of the incision site were warmer than the surroundings. The findings suggest that contact thermography may help in the early identification of a wound that is not healing according to expectations (Horzic, et al., 1996).

Pressure Ulcers:
- require dressings to maintain their physiologic integrity.
- require clean dressing rather than sterile in health care facilities AND in a home setting (USDHHS, 1994).
- normal saline is used to clean most ulcers, however mild cleaning agents that minimize irritation and dryness of skin can be used.
- hydrocolloid/alginate dressings have been found to help manage exudate, are easy to use, and comfortable for the patients (Barr, et al., 1995; Day, et al., 1995).

*Source: Used with permission from *New Mexico State University Department of Nursing Research-Based Skills Manual*, 1998, Las Cruces, NM.

practice on scientific knowledge. Because the credibility of the protocol procedure or policy depends on the validity of the research base, some clinical problems cannot be addressed by identifying a body of relevant research that can be transferred into practice because insufficient valid research is available. Also, although it may serve to provide clarifying information, science does not drive ethical decision-making, and a different frame of reference provides the appropriate rationale for action (Stetler et al., 1998).

● TOWARD EVIDENCE-BASED NURSING PRACTICE

Research utilization is a critical component of the broader process of evidence-based practice. Health care reform issues and the increasing focus on the delivery of effective health care services are the driving forces influencing not only medicine but nursing as well to demonstrate that they are evidence-based. Reference to evidence-based practice specific to nursing has been more common in the Canadian and English nursing literature and has only recently begun to appear in the American literature and at professional meetings. The Centre for Evidence-Based Nursing at the University of York in the United Kingdom co-edits the *Journal of Evidence-Based Nursing*, an international journal designed to provide access not only to nursing-related research but also to the most important evidence within nursing.

Historically, in the United States, evidence-based practice has been associated primarily with the clinical practice guidelines formulated by the Agency for Health Care Policy Research (AHCPR). Created at the federal level in 1989, the agency's primary goal is to enhance the quality, appropriateness, and effectiveness of health care services on a national basis. One of its functions has been to facilitate the development, periodic review, and updating of clinical practice guidelines designed to assist practitioners in preventing, diagnosing, and managing clinical conditions. Multidisciplinary panels comprising physicians, nurses, and other experts have conducted extensive literature searches related to the topic of the proposed guideline and have critically reviewed and synthesized the literature to evaluate empirical evidence and significant outcomes. Panel recommendations are based primarily on published scientific literature; when the scientific literature is incomplete or inconsistent in a particular area, recommendations reflect the professional judgment of panel members and consultants. The AHCPR has developed guidelines for acute pain management, urinary incontinence in adults, prediction and prevention of pressure ulcers in adults, and depression in primary care, among others. Patient-centered rather than provider-centered, these guidelines have been formulated with the goal of encouraging health care providers to change their practice behavior. "For nurses wanting to base their practice on scientific evidence, these guidelines provide a basis for reviewing nursing policies, procedures, and protocols related to these areas of care" (May-hew, 1993b, p. 336).

The guideline development panels were disbanded when the AHCPR ended its guideline program in the fall of 1996 and launched its Evidence-Based Practice Initiative, an initiative designed to develop evidence reports based on comprehensive reviews and rigorous analyses of relevant scientific evidence. The first evidence report (on colorectal cancer) was issued in January 1997.

What Constitutes Evidence-Based Practice?

It would be ideal to base clinical, educational, and administrative practice on the evidence of well-established research findings because this type of evidence "reflects verifiable, replicated facts and relationships that have been exposed to a stringent criteria of truth. . . In reality, however, the best evidence of well-established research findings often is not available to substantiate various decisions" (Stetler et al., 1998, p. 48). **Evidence-based practice** not only incorporates the use of well-established research findings but also goes beyond research utilization in incorporating other valid and relevant evidence as well:

> Evidence-based practice is essentially about using the best available evidence to ensure clinically effective and cost-effective treatment of patients, thereby increasing the proportion of clinical care shown by that evidence to be effective. Ideally, the evidence needs to be drawn from systematic research and detailed evaluations of health care interventions. However, it is also recognized that clinical expertise and patient preferences have a part to play. *(Gerrish & Clayton, 1998, p. 58)*

Stetler and colleagues (1998) have observed that the meaning of the term is not always clear, and offered the following summary definition:

> Evidence-based nursing deemphasizes ritual, isolated and unsystematic clinical experiences, ungrounded opinions and tradition as a basis for nursing practices . . .and stresses instead the use of research findings and, as appropriate, quality improvement data, other operational and evaluation data, the consensus of recognized experts and affirmed experience to substantiate practice. *(pp. 48–49)*

The present reality is that nurses are being urged more and more to identify evidence to justify their practice, and it is suggested that this is how they will be accepted as players within the evidence-based medicine/clinical effectiveness movement (Kitson, 1997).

We conclude this basic nursing research textbook with a final—and sobering—consideration that provides a clear mandate for the future of the nursing profession:

> A profession that fails to change its values and holds on to tradition and routine in the face of developing technologies, more knowledge, increased information and rising expectations, is a profession that is unlikely to survive in any recognizable form in the 21st century. *(Sullivan, 1998, p. 9)*

● SUMMARY

Conducting research and utilizing research are distinct yet complementary and interdependent processes; each is dependent on the other to further the development of a scientific basis for the practice of nursing. Even though knowledge seems to be expanding at a rapid rate, every discipline has a research–practice gap—that is, a major time lag between the scientific knowledge generated by research and its implementation in practice.

Barriers to research utilization fall into four major categories: those related to nurses' research values and skills, those related to limitations in the setting, those related to how the research itself is communicated, and those related to the quality of the research itself. Research utilization can be viewed as a collaborative effort on the part of the entire nursing profession—administrators, clinicians, educators, and researchers. Because research utilization must be based on the highest quality of research, a recurring theme in the nursing literature is the urgent need for more replication studies to build a stronger scientific basis for innovation.

Beginning in the 1970s, three large-scale research utilization projects received grant support from the Division of Nursing at the federal level. Each of these pioneering demonstration projects was designed to bridge the gap between the conduct of research and its use in clinical practice.

During the past 25 to 30 years, a number of research utilization models have been developed with the purpose of providing a process for bridging the gap between nursing research and nursing practice. Each of these models can be viewed as a form of prescriptive information that specifies the process by which research utilization should occur.

The research utilization process provides a step-by-step method that facilitates systematic movement from identifying a problem in need of a scientific basis through formulation and evaluation of research-based innovations in the practice setting.

Research utilization is a critical component of the broader process of evidence-based practice. Health care reform issues and the increasing focus on the delivery of effective health care services are the driving forces influencing not only medicine but nursing as well to demonstrate that they are evidence-based. Evidence-based practice not only incorporates the use of well-established research findings but also goes beyond research utilization in incorporating other valid and relevant evidence as well.

The following application activities should help you to evaluate your understanding of the material in this chapter.

REFERENCES

American Nurses Association. (1991). *Standards of clinical nursing practice.* Kansas City, MO: Author.

Baessler, C. A., Blumberg, M., & Cunningham, J. S. (1994). Medical-surgical nurses' utilization of research methods and products. *MedSurg Nursing, 2,* 113–121, 141.

Barnsteiner, J. H. (1996). Research-based practice. *Nursing Administration Quarterly, 20*(4), 52–58.

Brett, J. L. (1987). Use of nursing practice research findings. *Nursing Research, 36,* 344–349.

Coyle, L. A., & Sokop, A. G. (1990). Innovation adoption behavior among nurses. *Nursing Research, 3,* 176–180.

Crane, J. (1995). The future of research utilization. *Nursing Clinics of North America, 30,* 565–577.

Dracup, K. A., & Breu, C. S. (1978). Using nursing research findings to meet the needs of grieving spouses. *Nursing Research, 27,* 212–216.

Funk, S. G., Tornquist, E. M., & Champagne, M. T. (1995). Barriers and facilitators of research utilization. *Nursing Clinics of North America, 30,* 395–407.

Gerrish, K., & Clayton, J. (1998). Improving clinical effectiveness through an evidence-based approach: Meeting the challenge for nursing in the United Kingdom. *Nursing Administration Quarterly, 22*(4), 55–65.

Goode, C. J., Lovett, M. K., Hayes, J. E., & Butcher, L. A. (1987). Use of research-based knowledge in clinical practice. *Journal of Nursing Administration, 17*(12), 11–18.

Grady, P. A. (1998). Bringing research to life. *Applied Nursing Research, 11*(1), 1.

Horsley, J. A., Crane, J., Crabtree, M. K., & Wood, D. J. (1983). *Using research to improve nursing practice: A guide.* New York: Grune and Stratton.

Kajermo, K., Nordström, G., Krusebrandt, Å., & Björvell, H. (1998). Barriers to and facilitators of research utilization, as perceived by a group of registered nurses in Sweden. *Journal of Advanced Nursing, 27,* 798–807.

Ketefian, S. (1975). Application of selected research findings into nursing practice: A pilot study. *Nursing Research, 24,* 89–92.

Kirchoff, K. (1982). A diffusion survey of coronary precautions. *Nursing Research, 31,* 196–201.

Kitson, A. (1997). Using evidence to demonstrate the value of nursing. *Nursing Standard, 11*(28), 34–39.

Krueger, J., Nelson, A., & Wolanin, M. (1978). *Nursing research: Development, collaboration and utilization.* Germantown, PA: Aspen Systems.

Lindeman, C. A. (1975). Priorities in clinical nursing research. *Nursing Outlook, 23,* 693–698.

Mayhew, P. A. (1993a). The importance of the practicing nurse in nursing research. *MedSurg Nursing, 3,* 210–211.

Mayhew, P. A. (1993b). Overcoming barriers to research utilization with research-based practice guidelines. *MedSurg Nursing, 4,* 336–337.

Peugh, S., Betts, M., Hamlin, P., & Krause, B. (1998). Development of a research-based protocol for asthma management in elementary-school children (unpublished manuscript). Las Cruces, NM.

Rogers, E. M. (1983). *Diffusion of innovations.* New York: Free Press.

Stetler, C. B. (1994). Refinement of the Stetler/Marram model for application of research findings to practice. *Nursing Outlook, 42,* 15–25.

Stetler, C. B., Brunell, M., Giulano, K. K., Morsi, D., Prince, L., & Newell-Stokes, V. (1998). Evidence-based practice and the role of nursing leadership. *Journal of Nursing Administration, 28,* 45–53.

Sullivan, P. (1998). Developing evidence-based care in mental health nursing. *Nursing Standard Online, 12*(31).

Titler, M. G. (1997). Research utilization: Necessity or luxury? In J. C. McCloskey & H. K. Grace (Eds.), *Current issues in nursing* (pp. 104–117). St. Louis, MO: Mosby.

Tordoff, C. (1998). From research to practice: A review of the literature. *Nursing Standard Online, 12*(25).

White, J., Leske, J., & Pearcy, J. (1995). Models and process of research utilization. *Nursing Clinics of North America, 30*(3), 409–420.

BIBLIOGRAPHY AND SUGGESTED READINGS

Abdellah, F., & Levine, E. (1994). *Preparing nursing research for the 21st century.* New York: Springer.

Akinsanya, J. A. (1994). Making research useful to the practicing nurse. *Journal of Advanced Nursing, 19,* 174–179.

Beck, C. T. (1994). Replication strategies for nursing research. *Image, 26*(3), 191–194.

Beyea, S. C., & Nicoll, L. H. (1998). Developing clinical practice guidelines as an approach to evidence-based practice. *AORN Journal, 67*(5), 1037–1038.

Bueno, M. M. (1998). Promoting nursing research through newsletters. *Applied Nursing Research, 11*(1), 41–44.

Closs, S. J., & Cheater, F. M. (1994). Utilization of nursing research, culture, interest, and support. *Journal of Advanced Nursing, 19*, 762–773.

Crane, J. (1985). Using research in practice: Research utilization nursing models. *Western Journal of Nursing Research, 7*, 494–497.

Dunn, V., Crichton, N., Roe, B., Seers, K., & Williams, K. (1998). Using research for practice: A UK experience of the Barriers Scale. *Journal of Advanced Nursing, 26*, 1203–1210.

Gennaro, S. (1994). Research utilization: An overview. *JOGN, 4*, 313–319.

Good, C. J. (1995). Evaluation of research-based nursing practice. *Nursing Clinics of North America, 30*(3), 421–428.

Gray, J. A. M. (1997). *Evidence-based healthcare*. New York: Livingston.

Haines, A., & Jones, R. (1994). Implementing findings of research. *British Medical Journal, 308*, 1488–1492.

Hayes, P. (1997). Evidence-based practice. *Clinical Nursing Research, 5*(2), 123.

Hicks, C. (1995). The shortfall in published research: A study of nurses' research and publication activities. *Journal of Advanced Nursing, 23*, 594–604.

Hicks, C. (1996). A study of nurses' attitudes towards research: A factor analytic approach. *Journal of Advanced Nursing, 23*, 373–379.

Horn Video Productions. (1996). *Critiquing research for use in nursing practice* [CD-ROM]. Ida Grove, IA.

Kessenich, C. R., Guyatt, G. H., & DiCenso, A. (1997). Teaching nursing students evidence-based nursing. *Nurse Educator, 22*(6), 25–29.

Kitson, A. (1997). Using evidence to demonstrate the value of nursing. *Nursing Standard, 11*(2), 34–39.

Lacey, E. A. (1994). Research utilization in nursing practice: A pilot study. *Journal of Advanced Nursing, 19*, 987–995.

Larson, L. L., & Turston, N. M. (1997). Research utilization: Development of a central venous catheter procedure. *Applied Nursing Research, 10*(7), 44–51.

McGuire, D., & Harwood, K. (1996). Research interpretation, utilization, and conduct. In A. Harmic, J. Spross, & C. Hanson (Eds.), *Advanced nursing practice: An integrative approach*. Philadelphia: Saunders.

Mitchell, G. J. (1997). Questioning evidence-based practice for nursing. *Nursing Science Quarterly, 10*(4), 154–155.

Moch, S. D., Robie, D. E., Bauer, K. C., Pederson, A., Bowe, S., & Shadick, K. (1997). Linking research and practice through discussion. *Image, 29*(2), 189–191.

Moore, P. A. (1995). The utilization of research in practice. *Professional Nurse, 10*(8), 536–537.

Mulhall, A. (1995). Nursing research: Our world or theirs? *Journal of Advanced Nursing, 25*, 969–976.

Mulhall, A. (1995). Nursing research: What difference does it make? *Journal of Advanced Nursing, 21*, 576–583.

Nelson, D. (1995). Research into research practice. *Accident and Emergency Nursing, 3*, 184–189.

Oldnall, A. S. (1995). Nursing as an emerging academic discipline. *Journal of Advanced Nursing, 21*, 605–612.

Paladichuk, A. (1997). Bridging the research–practice gap. *Critical Care Nurse, 17*(1), 80–85.

Pearcey, P. A. (1995). Achieving research-based nursing practice. *Journal of Advanced Nursing, 22*, 33–39.

Radjenovic, D., & Chally, P. S. (1998). Research utilization by undergraduate students. *Nurse Educator, 23*(2), 26–28.

Regan, J. A. (1998). Will current clinical initiatives encourage and facilitate practitioners to use evidence-based practice for the benefit of their clients? *Journal of Clinical Nursing, 7*(3), 244–250.

Robinson, A. (1995). Research, practice and the Cochrane collaboration. *Canadian Medical Association Journal, 152*(6), 883–889.

Robinson, K. R. (1997). You + research = nursing practice program. *Western Journal of Nursing Research, 19*(2), 265–269.

Rogers, S. (1994). An exploratory study of research utilization by nurses in general medical and surgical wards. *Journal of Advanced Nursing, 20*, 904–911.

Shively, M., Riegel, B., Waterhouse, D., Burns, D., Templing, K., & Tomason, T. (1997). Testing a community-level research utilization intervention. *Applied Nursing Research, 10*(3), 121–127.

Stetler, C. B., Morsi, D., Rucki, S., et al. (1998). Utilization-focused integrative reviews in a nursing service. *Applied Nursing Research, 11*(4), 195–206.

U. S. Dept. of Health and Human Services, Agency for Health Care Policy and Research. (1995). *Using clinical practice guidelines to evaluate quality of care.* Washington, DC: Author (AHCPR Pub. No. 95-0046).

Warren, J. J., & Heerman, J. A. (1998). The research nurse intern program. *Journal of Nursing Administration, 28*(11), 39–45.

SELECTED REFERENCES FOR RESEARCH-BASED PROTOCOL

American Lung Association. (1998). *Open airways for schools program.* American Lung Association.

Asthma Information Center. (1997). Helping city children control asthma. *Journal of the American Medical Association, 277,* 1503–1504.

Caldwell, C. (1997). Management of acute asthma in children. *Emergency Nurse, 5*(7), 33–39.

Carruthers, P., Ebbutt, A. F., & Barnes, G. (1995). Teachers' knowledge of asthma and asthma management in primary schools. *Health Education Journal, 54*(1), 28–36.

Gleeson, C. (1994). Partnership in asthma care: The role of the school nurse. *Health Visitor, 67*(7), 228–229.

Gleeson, C. (1995). Assessing children's knowledge of asthma. *Professional Nurse, 10*(8), 517–521.

Ladebauche, P. (1997). Managing asthma: A growth and development approach. *Pediatric Nursing, 23*(1), 37–44.

National Institutes of Health. (1995). *Nurses: Partners in asthma care* (NIH Publication no. 95-3308). Washington, DC: U.S. Government Printing Office.

National Institutes of Health. (1997). *Expert panel report 2, Guidelines for the diagnosis and management of asthma* (NIH Publication no. 97-405). Washington, DC: U.S. Government Printing Office.

Sly, P., Cahill, P., Willet, K., & Burton, P. (1994). Accuracy of peak flow meters in indicating changes in lung function in children with asthma. *British Medical Journal, 308,* 572–574.

Schneider, S. L., Richard, M., Huss, K., et al. (1997). Moving health care education into the community. *Nursing Management, 28*(9), 40–43.

SELECTED REFERENCES FOR RESEARCH-BASED NURSING PROCEDURE

Barr, J. E. (1995). Principles of wound cleansing. *Ostomy Wound Management, 41*(7A), 5S–50S.

Barr, J. E., Day, A. L., Weaver, V. A., & Taler, G. M. (1995). Assessing clinical efficacy of a hydrocolloid/alginate dressing on full-thickness pressure ulcers. *Ostomy Wound Management, 41*(3), 28–40.

Day, A., Dombranski, S., Farkas, C., et al. (1995). Managing sacral pressure ulcers with hydrocolloid dressings: Results of a controlled, clinical study. *Ostomy Wound Management, 41*(2), 52–65.

Gates, J. L., & Holloway, G. (1992). A comparison of wound environments. *Ostomy Wound Management, 38*(8), 34–37.

Horzic, M., Bunoza, D., & Maric, K. (1996). Contact thermography in a study of primary healing of surgical wounds. *Ostomy Wound Management, 42*(1), 36–44.

Stotts, N. A., Barbour, S., Griggs, K., et al. (1997). Sterile versus clean technique in postoperative wound care of patients with open surgical wounds: A pilot study. *Journal of Wound, Ostomy, and Continence Nursing, 24*(1), 10–18.

U.S. Department of Health and Human Services. (1985). *Guideline for prevention of surgical wound infections* (PB 85-0923403). Atlanta, GA: Centers for Disease Control.

U.S. Department of Health and Human Services. (1994). *Pressure ulcer treatment* (AHCPR Publication No. 95-0653). Rockville, MD: Agency for Health Care Policy and Research.

Walker, D. (1996). Choosing the correct wound dressing. *American Journal of Nursing* [on-line]. Available at: http://www.ajn.org/ajn/1996/6.9

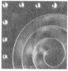

APPLICATION ACTIVITIES

1. Explain the relationship between conducting research and utilizing research in practice.

2. Discuss the relationship between research utilization and evidence-based nursing practice.

3. List at least three barriers to using research in practice that have been perceived by nurses.

4. Discuss at least three strategies that could be employed to facilitate research utilization in the practice setting.

5. It has been stated in the literature that research utilization is an organizational responsibility rather than the responsibility of the individual nurse. Do you agree or disagree with this statement? Defend your answer.

6. Explore one of your local health care agencies and describe the extent to which the nurses are using research to direct their practice.

7. Define the following terms:

   a. Research-based document

   b. Innovation

   c. Diffusion

   d. Evidence-based practice

8. Use the worksheet in Box 13-1 to summarize the pertinent information from each of the three studies you have already evaluated. List the findings from each study that could provide a research base to guide practice in the area of the clinical nursing problem you have identified. Determine whether there is a sufficient and relevant research base that could guide practice. If so, describe this research base. If not, you may need to locate additional studies that could strengthen the research base. Discuss your ideas about how you would develop a research-based protocol or procedure to address your nursing problem. Use the research utilization process to develop a research-based protocol or procedure.

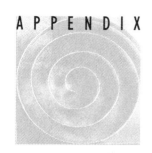

APPENDIX A

Example of a Quantitative Research Proposal

Compliance With Universal Precautions in Pediatric Settings

Jacquelyn C. Williams

INTRODUCTION AND STATEMENT OF THE PROBLEM
LITERATURE REVIEW
CONCEPTUAL FRAMEWORK
PURPOSE OF THE STUDY
DEFINITION OF TERMS
PLAN FOR DATA COLLECTION
PLAN FOR DATA ANALYSIS
LIMITATIONS OF THE STUDY
REFERENCES

● INTRODUCTION AND STATEMENT OF THE PROBLEM

Bloodborne pathogens, particularly human immunodeficiency virus (HIV) and hepatitis B (HBV), have been identified as significant threats to health care workers. To counter this threat consistently, the Occupational Safety and Health Administration (OSHA) issued definitive guidelines on Universal Precautions (UP) in 1991, delineating the responsibilities of both the employer and health care worker in avoiding exposure to body fluids which could serve as a vector for transmission of bloodborne diseases (Centers for Disease Control [CDC], 1997; OSHA, 1991). Employers were mandated to provide several critical elements: (1) education of employees in the use of UP, (2) provision of the protective equipment needed to implement the system, (3) engineering and work practice controls, and (4) follow-up (OSHA, 1991).

Health care workers (HCWs), however, have frequently failed to comply with UP guidelines (Gershon et al., 1995; Gould, Wilson-Barnett, & Ream, 1996; Hanrahan & Reutter, 1997; Khuri-Bulos et al., 1997; Ramsey & Glenn, 1996; Ramsey, McConnell, Palmer, & Glenn, 1996; Sulzbach-Hoke, 1996). Nurses have figured prominently in the concern about this phenomenon since nurses constitute the largest single group of HCWs who have experienced seroconversion to HIV and are significantly represented in the frightening numbers of HCWs who are infected with HBV and HCV (hepatitis C virus) annually (CDC [1996]; Hanrahan & Reutter; Sulzbach-Hoke). Studies conducted in specialized and general areas of clinical practice have yielded similar results and identified various reasons for noncompliance with UP (Ramsey & Glenn; Ramsey, McConnell, Palmer, & Glenn; Sulzbach-Hoke). A large body of evidence has accumulated about the role and occurrence of sharps injury as the major risk for acquiring bloodborne disease in health occupations, with nurses reporting the highest injury rate of all HCWs (Jagger, 1994, 1996; Patel & Tignor, 1997; Ramsey, McConnell, Palmer, & Glenn; Roy & Robillard, 1995).

After several years of involvement with teaching UP in and out of the hospital setting, the researcher became interested in observing nurses involved with pediatric patients, focusing in particular on the decreased attention to UP that is exhibited when nurses work with children in a general hospital setting. Informal inquiry into this observation indicated that the nurses were often sacrificing the safety of UP in an effort to increase efficiency because of their anxiety and desire to do procedures, such as venipuncture, as expediently as possible.

Although some studies have focused on practice areas where children may be seen, there is little data found in the literature that applies specifically to pediatric practice settings. Few investigators focused on ways the special problems of pediatric practice may influence risk-taking by nurses in this regard. Patel and Tignor (1997) classified pediatric areas as practice ". . . under difficult circumstances that resulted in high sharps injury rates for staff" (p. 77). In light of the fact that the threat of pathogens will continue and expand in all populations, evaluation of compliance rates as an important facet of monitoring the effectiveness of employee education and engineering/work practice controls is important to nursing administration, infection control, employee health, and education departments in health care organizations (Hanrahan & Reutter; Sulzbach-Hoke). The questions posed for this study are: (1) What are the rates of compliance to UP by registered nurses working with pediatric populations in hospital settings, and (2) How are the ages of the children, and the size and type of hospital related to compliance?

● LITERATURE REVIEW

In the recommendations of the CDC and OSHA, UP represents the minimal actions that can be taken by employers and HCWs to avoid exposure to bloodborne pathogens (CDC, 1997; OSHA, 1991). Compliance with UP, assuming that HCWs have knowledge of the system and are equipped with an adequate supply and quality of barrier equipment and engineering controls, is the responsibility of the individual. In 1996 the CDC replaced the term "universal precautions" with the term "standard precautions" in the release of new patient isolation guidelines that include the protection of HCWs from exposure to all contagion (CDC, 1996). However, the OSHA standards for control of exposure to bloodborne pathogens have not been altered at this point to reflect this change in nomenclature.

Studies in the past decade of HCWs, including nurses, can be grouped into two types: (1) those reporting on overall compliance rates and (2) those focusing on specific portions of UP (sharps usage, for example). In 1991 Gauthier, Turner, Langley, Neil, and Rush noted only one study on compliance rates in which more than two of the four aspects of UP protocols (barrier precautions, handwashing, handling of sharp instruments, and avoidance of unprotected mouth-to-mouth resuscitation) were assessed simultaneously. A survey of the literature since that date found only two new studies (Ramsey, McConnell, Palmer, & Glenn; Wright, Turner, & Daffin, 1997). Basically, two types of tools have been used by researchers to judge compliance rates: direct observation and retrospective, self-report surveys.

Building on the work done by investigators in the 1980's and early 1990's, several researchers have reassessed compliance with various facets of UP. Ramsey, McConnell, Palmer, and Glenn measured compliance of 140 nurses in Tennessee before and after the OSHA mandate in 1992. While they found an increase in UP use, there was still significant noncompliance with precautions. London researchers found hand decontamination performed only 49.85% of the time even after activities likely to result in heavy bacterial or viral contamination (Gould, Wilson-Barnett, & Ream). Glove use has increased and most researchers find gloves used appropriately but no relationship between the frequency or appropriateness of hand decontamination and glove use (Gould, Wilson-Barnett, & Ream; Gershon et al.). Ramsey and Glenn (1996), using evidence from several earlier studies for comparison, found continuation of a trend toward severe underreporting of exposures. Only 4.1% of 143 nurses completing a self-report survey had reported exposures, showing the most consistent concern for needle injuries. Body fluid splashes, by far the most common exposure, were the least likely to be reported. Although infection has been transmitted occupationally through mucous membrane and nonintact skin, parenteral exposure carries the greatest risk, resulting in epidemiological studies in recent years that focus on exposure to sharps injury (CDC, 1997; Jagger, 1994, 1996). The international nature of the problem is illustrated by the development of formal monitoring systems in numerous countries (Khuri-Bulos et al.; Patel & Tignor; Danchaivijitr, Tangtrakool, Chokloikaew, & Thamlikitkul, 1997; Puro, Petrosillo, & Ippolito, 1995).

The purposes for which studies on UP compliance are conducted reveal the complexity of the problem. Many studies attempt to identify how knowledge levels were related to behaviors (Gershon et al.; Gould, Wilson-Barnett, & Ream; Hanrahan & Reutter; Ramsey & Glenn; Sulzbach-Hoke; Wright, Turner, & Daffin). A second area of focus is identification of situations where exposure most often occurs so that education, institutional policy, and the engineering and provision of equipment could be altered to counter the threat (Gould, Wilson-Barnett, & Ream; Hanrahan & Reutter; Jagger, 1994, 1996; Patel & Tignor; Roy & Robillard).

Throughout the literature review there was widespread consensus that nurses generally have the knowledge to understand UP compliance and are choosing not to do so for a variety of poorly understood reasons. Researchers have identified some trends in reasons for noncompliance which involve a complex relationship between systems problems and personal risk taking (Gershon et al.; Hanrahan & Reutter; Ramsey & Glenn; Sulzbach-Hoke).

● CONCEPTUAL FRAMEWORK

In viewing the issue of nurses' compliance with UP, it is obvious that the problem has far-reaching implications. The employer is responsible for the training, supervision, and monitoring of adherence to UP. Institutional compliance with OSHA requirements has not been matched by compliance rates from individuals. Imogene King's open systems framework and its resultant theory of goal attainment are chosen for this study as a systematic way to analyze and evaluate UP compliance.

The open systems framework is a model envisioning all human relations, including nursing, as occurring within three interacting systems—personal, interpersonal, and social (King, 1995a). Certain key concepts occur in each of these systems.

The Personal System includes perception, self, growth and development, body image, space, and time. The Interpersonal System includes interaction, communication, transaction, role, stress, and coping. The Social System contains the social roles, the practices and the behaviors that are developed to maintain values; these include organization, authority, power, status, and decision making. By extension, knowledge of UP protocols resides within the personal system of the individual nurse, usage in a patient care situation occurs on an interpersonal level, and accountability for compliance is a function of the social system, such as a hospital, or more globally, the federal government through OSHA regulations.

King's application of the interacting systems model is represented by the goal attainment theory (King, 1995b). The overall goal of nursing is to assist individuals to maintain a state of health. Many of the problems revolving around the issues of bloodborne pathogens can be viewed more clearly in this context. If it were possible for patients and nurses to know one another's infection status, for example, bloodborne pathogens could be treated the same as other forms of contagion. But the peculiarities of the infection and the requirement of confidentiality make reliable identification of carriers of the infections impossible. The nurse is unable to *perceive* which individuals represent true risks because this vital bit of knowledge cannot be *communicated* between the nurse and patient in most situations. The concept of UP has been chosen to replace that knowledge. Operating on the assumption that any client or any care giver may be carrying a bloodborne disease, UP is utilized in all physical *transactions*, whether disease is actually present or not, to attain the goal of preventing transmission of the bloodborne disease.

Within the social system of a health care institution, the employer has a mandated ethical and fiscal responsibility to both clients and employees as a result of legal precedents and such global social agencies as OSHA. The hospital *perceives* the nurse to be at risk for exposure to bloodborne pathogens, *communicates* expectations, encourages feedback and information, provides resources, and oversees the mutual expectation of guarding the nurse and client alike against exposure.

This research proposal represents only a small segment of the complicated processes of monitoring UP compliance. It is an attempt to document how well nurses are complying with UP in a specific setting with a subset of the population in the social system of hospitals in the southwestern part of the United States. The information obtained from this study can be evaluated with the open systems framework, and that system can be used to suggest areas for further evaluation or action.

The subject of motivating nurses to follow UP guidelines may also be analyzed in better perspective when viewed within the interacting systems framework. For example, nurses indicated a need for institutions to get more input from them in making and carrying out policies in regard to many aspects of bloodborne disease policies and procedures (Gershon et al.; Ramsey, McConnell, Palmer, & Glenn; Sulzbach-Hoke). Viewed in the open systems framework, this represents a failure in the interpersonal realm of *communication* which may result in the social system *making decisions* which are not best suited for attaining the goal of providing the means and incentive for nurses to avoid exposure to bloodborne pathogens. "Reminder" campaigns were found to have transitory, rather than permanent, effects on compliance (Sulzbach-Hoke). Researchers also noted that knowledge alone was a poor predictor of compliance to UP. Studies indicated that situational factors have great influence on compliance rates and that mandated compliance policies may be more productive in achieving the goal of increased compliance than general knowledge (Gershon et al.; Gould, Wilson-Barnett, & Ream; Ramsey, McConnell, Palmer, & Glenn; Sulzbach-Hoke).

● PURPOSE OF THE STUDY

The purpose of this study is to describe the rates of compliance to UP by registered nurses working with pediatric populations in two different general hospitals and two different pediatric hospitals and to analyze how the age of the child may have an impact on compliance in these settings. It is important to know if some of the special challenges of working with pediatric age groups (such as difficult IV starts, the high acuity of hospitalized children, etc.) will be reflected in compliance rates. There is little published data on the trends for the southwestern United States; therefore this study can add to the body of knowledge concerning UP protocols.

● DEFINITION OF TERMS

The following definitions will be used:

- *Universal Precautions (UP)*—a system approved by the Centers for Disease Control which includes avoidance of exposure to blood and body fluids which can harbor hepatitis B and human immunodeficiency viruses. Fluids which always require UP are blood, semen, vaginal secretions, cerebral spinal, pleural, peritoneal, pericardial, synovial, and amniotic fluids. Fluids of mucous membranes are considered to require UP.
- *Compliance*—appropriate use of barrier equipment, handwashing, disposal of sharps, and resuscitation and ventilation devices to avoid exposure of the nurse to blood or body fluids of clients as outlined by UP.
- *Opportunity for compliance*—any action or interaction of the nurse in a client care situation which could result in an exposure and during which UP should be used as judged by a trained observer.
- *Exposure*—transfer of blood, or any of the body fluids listed under the definition of UP, into the blood stream, onto mucous membranes, or onto the nonintact skin of a nurse.
- *Pediatric patient*—a client age 18 years or younger.
- *General hospital*—one treating a wide range of ages and conditions and including pediatric services with at least one medical/surgical inpatient unit.
- *Pediatric hospital*—hospital in which all clients fall into the pediatric population.

● PLAN FOR DATA COLLECTION

This study will be conducted at four different hospitals in the southwestern United States and will include one or more pediatric medical/surgical units in each of the four hospitals. Medical/surgical units will be included due to the relatively high acuity seen there and because they can be found in both large and small hospitals. Two of the hospitals will be general hospitals with pediatric services and two will be pediatric hospitals. One general and one pediatric hospital will be approximately 250 beds, while the other general hospital and pediatric hospital will be greater than 500 beds.

The target population will be all registered nurses on pediatric medical/surgical units observed in their practice setting with pediatric clients in the four different hospitals selected for the study. The sample will consist of thirty registered nurses from each of the four hospitals and will be chosen by using a random numbers table where staffs are large enough to make observing all of them prohibitive.

The research team will include a project coordinator and individuals iden-tified by the infection control departments of the four hospitals in the study who will be trained to collect the observational data.

An adapted version of The Universal Precautions Assessment Tool (UPAT) devised by Dorothy Gauthier and colleagues at the University of Alabama at Birmingham School of Nursing will be used to collect the data. The tool is designed to collect data related to compliance with the four major compo-nents of UP—handwashing, barrier precautions, disposal of sharps, and use of resuscitation/ventilation devices. With permission of Dr. Gauthier, the cate-gory of "disposal sharps" is altered to reflect current knowledge that engi-neering and work practice controls require more than proper handling of sharps. It also requires selection of the safest available equipment for par-enteral treatments, such as needleless systems. Therefore, the selection of the most appropriate sharps device is considered an opportunity for compliance and an additional scoring category (D. K. Gauthier, personal communication, May 26, 1998). The UPAT is a one-page tool on which an observer records whether or not the proper procedure is followed by the nurse by marking the corresponding "yes" or "no" space on the checklist. The individual's score is obtained as a percentage of correct responses per number of opportunities noted for complying with UP while working with patients. A separate section records demographic data and will be modified from the original tool to add the age of the child (in months) in addition to the hospital unit, observation times, nurse code, observer initials, and final score. One score sheet per child will be used. Two observers will simultaneously score the same nurse caring for a child.

The UPAT can be used to assess compliance both individually and collec-tively. The authors of the tool established its consensual validity by submitting it for review to three experts in infection control during their two pilot stud-ies (Gauthier, Turner, Langley, Neil, & Rush, 1991). It is described as being able to analyze, by category, the strengths and weaknesses of personnel in compliance with UP. By adding space for the age of patient and category of hospital, the data can be further compared for these variables. Anonymity of both the nurse and patient will be preserved by using only codes on the score sheets.

Observers will be trained in the use of the instrument by the researcher. The original authors conducted tests of interrater reliability in two pilot tests by having observers simultaneously rate the same nurses and using an intra-class correlation coefficient to compare the scoring. The tool was found to have an interrater reliability score within the 95% confidence limits (Gauthier, Turner, Langley, Neil, & Rush). Interrater reliability scores will be calculated in the same way for this study.

Observers will spend 45 to 60 minutes either continuously or intermit-tently observing each of the study subjects during the nurses' regular shifts. To accustom the staff to the presence of the observers, members of the research team will spend some time on the unit in other infection control activities prior to beginning use of the UPAT. Because the hospitals have an obligation to monitor compliance to UP throughout their facility, individual informed consent will not be obtained. Gauthier et al. tested this instrument under these conditions by informing subjects prior to observations that the observers were noting either "patient care" or "nursing activities" and that the results were to be used in a study. The same information will be provided to the subjects of this study.

● PLAN FOR DATA ANALYSIS

The UPAT yields a series of compliance scores. Since there is an ideal individual level of compliance with UP (100%), the compliance scores for each subject will be expressed as percentages (e.g., nurse was observed to comply with UP 75% of the time). It will provide a score for each major category of UP (handwashing, use of barrier precautions, handling of sharps, and use of resuscitation/ventilation devices) as well as an overall score. The raw scores will be used in the statistical analysis. The chi-squared statistic will be used to determine if there are statistically significant differences in nurses' compliance with UP based on hospital setting and age of the child. The UPAT will also allow a comparison of compliance rates within the categories of UP itself. For example, handwashing use can be analyzed separately from the other three elements of UP. Table A-1 shows a sample (dummy) table.

King's open systems framework and its resultant theory of goal attainment will be used to provide a systematic analysis and evaluation of UP compliance.

● LIMITATIONS OF THE STUDY

The UPAT is a relatively new tool that has both advantages and limitations. One strength is its concise assessment of all the categories of UP. It avoids the

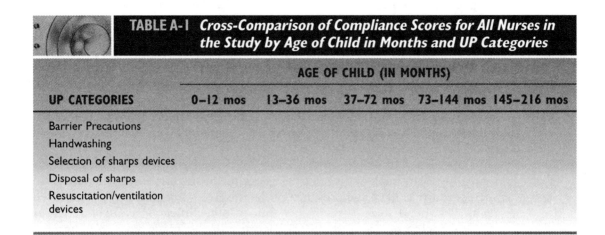

TABLE A-1 *Cross-Comparison of Compliance Scores for All Nurses in the Study by Age of Child in Months and UP Categories*					
	AGE OF CHILD (IN MONTHS)				
UP CATEGORIES	**0–12 mos**	**13–36 mos**	**37–72 mos**	**73–144 mos**	**145–216 mos**
Barrier Precautions					
Handwashing					
Selection of sharps devices					
Disposal of sharps					
Resuscitation/ventilation devices					

bias of self-reporting tools which have been associated with significant underreporting due to lack of awareness and poor recall over a period of time (Ramsey & Glenn).

This study has several limitations. The most significant is the Hawthorne effect, as all subjects will be aware they are being observed. Having members of the research team come from within the hospital and spend some preliminary time on the target unit can lessen but not eliminate this effect. Another limitation is that scoring will rely on the judgment of the observer. For example, CDC guidelines advise glove usage for phlebotomy when the phlebotomist perceives a risk to blood exposure to be probable. The authors of the UPAT suggest research teams will need to confer during the training phase to agree on ground rules for such situations to control for this possibility. A final limitation is that grouping the data for the proposed analyses (such as age group comparisons) may result in decreased cell sizes necessary for statistical testing and may affect determination of statistical significance.

REFERENCES

Centers for Disease Control. (1996). Hospital infection control practices advisory committee. Washington, DC: Author.

Centers for Disease Control. (1997). Guideline for infection control in health care personnel: Draft of second edition. Federal Register, 62 (pp. 47275–47327). Washington, DC: Author.

Danchaivijitr, S., Tangtrakool, T., Chokloikaew, S., & Thamlikitkul, V. (1997). Universal precautions: Costs for protective equipment. *American Journal of Infection Control, 25*(1), 44–50.

Gauthier, D. K., Turner, J. G., Langley, L. G., Neil, C. J., & Rush, P. L. (1991). Monitoring universal precautions: A new assessment tool. *Infection Control and Hospital Epidemiology, 12*(10), 597–601.

Gershon, R. M., Vlahov, D., Fleknor, S. A., Vesley, D., Johnson, P. C., & Delcios, L. R. (1995). Compliance with universal precautions among health care workers at three regional hospitals. *American Journal of Infection Control, 23*(4), 225–235.

Gould, B., Wilson-Barnett, J., & Ream, D. (1996). Nurses' infection-control practice: Hand decontamination, the use of gloves and sharp instruments. *International Journal of Nursing Studies, 33*(2), 143–160.

Hanrahan, A., & Reutter, L. (1997). A critical review of the literature on sharps injuries: Epidemiology, management of exposures and prevention. *Journal of Advanced Nursing, 25,* 144–154.

Hospital Infection Control Practices Advisory Committee, Centers for Disease Control. (1996). Guidelines for isolation precautions in hospitals. *Infection Control and Hospital Epidemiology, 16,* 53–80.

Jagger, J. (1994). Risky procedure, risky device, risky job. *Advances in Exposure Prevention, 1*(1), 4–6.

Jagger, J. (1996). Reducing occupational exposures to bloodborne pathogens: Where do we stand a decade later? *American Journal of Infection Control, 25,* 22–24.

Khuri-Bulos, N. A., Toukan, A., Mahafzah, A., Adham, M. A., Faori, I., Khader, I. A., & Rumeileh, Z. I. (1997). Epidemiology of needlestick and sharp injuries at a university hospital in a developing country: A 3-year prospective study at the Jordan University Hospital, 1993–1995. *American Journal of Infection Control, 25*(4), 322–329.

King, I. M. (1995a). A systems framework for nursing. In M. A. Frey & C. L. Sieloff (Eds.), *Advancing King's systems framework and theory of nursing* (pp. 14–21). Thousand Oaks, CA: Sage.

King, I. M. (1995b). The theory of goal attainment. In M. A. Frey & C. L. Sieloff (Eds.), *Advancing King's systems framework and theory of nursing* (pp. 23–32). Thousand Oaks, CA: Sage.

Occupational Safety and Health Administration. (1991). Occupational exposure to bloodborne pathogens: Final rule. *Federal Register, 56* (pp. 64004–64174). Washington, DC: Author.

Patel, N., & Tignor, G. H. (1997). Device-specific sharps injury and usage rates: an analysis by hospital department. *American Journal of Infection Control, 25*(2), 77–84.

Puro, V., Petrosillo, N., & Ippolito, G. (1995). Risk of hepatitis C seroconversion after occupational exposures in health care workers. *American Journal of Infection Control, 25*(5), 273–277.

Ramsey, P. W., & Glenn, L. L. (1996). Nurses' body fluid exposure reporting, HIV testing and hepatitis B vaccination rates before and after implementing universal precautions regulations. *AAOHN Journal, 44*(3), 129–137.

Ramsey, P. W., McConnell, P., Palmer, B. H., & Glenn, L. L. (1996). Nurses' compliance with universal precautions before and after implementation of OSHA regulations. *Clinical Nurse Specialist, 10*(5), 234–239.

Roy, E., & Robillard, P. (1995) Underreporting of accidental exposures to blood and other body fluids in health care settings: An alarming situation [abstract]. *Advances in Exposure Prevention, 1*(4), 11.

Sulzbach-Hoke, L. M. (1996). Risk taking by health care workers. *Clinical Nurse Specialist, 10*(1), 30–37.

Wright, B. J., Turner, J. G., & Daffin, P. (1997). Effectiveness of computer-assisted instruction in increasing the rate of universal precautions-related behaviors. *American Journal of Infection Control, 25*(5), 426–429.

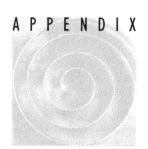

APPENDIX B

Example of a Qualitative Research Proposal

Homeless Persons With AIDS Living in a Congregate Facility: An Ethnographic Study

Suzan E. Norman Jaffe

● INTRODUCTION AND STATEMENT OF THE PROBLEM

Acquired immunodeficiency syndrome (AIDS) is now the leading cause of death in the United States in men under 45 years of age. It is reported that over 600,000 persons in the United States have been diagnosed as having AIDS. Nearly half of these persons with AIDS (PWAs) have died (Centers for Disease Control, 1998).

Most PWAs are not hospitalized until an AIDS-related infection with serious physical or psychological debilitation necessitates admission. As such, most PWAs live at home, alone, with friends or family (Kadushin, 1996). The financial burden to PWAs is often unmanageable. It can be devastating to someone who, prior to diagnosis, had inadequate insurance coverage. For PWAs without insurance or family support, the ramifications of having AIDS are overwhelming and can result in one's becoming homeless.

Even though there has been some funding for housing for PWAs, there are not enough shelters or congregate living facilities in the United States that offer food and shelter for homeless PWAs (Sabados, 1997; Takahashi, 1997). Having AIDS is saturated with its own unique set of physical, psychological, and social puzzles. Being homeless is accompanied by a multitude of problems. Being a homeless PWA is a contemporary condition, and the needs of this group have not been clearly identified.

There are over 5 million homeless in the United States. The typical homeless person has a high school education, a family to support, a drug and/or alcohol problem, and nowhere to turn for help. There are thousands of individuals who, despite their "homelessness," do not fit the stereotypical "skid row" street bums. Many are families headed by single women (Clarke, Williams, Percy, & Kim, 1995). A large percentage suffer from untreated psychiatric illnesses or have untreated drug and alcohol addictions (U.S. Department of Housing and Urban Development and U.S. Department of Health and Human Services, 1996; Waterson, 1997). It is estimated that between 2.5 and 15 percent of the homeless have AIDS (Regional Task Force on Homelessness, 1997; Seattle-King County, WA, Dept. of Public Health, 1997).

Despite the apparent interest and the abundance of published information on and about PWAs and homelessness, the literature has focused on the person either caring for PWAs or on those persons living with PWAs. Literature describing what it is like to be a homeless PWA from the PWA's perspective is lacking, but is a necessary first step in addressing the needs and planning appropriate interventions for this growing population.

● LITERATURE REVIEW

The literature describes HIV-infected individuals from a multiplicity of ethnic cultures and subcultures within these ethnic groups. Even though issues pertaining to specific cultural groups are mentioned, the predominant discussion and source of knowledge is not from an emic perspective (that of the participant). For example, what it is like to live in the United States as a black American male intravenous drug user may change dramatically once this male becomes infected with HIV or is labeled as having AIDS. The cultural rules and expected behaviors may be significantly transformed. How this individual perceives his world may also be modified.

Physicians' attitudes towards AIDS patients have been examined in the literature with the conclusion that willingness to treat PWAs was related to the physician's attitudes toward social stigma, homophobia and fear of infection (Carter, Lantos, and Hughes, 1996; Fournier, Baldor, Warfield, & Frazier, 1997). Caregivers of children with AIDS also face the problems of "isolation, shame, anger, stigmatization, ostracism" (Hansell et al., 1998, p. 79). Discussions of AIDS and treatments for HIV have often been politicized (Epstein, 1996).

Freidson (1988) noted that individuals with sexually transmitted diseases were often held in lower respect by medical professionals. The attitude of health care workers has reinforced the stigma of AIDS, with the result that high-risk groups (regardless of their seropositivity status) are even further feared by society. If an illness is discredited by the medical (professional) community, there appears to be more likelihood of stigmatization of the affected persons.

Almost all aspects of AIDS can be considered a social phenomenon. The characterization of high-risk individuals as being primarily the homosexual and drug addict groups made AIDS a stigmatized disease almost immediately. The uncertainties of AIDS are endless, and being labeled as an HIV-infected individual or a PWA may be an obstacle to social interaction, employment, and insurance qualification. As such, the positive characteristics of an individual may be ignored.

Not since the plagues of the sixteenth century and the views of syphilis during the seventeenth century has a disease earned so much social consequence. The social response to AIDS has been such that even highly educated health care professionals interpret the disease as a punishment for social and sexual deviance (Danziger, 1996). In twentieth-century America, AIDS has clearly been related to certain types of antisocial behavior. Fear generated by the uncertainties of AIDS is a common emotional response of all groups. Children with AIDS made headlines and were banned from attending public school. Headlines have fashioned AIDS into a highly stigmatized disease. Persons infected with HIV, as well as suspected (by the public) of infection, have been openly shunned and alienated. The media has often referred to the blameless innocent victims (children and hemophiliacs) being infected by the guilty (homosexuals and intravenous drug abusers).

In Goffman's (1963) classic work, *stigma* was defined as an attribute, an undesired differentness, that discredits or disqualifies the individual from full social acceptance. This "differentness" was not in itself cause for social disqualification, but rested upon an interactional process through which this differentness was given social significance and meaning. It was the public's reaction, therefore, that measured the inner strength of a social norm (Shoham and Rahav, 1970).

Some diseases are clearly more biophysically discrete or recognizable. Venereal diseases have been associated with clandestine or immoral sexual activities. Freidson (1988) states that in certain cases, such as venereal disease, there is a moralistic judgment of blame and the indisposed is held responsible for the diseased state. The concept of stigma as some type of repercussion of norm violation is almost universal. The interpretation of such marks or signs is culturally defined, and the position of the one doing the stigmatizing is influential.

Research reports and articles in the medical, nursing, and behavioral sciences are saturated with articles about AIDS, its etiology and pathogenesis; its impact on sexual behaviors and practices, drug addiction, health care delivery, employment, and discrimination issues. These reports, however, have only minimally addressed the perspectives and attitudes of PWAs.

● PURPOSE OF THE STUDY

The purpose of this study is to describe what it is like to be a homeless PWA living in a congregate facility. Ethnographic methodology will be the approach used to conduct this investigation.

● PLAN FOR DATA COLLECTION

Study Design

Ethnography is a method by which a culture or subculture can be described. The final product of the ethnographic method is a written report based on the description and analysis of the culture of concern. Ethnography has been defined in the nursing literature as the systematic process of observing, detailing, describing, documenting, and analyzing the lifeways or particular patterns of a culture (or subculture) (Leininger, 1985). Ethnographic methodology is an ideal way to identify behaviors and generate knowledge that will establish the groundwork for further research. Homeless PWAs living in a congregate facility can be considered a subculture whose lifeways are as yet unidentified. The ethnographic approach provides the most appropriate means for describing what living in the congregate setting is like from the perspective of PWAs.

Setting

A church-affiliated congregate living facility in a large metropolitan area in the Southeastern United States has been selected as the field setting for the researcher's ethnographic study. This congregate residence accepts PWAs who have nowhere else to go and who otherwise would probably be forced to live on the streets. All persons living in this setting have a diagnosis of AIDS or have had an AIDS-related infection or complication. For anonymity, this residence will be given the fictional name "Sunrise Manor."

Sample

The sample will be drawn from those PWAs living full time at Sunrise Manor. The sampling approach will be a purposive sample of convenience. Residents' charts, containing medical, family, and social histories, will be available for the investigator's review. To avoid preconceived views toward residents and the risk of biasing sample selection, the investigator will not review the charts until after the participants have been selected.

Four to six residents (male and female) will be interviewed in a series of in-depth interviews. It is also anticipated that the staff will be observed as they interact with the residents and will be spoken with informally. It is contemplated that the investigator will spend 15 to 30 hours a week in the field setting.

Data Collection Techniques

Data will be obtained primarily by observation and participant observation. Participant observation will combine straight observation and both unstructured and structured interviews. An interview schedule will be developed before each formal interview. After analysis of each interview, new questions will be generated and, if possible, follow-up interviews will be scheduled. Questions will be of the grand-tour and mini-tour variety (as discussed in Spradley, 1979). An example of the initial interview schedule is attached (Appendix A).

A tape recorder will be used whenever possible during formal and informal interviews. Once transcribed, the tapes will be kept for review in order to listen to the residents' articulation and exclamation and in order to facilitate a further appreciation of their moods. At the completion of this study, the tapes will be erased.

Because the investigator anticipates the use of photography as adding an important dimension to the data base and as facilitating content analysis, a camera will be used (when permitted and appropriate) to capture germane scenes. Photographs allow the researcher to witness an event, situation, or condition through the camera and simultaneously to become a participant observer. All photographs, including negatives, will be destroyed upon completion of the study. In addition to photographs, hand-drawn sketches, and maps and floor plans of the living quarters and private and public areas of Sunrise Manor will be interpreted throughout the data presentation process to better orient the reader to the setting.

PLAN FOR DATA ANALYSIS

According to Lincoln and Guba (1985), within the ethnographic paradigm, data analysis is not a matter of reduction but of induction. Inductive analysis begins with the data analysis, rather than from established theories or hypotheses. The investigator will use the transcriptions of the interviews and field notes as the source of data analysis. Words and word combinations will be selected so that the researcher can identify the significant area for analysis. Recurrent combinations will generate conceptualizations, understandings, and trends from the perspective of PWAs living in Sunrise Manor.

LIMITATIONS OF THE STUDY

Since the sample will be drawn from a group of homeless PWAs living in a specific setting, the conclusions cannot be generalized to all PWAs living in congregate facilities, or to all homeless.

● ETHICAL CONSIDERATIONS

The protocol for this research study, initial interview schedule, and informed consents will be submitted to the appropriate institutional review boards responsible for the protection of human subjects involved in research. Three different consent forms will be written: one will be for resident participation in the ethnographic study; two will be for permission to be photographed (resident and staff forms). A copy of the resident participation informed consent form can be found in Appendix B.

All study participants will be asked to sign informed consents prior to formal interviews and photograph sessions. Confidentiality of the subjects and informants (staff) will be maintained by not identifying them by name. Data will be recorded with special code names, so that there is no link between these codes and the subject's identity. Names of the subjects and informants will be known only to the investigator, who will hold this information in the strictest confidence, coded, and securely stored in a locked file (in the home of the investigator) for a period of not less than three years.

Once agreeing to participate in this study, all participants will be informed that they are free to withdraw from the study at any time. They will also be informed that if the content of the interviews causes emotional discomfort or stress, they are free to terminate the interview at that time and also are at liberty to refuse to answer any question. All participants will be informed that their participation in this study or their wish not to participate will not, in any way, affect their status at Sunrise Manor.

● NURSING IMPLICATIONS

Being homeless is accompanied by a multitude of problems. Having AIDS is saturated with its own distinctive set of physical, psychological, and social puzzles. The medical, especially the neurological, problems that are common in AIDS further increase and aggravate the existing gravity of the person's life prior to becoming homeless.

Being a homeless PWA is a "contemporary condition," and it is anticipated that the description derived from this ethnography will present new dilemmas for health care professionals and society. Finding answers to such dilemmas will necessitate that the nurse look beyond the health care setting for practical answers.

As the numbers of AIDS cases multiply, the need for facilities such as Sunrise Manor will undoubtedly increase. AIDS is not a problem that lends itself to simple or immediate solutions, and descriptions of homeless PWAs in other parts of the country are necessary to understand the magnitude and intricacies of the AIDS dilemma. The intent of this study is to establish the first description of what it is like to be a homeless PWA living in a congregate facility from the PWA's perspective. The findings from this investigation will enhance the knowledge base of the nursing profession with regard to the needs of this population and assist with planning appropriate interventions.

The author wishes to thank Dr. Lydia DeSantis, Professor, University of Miami School of Nursing, Coral Gables, Florida, for her professional guidance and editorial assistance in preparing this proposal.

APPENDIX A: INTERVIEW SCHEDULE
1. What is it like for you to live in Sunrise Manor?
2. What was it like for you before you moved in?
3. How are things here compared to where you were before?
4. How do you spend the day?

APPENDIX B: INFORMED CONSENT FORM:
LIVING IN SUNRISE MANOR
1. **Purpose:** You are being asked to participate in a research study in which you will be asked to describe your thoughts and feelings as a person living in Sunrise Manor. The reason for conducting this study is to understand what it is like to live in Sunrise Manor and to determine how the experience can be made more beneficial to the residents.
2. **Procedure:** The study will consist of three to five interviews that the Investigator will conduct over a period of 2–3 months. The interviews will last approximately 60 minutes. You will be asked to respond to questions about what it is like to live in Sunrise Manor and what things were like for you before you moved in. The interviews will be tape recorded and the tape recordings will be erased once the tapes have been typed. At your request, the tape recorder will be turned off at any time during the interview(s). Toward the end of this study, a request may be made to take photographs of resident activities in Sunrise Manor. The photographs will be used to assist in describing the residence and its social activities. The photographs will not be published or displayed in any manner. The photographs will be destroyed at the end of the study. Only persons granting permission to be included in photographs will be.
3. **Risks:** There are no anticipated physical risks involved by participating in this study. If you feel that the content of an interview is causing you feelings of stress or emotional discomfort, please know that you may end the interview.
4. **Benefits:** There is no direct benefit to you for participating in this study. The results of this study may help health care providers gain understanding and make necessary changes to improve your living environment while in Sunrise Manor.
5. **Confidentiality:** Names will not be used in the reporting of any information you tell the investigator. All information which refers to or can be identified with you will remain confidential to the extent permitted by law. The results of this study will be reported as group results.

6. **Participation is voluntary:** Your participation in this study is voluntary. If you decide to participate and later decide that you do not wish to continue, you may at any time withdraw your consent and stop your participation, without affecting your status at Sunrise Manor. You may refuse to answer any question without affecting your status at Sunrise Manor or your continued participation in this study.

7. **Whom to contact for answers:** If there are any questions at any time regarding this study or your participation in it, you are always free to consult with the investigator [*investigator's phone number was provided*].

8. I have read and received a copy of this informed consent form.
   SIGNATURE OF INVESTIGATOR: DATE
   SIGNATURE OF PARTICIPANT: DATE
   SIGNATURE OF WITNESS: DATE

REFERENCES

Carter, D., Lantos, J., & Hughes, J. (1998). Reassessing medical students' willingness to treat HIV-infected patients. *Academic Medicine, 71*(11), 1250–1252.

Centers for Disease Control. (1998). *HIV/AIDS surveillance report.*

Clarke, P. N., Williams, C. A., Percy, M. A., & Kim, Y. S. (1995). Health and life problems of homeless men and women in the southeast. *Journal of Community Health Nursing, 12*(2), 101–110.

Danziger, R. (1996). HIV infection must be destigmatized [Letter to the Editor]. *British Medical Journal, 312*(7045), 1541.

Epstein, S. (1996). *Impure science: AIDS, activism, and the politics of knowledge.* Berkeley, CA: University of California Press.

Fournier, P. O., Baldor, R. A., Warfield, M. E., & Frazier, B. (1997). Patients with HIV/AIDS: Physicians' knowledge, attitudes, and referral practices. *Journal of Family Practice, 44*(1), 85–89.

Freidson, E. (1988). *Profession of medicine: A study of the sociology of applied knowledge* (2nd ed.). Chicago: University of Chicago Press.

Goffman, E. (1963). *Stigma.* New York: Simon and Schuster.

Hansell, P. S., Hughes, C. B., Caliandro, G., Russo, P., Budin, W. C., Hartman, B., & Hernandez, O. C. (1998). The effect of a social support boosting intervention on stress, coping, and social support in caregivers of children with HIV/AIDS, *Nursing Research, 47*(2), 79–86.

Kadushin, G. (1996). Gay men with AIDS and their families of origin: An analysis of social support. *Health and Social Work, 21*(2), 141–149.

Leininger, M. M. (1985). *Qualitative research methods in nursing.* New York: Grune & Stratton.

Lincoln, Y. S., & Guba, E. G. (1985). *Naturalistic inquiry.* Beverly Hills, CA: Sage Publications.

Regional Task Force on Homelessness. (1997). *AIDS and homelessness.* San Diego, CA: Author.

Sabados, R. (1997, January 17). San Francisco's AIDS housing crisis. *Bay Area Reporter,* p. 1.

Seattle-King County, WA, Dept. of Public Health. (1997). *Facts about HIV/AIDS in homeless people.* Seattle, WA: Author.

Shoham, S. G., & Rahav, G. (1970). *The mark of Cain.* St. Lucia: University of Queensland Press.

Spradley, J. P. (1979). *The ethnographic interview.* New York: Holt, Rinehart & Winston.

Takahashi, L. M. (1997). The socio-spatial stigmatization of homelessness and HIV/AIDS: Toward an explanation of the NIMBY syndrome. *Social Science Medicine, 45*(6), 903–914.

U.S. Department of Housing and Urban Development & U.S. Department of Health and Human Services. (1996). *Addressing the needs of homeless persons living with HIV/AIDS who also have a serious mental illness and/or alcohol and/or drug abuse problems.* Washington, DC: Author.

Waterson, A. (1997). Anthropological research and the politics of HIV prevention: Towards a critique of policy and priorities in the age of AIDS. *Social Science Medicine, 44*(9), 1381–1391.

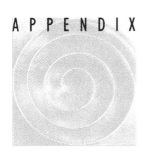

APPENDIX C

Example of a Quantitative Research Report

The Effect of a Social Support Boosting Intervention on Stress, Coping, and Social Support in Caregivers of Children with HIV/AIDS

Phyllis Shanley Hansell, Cynthia B. Hughes, Gloria Caliandro, Phyllis Russo, Wendy C. Budin, Bruce Hartman, and Olga C. Hernandez

ABSTRACT

Background: Caring for the human immunodeficiency virus (HIV)-infected child is challenging and affects the entire family system. Studies have shown that social support can mitigate caregiver stress and enhance coping; however, social support may not always result in a positive outcome for the recipient.

Objectives: To measure caregiver stress, coping, and social support, and to test the effect of a social support boosting intervention on levels of stress, coping, and social support among caregivers of children with HIV/acquired immune deficiency syndrome (AIDS).

Methods: An experimental design was used with monthly social support boosting interventions implemented. The stratified randomized sample included 70 primary caregivers of children with HIV/AIDS. The sample strata were seropositive caregivers (biological parents) and seronegative caregivers (foster parents and extended family members). Study measures included the Derogatis Stress Profile, Family Crisis Oriented Personal Evaluation Scale, and the Tilden Interpersonal Relationship Inventory. Data were analyzed using descriptive statistics and repeated measure MANOVA.

Results: Statistically significant differences between the experimental and control groups were found on changes in the dependent variables over time when caregiver strata were included as a factor in the analysis; no statistically significant results were found when caregiver strata were combined. Univariate *F* tests indicated that the level of social support for caregivers who were seronegative in the experimental group was significantly different from seronegative caregivers in the control group and seropositive caregivers in both groups. No significant treatment group differences were found for seropositive caregivers.

Conclusions: Seronegative caregivers derived substantial benefit from the social support boosting intervention. Seronegative caregivers who acquire a child with HIV/AIDS are confronted with a complex stressful situation; the critical need to enhance their social support is achievable through the intervention tested in this study.

Key Words: social support; stress; coping; caregivers

The human immunodeficiency virus (HIV) infects 1,300 to 2,000 children annually in the United States (Centers for Disease Control, 1997). In children, HIV progresses rapidly to acquired immune deficiency syndrome (AIDS). These children experience impaired growth and development and frequent infections owing to immune system immaturity (Pediatric HIV Disease, December 1995). Most HIV infection in children occurs through perinatal transmission; thus, HIV/AIDS in children has implications for the entire family system (Pediatric AIDS, June 1996).

Caring for the HIV-infected child includes the challenges of caring for a seemingly well and developing child, while simultaneously dealing with episodes of recurrent acute illnesses (Larson & Bechtel, 1995). As Andrews, Williams, and Neil (1993) reported, guilt, grief, emotional pain, and exhaustion can overwhelm mothers of HIV-positive children, severely compromising available resources needed to meet the demands of their daily lives while affecting their mental-emotional responses to stressful situations. Others (Wiener, Theut, Steinberg, Riekert, & Pizzo, 1994) found that parents of HIV-infected children experience clinically significant elevations of depression and anxiety. Caregiver problems associated with HIV-positive children include: isolation, shame, anger, stigmatization, ostracism, disclosure, uncertainty, terminal illness, and preparation for the HIV-positive child's death (Brown & Powell-Cope, 1991; Cohen, Nehring, Malm, & Harris, 1995; Mayers & Spiegel, 1992; Sherwen & Boland, 1994).

Studies have shown that social support can mitigate caregiver stress and enhance coping. Black, Nair, and Harrington (1994) reported that HIV-positive mothers benefited more from a social support intervention given at home than HIV-negative mothers by demonstrating more positive attitudes and behaviors toward parenting. These HIV-positive mothers also reported decreased levels of child-related stress and more positive involvement with their children.

Social support may not always result in a positive outcome for the recipient. Critical aspects of social support are: timing, amount of support, provider mode of behavior, and the relationship between the provider and the recipient (Vaux, 1988). One of the most important determinants of satisfaction with support is the person's perception of support (Baille, Norbeck, & Barnes, 1988; Fondacaro & Moos, 1987; Hobfoll, Nadler, & Lieberman; 1987;

Schulz, Tompkins, Wood, & Decker, 1987; Vinokur, Schul, & Caplan, 1987). Individuals with a negative outlook toward support may repel it, receiving and perceiving less social support (Vinokur et al., 1987).

The conceptual framework for this study is based on the work of Thoits (1986). Thoits links the major constructs of this study—stress, coping, and social support—by drawing on the work of Lazarus and Folkman (1984). Thoits states that stressors are aspects of one's lives viewed as undesirable consequences. Within this context, negative life events and chronic strains that produce stress interfere with an individual's performance of role-related activities. Thus, when confronted with stressors that exceed individual resources, cognitive and behavioral efforts are needed to cope with the stressors.

Two major ways of coping are problem-focused and emotion-focused coping. Problem-focused coping includes taking action on the environment or the self to remove or alter stressful situations. Emotion-focused coping aims to help individuals better understand their feelings and responses to stressful situations and to change their behavior as needed. Thoits states that social support (aid given to the distressed individual by significant others such as family, friends, relatives, and neighbors) may enable the individual to cope more successfully. Thoits (1986) stated that social support and coping are influenced by an individual's perception of them and have many functions in common because both are directed at changing or managing stressful situations. Coping and social support may eliminate or change demands and alter an individual's response to the demands; thus, social support is conceptualized as coping assistance.

The objectives for this study were twofold: (1) to measure caregiver stress, coping, and social support and (2) to test the effect of a social support boosting intervention on levels of stress, coping, and social support among caregivers of children with HIV/AIDS.

● METHODS

Sample

Caregivers who participated in the study met the following criteria: identified themselves as the biological parent, blood relative, or foster parent of a child with HIV/AIDS; were legally assigned as the primary caregiver of a child who has symptomatic HIV/AIDS infection (Centers for Disease Control, 1997); resided in the New York/New Jersey metropolitan area; could read and write in English or Spanish.

Caregivers were recruited from clinics and outreach centers that provide care for women and children with HIV/AIDS. Caregivers were stratified a priori according to caregiver type (biological parent, extended family member, or foster parent) using computer-generated random numbers and then randomly assigned to study groups. Stratification of the sample by caregiver type was conducted to achieve equal distribution of caregiver type between the experimental and control study groups in proportion to the study population. All biological parents were seropositive and all extended family and foster caregivers were seronegative. One hundred twenty-two caregivers were entered into the study. The final sample consisted of 70 caregivers who completed all interventions and measures at the 6-month data collection. These caregivers included biological parents (n = 39, 56%), extended family members (n = 12, 17%), and foster parents (n = 19, 27%). Because of progressive illness in the caregiver, death of a child or caregiver, or change in caregiver status, attrition was substantial. Children of participants were often moved to foster care, and some were returned to their biological parent. Many participants had a history of intravenous drug use and most of the caregivers were receiving public assistance. The caregivers who did not remain in the study did not differ from those who remained in the study on demographic variables or baseline measures.

All caregivers in the final sample (N = 70) were between 18 and 61 years of age (M = 36, SD = 10.42). The ethnic background of participants was largely minority (African American, n = 52, 74%; Hispanic, n = 9, 13%; White, n = 9, 13%). The majority of caregivers reported being nonpartnered (single, n = 27, 39%; separated or divorced, n = 18, 26%; widowed, n = 4, 5%). The remaining 30% were either partnered (n = 9, 13%) or married (n = 12, 17%). Nearly half the sample (n = 29, 41%) had not completed high school. Social status of almost all of the participants (n = 64, 96%) fell within the lowest three levels of the Hollingshead Index of Social Position. Thirty-one (44%) of the caregivers were seronegative (HIV-) and 39 (56%) were seropositive (HIV+). No significant differences were found in demographic characteristics between participants in the experimental and control group. However, when comparing demographics between the seropositive caregivers and the seronegative caregivers, there were some significant differences (Table 1). The seronegative caregivers were significantly older (M = 42 years) than the seropositive caregivers (M = 32 years) (t = -5.2, p < .001). The seronegative caregivers were also of a higher educational level and a higher social status. However, no differences were noted in racial background or marital status between the seropositive and seronegative caregivers.

Procedures

Eligible participants were approached and given complete information regarding the study protocol, risks, and benefits of the study. Interested participants provided written consent and were also given a copy of the informed consent. Consent forms and instruments were available in both English and Spanish.

The study was originally proposed as a four-group experimental design with repeated measures to compare a social support boosting intervention, a respite intervention, and a social support with respite intervention to a control group. Early in the study it was noted that the respite intervention was not

TABLE C-1 *Sample Characteristics According to Caregiver HIV Status*				
	SERO-NEGATIVE	**SERO-POSITIVE**	**TOTAL SAMPLE**	
	(n = 31)	*(n = 39)*	*(n = 70)*	
VARIABLE	*n*	*n*	*n*	*%*
Ethnic background				
African American	26	25	51	73
White	5	4	9	13
Hispanic	7	2	9	13
Marital status				
Single	18	9	27	39
Separated/divorced	7	11	18	26
Widowed	2	2	4	5
Partnered	8	1	9	13
Married	4	8	12	17
Educational level				
<7th grade	2	0	2	3
Junior HS	6	2	8	11
Partial HS	14	5	19	27
HS graduate	8	6	14	20
Partial college	8	12	20	29
College graduate	1	6	7	10
Hollingshead Index				
Social Status 1	26	5	31	44
Social Status 2	6	12	18	26
Social Status 3	7	8	15	22
Social Status 4	0	2	2	3
Social Status 5	0	3	3	4
Missing data			1	1

under investigator control as many caregivers received respite from a variety of sources, such as family members, day care, employment, and/or hospitalization. It was therefore determined to count respite hours for all participants and to control the respite variable through statistical analyses. When statistical analyses showed that the number of respite hours across study groups did not differ or correlate with any of the study outcome variables, the four-study group design was collapsed into a two-group design. The two-group design compared participants who received social support boosting to those participants who did not receive the social support boosting intervention.

Data analyses were performed using a two-group experimental design with repeated measures at baseline, 6 months, and 12 months to test the effect of the intervention. The experimental group received a social support boosting intervention, and the control group received standard care. The social support boosting intervention was implemented over a 12-month period through monthly contacts between an investigator and the caregiver. Each contact for the social support boosting intervention lasted between 30 minutes and 1 hour based on individual caregiver needs.

Conceptually, the social support boosting intervention integrated the work of Vaux (1988) and Thoits (1986). Vaux (1988) identified social support as consisting of support network resources, specific supportive behaviors, and subjective appraisal of support, all of which were incorporated into the social support boosting intervention. Social support was conceptualized as coping assistance that aims to reduce stress (Thoits, 1986). Coping assistance in this study's intervention was both problem focused and instrumental and included the caregiver's appraisal of the support.

Specifically, the social support boosting intervention used a modified case management approach to enhance the coping ability of caregivers of children with HIV/AIDS and reduce stress by using social support network resources directed at changing or managing problems identified as stressful. According to the social support boosting (coping assistance) intervention protocol, the caregiver and the investigator together focused on the identification of the caregiver's stressful problems and network resources to achieve more of a positive, subjective appraisal of social support to enable its mobilization to deal with caregiver stress. The caregiver with the investigator set mutual, objective goals to facilitate caregiver problem solving. Based on this assessment, the investigator and the caregiver identified potential formal and informal social support network resources for achieving caregiver goals and developed a plan for using social support network resources. Social support boosting strategies included the identification of individuals from the caregiver's social support network who would help to provide resources that meet the individual's support needs. Social support included emotional support, cognitive support, and material support (Cohen & Willis, 1985; Thoits, 1982). Emotional support consisted of behaviors that generated feelings of respect, comfort, and a sense of worth. Cognitive support refers to knowledge and information. Material or instrumental support refers to services and goods that facilitate problem solutions. The intervention aimed at helping caregivers identify and access network resources that could provide all three types of social support.

At monthly intervals, the investigator and the caregiver met for the intervention, and the effectiveness of the plan was evaluated and revised as necessary. Problems, resources, goals, plans for meeting goals, and the evaluation of the plan were all recorded using a structured flow sheet used to monitor the intervention continuously. The flow sheet incorporated subjective (caregiver evaluation) and objective evaluation (investigator evaluation) of intervention outcomes.

Participants in the control group received standard care that included a multidisciplinary team approach in which the children of the participants received medical treatment and nursing care, and the caregiver received social services and caregiver respite. The major difference between the study groups was the social support boosting protocol implemented with only the experimental group. All participants were paid $50.00 for completing the measures at 6 months and 12 months.

Instruments

All caregivers were asked to complete the study measures at baseline, 6 months, and 12 months. All instruments used in this study were pilot tested on a small group of AIDS caregivers and were found appropriate for use with this particular study group.

The Derogatis Stress Profile (DSP) (Derogatis, 1986) is a 77-item multidimensional self-report instrument, which was derived from the interactional theory of stress proposed by Lazarus and Folkman (1984). Within this instrument, stress is represented as a hierarchical model containing 11 primary stress vectors subsumed under the three principal stress domains: (a) environmental events domain; (b) emotional response domain involving anxiety, hostility, and depression; and (c) personality mediators. For scoring purposes, the total stress score of the DSP was used. Reliability assessment of the DSP has included test–retest reliability ranging from .79 to .93, indicating good temporal stability for the instrument. Internal consistency coefficients ranged from .79 to .93, indicating respective levels of item homogeneity for the various domains of the DSP. The validity of the DSP has been previously assessed through hypothesis testing, factor analysis, and tests for prediction validity. In this study the Cronbach's alpha coefficient evaluating internal consistency of the total DSP score was .85.

The Tilden Interpersonal Relationship Inventory (Tilden, 1991) is a 39-item multidimensional measure of interpersonal relationships that contains an index of network structure and three subscales of network function: interpersonal support, reciprocity, and conflict. Cronbach's alpha coefficients range from .83 to .92 for the subscales, and test–retest reliability coefficients range from .81 to .91. Validity was assessed sufficiently through three approaches: theory testing, contrasted groups, and a multi-trait, multi-method approach. This instrument has been used with a wide variety of adult populations including cancer patients, adult women in the community, and battered women. In this study the Cronbach's alpha coefficients ranged from .73 to .87; the interpersonal support subscale was used as the measure of social support appraisal. The reciprocity and the conflict scales were not used. The 13-item interpersonal support measure was consistent with the conceptual definition of social support identified as described in the framework. The items on the interpersonal support subscale measure perceived availability or enactment of helping behaviors by persons with whom one is engaged in relationships that are usually informal or noncontractual. Items on this subscale tap into aspects of emotional support ("makes me feel confident"); cognitive support ("talk things over"); and material support ("neighbors who help").

Family Crisis Oriented Personal Scales (F-COPES) (McCubbin & Thompson, 1987) is a 30-item self-report instrument that assesses internal and external family coping. Its purpose in this study was to measure effective problem solving and behavioral coping strategies used by an individual member of a family encountering difficult situations. The F-COPES instrument was evaluated for both reliability and validity on a sample of 199 graduate and undergraduate students and sample that included single parents. Internal consistency reliability using Cronbach's alpha coefficient for the overall scale was .86 for the first sample and .87 for the second sample. Values for test–retest reliability ranged from .61 to .95. In this study Cronbach's alpha coefficient was .82. Coping strategies assessed among the subscales of the F-COPES included (a) acquiring social support, (b) reframing, (c) seeking spiritual support, (d) mobilizing family to acquire and accept help, and (e) passive appraisal. The total or overall F-COPES score that is a sum of the items on all subscales was used to assess coping in this study.

All caregivers were also evaluated for social status using the two-factor Hollingshead Index of Social Position (1957). This index combines two 7-point scales—educational level and occupational level of the individual—to determine the social stratum that the individual occupies. Scale raw scores are each multiplied by a weighted factor, summed, and then transformed into a scale score to determine social status. Social strata range from 1 (the lowest) to 5 (the highest).

● RESULTS

The findings presented are for the 6-month ($N = 70$) data collection. Because of attrition, the number of participants remaining at 12 months ($N = 39$) did not provide sufficient power to conduct the appropriate statistical analyses on these data. Descriptive statistics, including ranges, means, and standard deviation, were computed for the three dependent variables of stress, coping, and social support at Data Collection Time 1 (DC1, baseline) and at Data Collection Time 2 (DC2, 6 months) (Table 2).

Before data analysis, the main study variables were examined for univariate and multivariate outliers and evidence of normal distribution. Based on these results, no data transformations were necessary. Repeated measures multivariate analysis of variance (MANOVA) were performed to determine significant differences in change over time between the experimental and control study groups on the three dependent variables: stress, coping, and social support. No significant differences were found in change over time between the experimental and control groups on any of the dependent variables.

Further analyses were then performed to adjust for HIV status within experimental and control groups. These analyses were based on the results of a preliminary data analysis of the baseline data that indicated significant differences between the HIV-negative and HIV-positive caregivers on stress and coping levels. HIV-infected caregivers (biological parents) had significantly greater stress levels and use fewer coping strategies as compared with HIV-negative caregivers (extended family members and foster parents) (Hansell et al., 1993).

TABLE C-2 *Descriptive Statistics for Stress, Coping, and Social Support at Baseline (DCI) and at 6 Months (DC2)*

	DCI			DC2		
	X	(SD)	Range	X	(SD)	Range
Total sample (N = 70)						
Stress	529	(73.4)	263–665	530	(54.6)	423–665
Coping	106	(16.6)	70–142	106	(14.6)	68–138
Social support	4.1	(.6)	2.0–5.0	3.9	(.66)	1.7–5.0
Experimental group (n = 34)						
Stress	513	(68.7)	364–661	520	(50.9)	423–612
Coping	104	(16.4)	70–138	105	(12.9)	70–129
Social support	4.23	(.57)	1.7–4.9	4.07	(.7)	1.7–4.9
Control group (n = 36)						
Stress	544	(75.6)	263–665	540	(56.9)	431–665
Coping	108	(16.78)	74–142	106	(16.2)	68–138
Social support	4.04	(.62)	2.7–5.0	3.91	(.62)	2.7–5.0

Note: Stress was measured by the total score of the Derogatis Stress Profile. Coping was measured by the total score of the F-COPES, and Social Support was measured by the interpersonal support scale of the Tilden Interpersonal Relationship Inventory.

The subsequent analyses performed in the present study tested the effect of a social support boosting intervention on the dependent variables of stress, coping, and social support. A repeated measures MANOVA was used to test for a group by HIV status interaction. The combined dependent variables were significantly related to the interaction of group by HIV status over time (F [1,66] = 3.47, p = .02).

To investigate further the nature of the relationship among the independent variables and the dependent variables, univariate F values were examined (Table 3). Although no statistically significant differences were found for stress (F [1,66] = .197, p = .658) or coping (F [1,66] = 3.27, p = .075), there were

TABLE C-3 *Univariate Analyses of Variance of Three Dependent Variables for Effects of Group by HIV Status Interaction Over Time*

VARIABLE	F	P
Stress	.197	.658
Coping	3.276	.075
Social support	10.391	.002

Note: Univariate F test with (1,66) df.

significant differences in measures of social support between the experimental and control groups when adjusting for HIV status of the caregiver (F [1,6] = 10.39, p = .002) (Figs. 1 to 3).

The change in levels of social support over time in the seronegative caregivers in the experimental group was significantly different from those of seronegative caregivers in the control group and seropositive caregivers in both groups. The results suggest that the social support boosting intervention resulted in significantly increased levels of social support for seronegative caregivers who were in the experimental group.

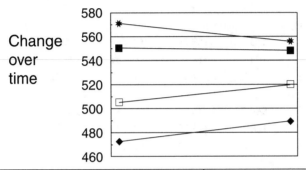

	Data Collection 1	Data Collection 2
Exp. (sero+) ■	550	548
Exp. (sero–) ◆	472	489
Control (sero+)✳	571	555
Control (sero–)☐	506	519

F (1,66) = .197, p = .658

FIGURE C-1. Changes in mean stress levels over time.

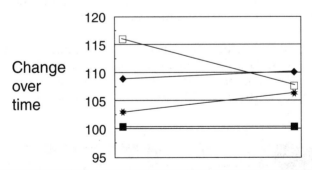

	Data Collection 1	Data Collection 2
Exp. (sero+) ■	100.38	100.33
Exp. (sero–) ◆	108.60	110.00
Control (sero+)✳	103.23	106.04
Control (sero–)☐	116.10	107.00

F (1,66) = 3.27, p = .075

FIGURE C-2. Changes in mean coping levels over time.

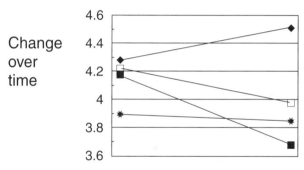

	Data Collection 1	Data Collection 2
Exp. (sero+) ■	4.18	3.68
Exp. (sero−) ◆	4.27	4.50
Control (sero+)✳	3.90	3.85
Control (sero−)□	4.22	3.97

$F (1,66) = 10.39$, $p = .002$

FIGURE C-3. Changes in mean social support levels over time.

● DISCUSSION

A major finding of this study was that seronegative caregivers in the experimental group had significantly increased levels of social support over time after six monthly interventions. Upon entry into the study at the baseline, seronegative caregivers in both groups had higher mean levels of social support than seropositive caregivers in both groups. At the 6-month data collection the only increased levels of social support were measured in seronegative caregivers in the experimental group. Seronegative caregivers in the control group experienced a decrease in social support level, as did seropositive caregivers in the experimental and control groups. Interestingly, the lowest levels of social support at 6 months were experienced in seropositive caregivers in the experimental group.

The social support boosting intervention's effectiveness for the seronegative group of caregivers has significance from both a research and practice perspective. Seronegative caregivers in the study included foster parents and extended family members. For many of these individuals, caregiving responsibilities for a child with HIV/AIDS was a new experience requiring substantial role redefinition and adjustment for the caregiver. Problems regarding confidentiality issues about the HIV status of the child were a common experience, distancing many of these caregivers from members of their social support network. Because of the study intervention, seronegative caregivers in the experimental group could more effectively deal with their problems. The use of the social support boosting intervention ultimately increased appraisal of social support for seronegative caregivers.

The experience of the seropositive caregivers was quite different. For them, HIV/AIDS is both a personal health crisis and a caregiver crisis. For the seropositive caregivers in both the experimental and control groups, the mean social support appraisal values decreased. Control group social support means between baseline and 6 months remained relatively flat, whereas the mean level of social support of participants in the seropositive experimental groups decreased to the lowest level in the study.

The study intervention may have been more congruent with the higher educational level and prior use of social support for the seronegative care-givers in the experimental group. Perhaps these caregivers could more effectively deal with their problems with the use of the social support boosting intervention. It is also possible that increased stress levels experienced by these caregivers over time may have increased their receptiveness, need, and thus their use of social support resources. A third possibility is that the seropositive caregivers in the experimental group were using other coping strategies not captured by the F-COPES instrument.

For the dependent variable stress, the levels for the experimental and control group remained relatively flat with very little change over time. Both in the experimental and control groups, seropositive caregivers reported higher stress levels at entry into the study than the seronegative caregivers. This finding suggests that the stress levels of these caregivers are separate from care-giver social support levels and probably arise from multiple sources. Individualized interventions may need to be designed for these two distinct groups, although some characteristics of the caregivers are similar.

Coping levels as measured at 6 months also were not significantly different between the baseline and the 6-month data collection. When these data were analyzed incorporating HIV status, the highest coping scores at 6 months were reported by the seronegative caregivers in the experimental group. The lowest levels of coping were experienced by the experimental seropositive group, with the control group for seropositive and seronegative caregivers falling between the seronegative and seropositive caregivers in the experimental group. This result is congruent with the reports of increased social support appraisal in the seronegative experimental group because some items on the F-COPES instrument measure acquiring social support and mobilizing family to acquire and accept help as coping strategies.

The results of this study document the effectiveness of the social support boosting intervention through significantly increased social support levels for seronegative caregivers. Although social support was enhanced at a statistically significant level, stress levels and coping levels were not affected to the same extent. Thus, these results are not conceptually congruent with the work of Lazarus and Folkman (1984) relative to the interactive theory of stress as to the buffering effect of social support on stress by enhancing coping. These findings suggest that stress and coping for the caregiver of a child with HIV/AIDS are not significantly buffered by increased levels of social support. As Wiener et al. (1994) found, parents of HIV-infected children experienced clinically significant elevations of depression and anxiety but not a direct relationship between the child's degree of debilitation and parental psychological stress. Thus, stress for these caregivers is constant, complex, and ever-present with limited opportunity for coping.

Stress and coping in caregivers of children with HIV/AIDS presents nursing with a highly complex patient care situation, with stressors occurring over time that are erratic and unpredictable. However, providing these caregivers with a social support boosting intervention has been shown in this study to significantly increase levels of social support appraisal in seronegative caregivers that eventually should provide some level of relief.

Seropositive caregivers as a group present with multiple problems and a more complex situation. As a group the seropositive caregivers identified problems related to health status of the child, self, or family; health care services; transportation; finances; housing; food; schools; employment; clothing; counseling for the child, self, and family; prescription medications; recreation and rest (Hansell et al., 1992). These many sources of stress challenge these caregivers' ability to make it from day to day. These seropositive caregivers must focus on the needs of the ill child; at the same time they must cope with the experience of being ill from a progressive illness with an unpredictable course. Nursing implications for this study are to incorporate the social support network of the caregiver into the plan of care and to recognize the complexity of the needs of the AIDS caregiver.

The results of this study need to be understood within the context of the study's limitations. The caregivers who participated in this study were a highly challenging group of individuals, encountering stressors that were numerous, complex, and erratic. Because of the unpredictable course of HIV/AIDS, maintaining a sample over time was extremely difficult. One hundred twenty-two caregivers were entered into the study; at 6 months, 70 remained, and at 12 months, 39 remained. Attrition was 47% from entry into the study to the 6-month period and unacceptably high (68%) at the 12-month period, primarily because of progression of the illness. Other factors affected sample retention as well. Many participants became too ill to participate; some were hospitalized; dementia precluded participation; children seroreverted; children died, caregivers died, and caregiver status changed. Some caregivers were imprisoned; some were not able to continue to participate because of drug dependence; and some were lost to clinic care and to the study as well for unknown reasons. Many second-order changes that affected the entire system were factors in this population. Retention of participants in longitudinal studies is challenging in all research but was particularly difficult with this population.

This study has been helpful to identify the effectiveness of a social support boosting intervention for seronegative caregivers. Another important aspect identified is the serious complex needs of the seropositive caregiver who may be well advanced in the progress of HIV/AIDS. It is important that further research efforts focus on HIV caregivers, particularly those who are HIV-positive. Furthermore, the social support boosting intervention has the potential to be broadly applicable and needs to be tested with other caregiver groups such as those caring for adults with HIV/AIDS and individuals with cancer, Alzheimer's disease, and other terminal illnesses.

Acknowledgments

The participation of the AIDS Resource Foundation for Children, Newark, NJ; Jersey City Medical Center, Jersey City, NJ; and Newark Beth Israel Medical Center, Newark, NJ are gratefully acknowledged. Supported by a grant received from the National Institute of Nursing Research, National Institutes of Health (5R01 NRO 2903-03). Address reprint requests to Phyllis Shanley Hansell, EdD, College of Nursing, Seton Hall University, South Orange, NJ 07079.

REFERENCES

Andrews, S., Williams, A. B., & Neil, K. (1993). The mother-child relationship in the HIV-1 positive family. *Nursing Research, 25,* 193–198.

Baille, V., Norbeck, J. A., & Barnes, L. E. A. (1988). Stress, social support, and psychological distress of family caregivers of the elderly. *Nursing Research, 37*(4), 217–222.

Black, M. M., Nair, P., & Harrington, D. (1994). Maternal HIV infection: Parenting and early child development. *Journal of Pediatric Psychology, 19*(5), 595–616.

Brown, M. A., & Powell-Cope, G. M. (1991). AIDS family caregiving: Transitions through uncertainty. *Nursing Research, 40,* 338–345.

Centers for Disease Control. (1997). Revision of the CDC surveillance case definition for acquired immunodeficiency syndrome. *MMWR, 36,* 1–155.

Cohen, F. L., Nehring, W. M., Malm, K. C., & Harris, D. M. (1995). Family experiences when a child is HIV positive: Reports of natural and foster parents. *Pediatric Nursing, 21*(3), 248–254.

Cohen, S., & Willis, T. (1985). Stress, social support, and the buffering hypothesis. *Psychological Bulletin, 98,* 310–357.

Derogatis, L. (1986). *The Derogatis stress profile (DSP): A summary report.* Baltimore, MD: Clinical Psychometric Research.

Fondacaro, M. R., & Moos, R. H. (1987). Social support and coping: A longitudinal analysis. *American Journal of Community Psychology, 15*(5), 653–673.

Hansell, P., Hughes, C., Caliandro, G., Russo, P., Budin, W., & Hartman, B. (1993). *Stress, coping, social support and problems experienced by caregivers of HIV-infected children: A comparison of HIV-infected caregivers to non-HIV-infected caregivers.* Paper presented at Ninth International Conference on AIDS, Berlin, Germany.

Hansell, P., Hughes, C., Caliandro, G., Russo, P., Budin, W., Hartman, B., Zealand, T., & Zealand, F. (1992). *Problems identified by caregivers of children with HIV/AIDS.* Poster presented at the Eighth International AIDS Conference, Amsterdam.

Hobfoll, S. E., Nadler, A., & Lieberman, J. (1987). Satisfaction with social support during crisis: Intimacy and self-esteem as critical determinants. *Journal of Personality and Social Psychology, 51*(2), 296–304.

Hollingshead, A. B. (1957). *Two factor index of social position.* New Haven: Yale University Press.

Larson, T., & Bechtel, L. (1995). Managing the child infected with HIV. *Primary Care, 22*(1), 23–50.

Lazarus, R. S., & Folkman, S. (1984). *Stress, appraisal and coping.* New York: Springer.

Mayers, A., & Spiegel, L. (1992). A parental support group in a pediatric AIDS clinic: Its usefulness and limitations. *Health and Social Work, 17*(3), 183–191.

McCubbin, H., & Thompson, A. (1987). *F-COPES: Family assessment inventories for research and practice.* Madison: University of Wisconsin Press.

Pediatric AIDS [Electronic Database] (June 1996). Bethesda, MD: National Institute of Allergy and Infectious Diseases [producer and distributor].

Pediatric HIV Disease [Electronic Database] (December 1, 1995). Bethesda, MD: National Institute of Allergy and Infectious Diseases [producer and distributor].

Schulz, R., Tompkins, C. A., Wood, D., & Decker, S. (1987). The social psychology of caregiving: Physical and psychological costs of providing support to the disabled. *Journal of Applied Social Psychology, 17*(4), 401–428.

Sherwen, L. N., & Boland, M. (1994). Overview of psychosocial research concerning pediatric human immunodeficiency virus infection. *Developmental and Behavioral Pediatrics, 15*(3), S5–S11.

Spiegel, L., & Mayers, A. (1991). Psychosocial aspects of AIDS in children and adolescents. *Pediatric Clinics of North America, 38*(1), 153–167.

Thoits, P. A. (1982). Conceptual, methodological, and theoretical problems in studying social support as a buffer against life stress. *Journal of Health and Social Behavior, 23*, 145–159.

Thoits, P. A. (1986). Social support as coping assistance. *Journal of Consulting and Clinical Psychology, 54*(4), 416–423.

Tilden, V. P. (1991). *The interpersonal relationship inventory (IPRI): Instrument development summary.* Portland, OR: Oregon Health Science, University School of Nursing.

Vaux, A. (1988). *Social support: Theory research and intervention.* New York: Praeger.

Vinokur, A., Schul, Y., & Caplan, R. D. (1987). Determinants of perceived social support: Interpersonal transactions, personal outlook, and transient affective states. *Journal of Personality and Social Psychology, 53*(6), 1137–1145.

Wiener, L., Theut, S., Steinberg, S. M., Riekert, K. A., & Pizzo, P. A. (1994). The HIV-infected child: Parental responses and psychosocial implications. *American Journal of Orthopsychiatry, 64*(3), 485–492.

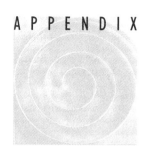

APPENDIX **D**

Example of a Quantitative Research Report

Correlates of Pain-Related Responses to Venipunctures in School-Age Children

Marie-Christine Bournaki

● ABSTRACT

Guided by the Roy Adaptation Model of Nursing, the relationship of children's age, gender, exposure to past painful experiences, temperament, fears, and child-rearing practices to their pain responses to a venipuncture was examined. A sample of 94 children aged 8 to 12 years and their female caregivers were recruited from three outpatient clinics. During the venipuncture, children's behavioral and heart rate responses were monitored; immediately after, their subjective responses were recorded. Canonical correlation revealed two variates. In the first, age and threshold (temperamental dimension) correlated with pain quality, behavioral responses, and heart rate responses, explaining 12% of the variance. In the second, age, the temperamental dimensions of distractibility and threshold, and medical fears explained only 5.7% of the variance in pain quality and heart rate magnitude. Significant correlations between pain intensity, quality, behavioral responses, and heart rate responses support the multidimensionality of pain.

Venipunctures are described as painful procedures by hospitalized children (Van Cleve, Johnson, & Pothier, 1996; Wong & Baker, 1988) and the most difficult to deal with by adolescent oncology survivors (Fowler-Kerry, 1990). However, not all children respond similarly to venipunctures. Between 4% and 17% of school-age children rated their pain intensity to a venipuncture as severe (Fradet, McGrath, Kay, Adams, & Luke, 1990; Harrison, 1991), and 38% of children ages 3 to 10 had to be physically restrained during a venipuncture (Jacobsen et al., 1990). Manne, Jacobsen, and Redd (1992) reported that the pain intensity and behavioral responses of 3- to 10-year-old children were moderate. In a recent study by Van Cleve et al., hospitalized school-age children were found to rate venipuncture or intravenous cannulation as moderately painful.

Factors that account for variability in children's responses to venipunctures have not been fully identified. The purpose of this study, therefore, was to examine the relationship of a set of correlates, including age, gender, past painful experiences, temperament, general and medical fears, and child-rearing practices, on school-age children's subjective, behavioral, and heart rate responses to a venipuncture.

● BACKGROUND

Conceptual Framework

The Roy Adaptation Model of Nursing (RAM) (Roy & Andrews, 1991) and the research literature on children's responses to painful procedures guided this study. According to the RAM, the goal of nursing is to facilitate adaptation between the person and the environment through the management of stimuli (Roy & Corliss, 1993). One of the assumptions of adaptation-level theory is that the person's "adaptive behavior is a function of the stimulus and adaptation level, that is, the pooled effects of the focal, contextual, and residual stimuli" (Roy & Corliss, 1993, p. 217). The focal stimulus immediately confronts the person; the contextual stimuli contribute to the effect of the focal stimulus; and residual stimuli are factors whose effects on the person's adaptation have not been clearly determined.

The focal and contextual stimuli are processed through coping mechanisms, such as the regulator and cognator subsystems. The regulator subsystem induces physiological responses through neural, chemical, and endocrine processes. The cognator subsystem elicits responses through perceptual/information processing, learning, judgment, and emotion processes (Andrews & Roy, 1991a). Outcomes of these coping mechanisms are the person's responses in four modes: self-concept, role function, interdependence, and physiological. The self-concept mode relates to feelings about one's personal and physical self. The role-function mode is associated with the need for social integrity based on roles assumed within society. The interdependence mode focuses on interactions that fulfill the need for affectional adequacy and support. The physiological mode is described as the person's physical responses to stimuli from the environment. In accordance with the proposition that stimuli serve as inputs to the person to elicit a response, children's pain-related responses were tested as a function of the pooled effects of the focal stimulus, the venipuncture, and the contributory effects of the contextual stimuli congruent with the RAM and the empiric pediatric pain literature. Contextual stimuli relate to culture, family, developmental stage, and cognator effectiveness, as well as those factors that have an effect on the person's adaptive responses in any of the modes (Andrews & Roy, 1991b). The pooled effects of a venipuncture, children's age, gender, exposure to past painful experiences, temperament, fears, and child-rearing practices were studied in relation to children's pain-related responses to the venipuncture.

Roy (1991) defined pain within the physiological mode as a sensory experience of acute or chronic nature, coded into the somatosensory pathways. Acute pain refers to "discomfort which is intense but relatively short-lived and reversible" (p. 166). Using principles from neurophysiology, Roy stated that a sensory experience such as pain involves the transmission of neural activity through specialized receptors, and transmission of information from sensory pathways to the cerebral cortex. A sensation results from receptors' activity and is converted into perceptual activity involving mental representations and interpretations. Thus, pain can be understood to be both a sensory and perceptual experience.

As a manifestation of the regulator subsystem activity, the sensory dimension was represented in this study by children's behavioral and heart rate responses. The perceptual dimension of pain, which is the response to the cognator subsystem activity, was portrayed by children's subjective responses about the location, intensity, and quality of pain.

Review of the Literature

Empirical evidence supports a negative relationship between the contextual stimulus of children's chronological age and pain intensity (Fradet et al., 1990; Lander & Fowler-Kerry, 1991; Manne et al., 1992) and behavioral responses to venipunctures (Fradet et al., 1990; Humphrey, Boon, van Linden van den Heuvell, & van de Wiel, 1992; Jacobsen et al., 1990). Mean pain intensity responses to a venipuncture or intravenous cannulation were found to be greater in preschoolers than in school-age children; however, it is not clear whether this difference was statistically significant (Van Cleve et al., 1996). Gender has been believed to be a mediator in pain experiences (Katz, Kellerman, & Siegel, 1980). However, researchers have shown that gender has no effect on pain intensity responses (Fowler-Kerry & Lander, 1991; Fradet et al., 1990; Manne et al., 1992) and behavioral responses to venipunctures (Fradet et al., 1990; Humphrey et al., 1992; Jacobsen et al., 1990). In view of the influence of socialization on school-age children's sex-role stereotypes, it was relevant to reexamine the effects of gender on pain responses.

Several researchers have reported that children's exposure to past painful procedures is inversely related to their behavioral responses to a venipuncture (Fradet et al., 1990; Jacobsen et al., 1990). However, in another study, this relationship did not reach statistical significance (Manne et al., 1992). The effects of past exposure to venipunctures on children's subjective, behavioral, and heart rate responses to a venipuncture remain unclear.

The contextual stimulus of temperament may explain the individual variability of responses across situations. According to Thomas and Chess (1977), temperament is the result of an interactive process between child and parent and consists of nine temperamental dimensions: activity, rhythmicity, approach/withdrawal, sensory threshold, intensity of reaction, quality of mood, distractibility, and attention span/persistence, and adaptability. Although the predictive effects of temperament have been studied in children's adaptation to chronic illness (Garrison, Biggs, & Williams, 1990; Wallander, Hubert, & Varni, 1988), the relationship between temperament and pain related to invasive procedures has only been examined in preschool children. Young and Fu (1988) found that a child's rhythmicity had a small effect on pain intensity and that approach accounted for 7% of children's behavioral responses to venipunctures. In view of the brevity of the venipuncture, the theoretical relevancy of each temperamental dimension, and school-age children's increased behavioral mastery, only sensory threshold, intensity, and distractibility were judged important in this study. Sensory threshold reflects sensitivity to stimulation and may be important in self-regulation and defense mechanisms (Rothbart & Derryberry, 1981). Intensity is the energy level of a response irrespective of the direction (Thomas & Chess, 1977). Distractibility, a measure of how sensitive one's attention is to environmental stimulation, may be relevant in children's coping mechanisms and adaptive responses.

Children fearful of medical procedures report higher pain intensity to venipunctures (Broome, Bates, Lillis, Wilson, & McGahee, 1990) and display more behavioral responses (Jacobsen et al., 1990). Nevertheless, investigators have not examined the contextual stimulus of children's medical fears in relation to a multidimensional view of the pain experience or accounted for another contextual stimulus, children's general fears. While fear is an immediate response to a threatening situation, general fears may serve as a context for the development of medical fears.

The family's influence on children's behaviors through the provision of structure and discipline is relevant in the study of children's responses to painful situations (Melamed & Bush, 1985). Parental restrictiveness and nurturance toward a child's behavioral expressiveness may help in understanding children's responses to pain. The contextual stimulus of child-rearing practices was examined in the situation of immunizations (Broome & Endsley, 1989). Children of authoritative (high-control, high-warmth) parents exhibited significantly fewer behavioral responses than those of authoritarian (high-control, low-warmth), permissive (low-control, high-warmth), and unresponsive (low-control, low-warmth) parents. This study extended examination of the influence of child-rearing practices to children's pain responses to venipunctures.

Previous studies of the effects of multiple variables on children's pain intensity and behavioral responses to venipunctures have been informative. However, children's pain has not been measured in a comprehensive fashion. The relationship between children's behavioral display and reported pain intensity has been found to be moderate in school-age children during venipunctures (Fradet et al., 1990; Humphrey et al., 1992; Manne et al., 1992) and during bone marrow aspirations (Jay & Elliott, 1984; Jay, Ozolins, Elliot, & Caldwell, 1983). Inasmuch as pain intensity represents one aspect of the pain experience, children's behavioral responses needed to be examined in relation to a global assessment of pain. Though not specific to pain, physiological responses have been described in acute pain experiences. However,

studies involving cardiac rate during painful procedures have yielded equivocal results. Broome and Endsley (1989) found no relationship between
preschoolers' behavioral responses and heart rate during a finger stick procedure, whereas Jay and Elliot (1984) reported a moderate correlation between
behaviors and heart rate of school-age children and adolescents during bone-
marrow aspirations. These findings support the need to reexamine the role of
sympathetic responses of heart rate combined with other pain measures during an invasive procedure. Based on the RAM and the empirical pediatric pain
literature, the hypothesis tested was that there is a relationship between the
set of independent variables age, gender, past painful experiences, temperament, medical fears, general fears, and child-rearing practices and the set of
school-age children's responses to venipuncture: pain location, pain intensity,
pain quality, observed behaviors, and heart rate.

● METHOD

Sample

The sample consisted of 94 children and their female caregivers recruited
from three outpatient clinics (gastroenterology, nephrology, and preoperative)
at a large pediatric hospital in a mid-Atlantic state. An initial power analysis
for multiple regression with 9 independent variables, a power of .80, a
medium effect size, and an alpha level of .05 revealed that 119 subjects were
necessary (Cohen, 1988). However, the actual obtained power of the main
analysis performed to test the study hypothesis was so low that an increase in
sample size would not have yielded more meaningful results. Consequently,
the study sample was judged sufficient.

Children between 8 and 12 years of age, cognitively normal for their
school grade, accompanied by a female caregiver, and expected to receive a
venipuncture during their clinic visit were asked to participate. Of the 121
subjects who were approached, 10 refused (8%) for lack of time or personal
reasons. Of those who agreed, 17 (15%) were excluded for various reasons; 4
children had cognitive deficits, 2 were not accompanied by a female caregiver,
7 did not require a venipuncture, and 4 caregivers did not have time to complete the questionnaires. Children's mean age was 10.3 (*SD* = 1.4). The majority of the children were female (54.3%) and white (86.2%).

Instruments

The Child Information Sheet (CHILDIS) was used to record information
about the child's gender, age, school grade, number of past hospitalizations,
and number of past venipunctures and other painful procedures. The Caregiver Information Sheet (CIS) was used to record demographic information
about the caregiver, including age, gender, ethnicity, marital status, education
level, employment status, and family income. Caregivers' perceptions about

the child's experiences with past hospitalizations and painful procedures were also requested.

The Middle Childhood Temperament Questionnaire (MCTQ) (Hegvik, McDevitt, & Carey, 1982) was used to measure temperament of children 8 to 12 years old. The MCTQ is a 99-item parent report using a 6-point scale from 1 (almost always) to 6 (almost never) for each of nine temperamental dimensions. Three dimensions, distractibility, intensity, and threshold, were included in this study. Higher scores are indicative of higher distractibility and intensity but lower sensory threshold. Satisfactory criterion-related validity was evidenced in comparisons of children's temperament at ages 7 and 12 (Maziade, Cote, Boudreault, Thivierge, & Boutin, 1986). For this study, the Cronbach's alpha internal consistency reliability coefficients were threshold, .68, distractibility, .75, and intensity, .81.

The Child Medical Fears Scale (CMFS) (Broome, Hellier, Wilson, Dale, & Glanville, 1988) is used to measure children's levels of reported fears related to medical personnel and diagnostic or therapeutic procedures. Children rate their level of fear for 17 items on a scale of 1 (not at all), 2 (a little), and 3 (a lot afraid), with higher scores indicating greater fear. Total scores range from 17 to 51. The content validity index for the CMFS is 78% (Broome et al., 1988). Criterion validity was established with the original Fear Survey Schedule (Scherer & Nakamura, 1968), with a correlation of .71 (Broome et al., 1988). The Cronbach's alpha internal consistency reliability coefficient was .87 for this study sample.

The Revised Fear Survey Schedule for Children (R-FSSC) (Ollendick, 1983) is an 80-item questionnaire used to measure children's general fears. Children rate their level of fear to the unknown, supernatural events, bodily injury, small animals, and death on a 3-point scale of 1 (none), 2 (some), and 3 (a lot). Total scores range from 80 to 240, with higher scores indicating greater fear. Construct validity was established by discriminating fears of phobic and normal children (Ollendick, 1983) and by supporting a decline in children's fears with age (King, Gullone, & Ollendick, 1991). The generalizability of a five-factor structure has been shown across cultures (Ollendick & Yule, 1990). The Cronbach's alpha internal consistency coefficient for the present study was .95.

The Modified Child-Rearing Practices Report (M-CRPR) (Dekovic, Janssens, & Gerris, 1991; Rickel & Biasatti, 1982) was used to measure two parental attitudes toward child rearing: parental restrictiveness, characterized by a high degree of control and endorsement of strict rules and restrictions, and parental nurturance, characterized by the willingness of parents to share feelings with their children and to show responsiveness to the child's needs. The M-CRPR consists of 40 statements with a 6-point response format, from 1 (not at all descriptive of me) to 6 (highly descriptive of me). Two scores are obtained, with lower scores indicative of low restrictiveness (range 0 to 22) and low nurturance (range 0 to 18). The validity of the M-CRPR was supported by discriminating the child-rearing practices of parents of rejected and highly sociable children (Dekovic et al., 1991) and by factor-structuring the scale (Dekovic et al., 1991; Rickel & Biasatti, 1982). In this study, the Cronbach's alphas for the restrictiveness and nurturance subscales were .90 and .92, respectively.

The Adolescent Pediatric Pain Tool (APPT) (Savedra, Tesler, Holzemer, & Ward, 1992) is a self-report measure of location, intensity, and quality of pain in children aged 8 to 17 years. Pain location is measured using a body outline figure on which children are instructed to mark the location(s) of their current pain. The number of locations is summed, with scores ranging from 0 to 43 (Savedra, Tesler, Holzemer, Wilkie, & Ward, 1989). Criterion-related validity of the pain location scale was documented when children's markings and investigators' observations reached an agreement of at least 80% (Savedra, Tesler, Holzemer, Wilkie, & Ward, 1990). A postoperative decrease in pediatric surgical patients' pain sites was found, thus supporting construct validity (Savedra et al., 1990). Intrarater reliability estimates of the agreement between subjects' markings and pointings ranged from 83% to 94% (Savedra et al., 1989).

Pain intensity was measured using a 100-mm word-graphic rating scale, with scores ranging from 0 to 100. A decline in postoperative pain intensity scores supported construct validity (Savedra et al., 1990). Criterion-related validity was established through correlations with four other pain intensity scales (Tesler et al., 1991). Test–retest reliability was .91 (Tesler et al., 1991).

Pain quality was measured using a list of 67 words that relate to the sensory, affective, evaluative, and temporal experiences of pain (Tesler, Savedra, Ward, Holzemer, & Wilkie, 1988). Based on a factor analysis that confirmed only three factors (Wilkie et al., 1990), scores, which range from 0 to 56, are reported only for sensory, affective, and evaluative subscales. Criterion-related validity was evidenced by correlations with pain intensity scores (Savedra et al., 1990). A significant decrease in the number of words used by recovering pediatric surgical patients (Savedra et al., 1990; Savedra, Holzemer, Tesler, & Wilkie, 1993) supported construct validity. Test–retest reliability of total, sensory, affective, and evaluative scores of surgical patients revealed high correlations, .95, .91, .97, and .78, respectively (Tesler et al., 1991).

The Observed Child Distress (OCDS) (Jacobsen et al., 1990; Manne et al., 1992) was used to measure six behavioral responses to venipunctures: pain verbalizations, cry/scream, request for termination of procedure, refusing to assume body position, muscular rigidity, and requiring physical restraint. These behaviors are observed during three phases of the venipuncture (phase 1, from sitting in the chair until the tourniquet is applied; phase 2, from tourniquet application until needle is to be inserted; and phase 3, from piercing the skin to bandage application). They are rated for their presence (1) or absence (0), for a total score ranging from 0 to 18. Construct validity of the OCDS was supported by a positive correlation between behavioral scores and self-reports of pain intensity (Manne et al., 1992). Cronbach's alpha internal consistency coefficient for the study sample was .83.

A Nellcor electronic pulse oximeter (N-10; Haywood, CA) was used to measure heart rate during the venipuncture through a taped sensor to a finger. Heart rate was measured at rest and monitored every 10 seconds throughout the venipuncture. The magnitude of heart rate change (highest heart rate during phase 3 relative to baseline heart rate) was calculated for each child.

Procedure

All subjects were recruited before their clinic appointments. Participation in the study was voluntary, and informed consents from female caregivers and children's assents were obtained in accordance with the institution's Committee for Protection of Human Subjects.

During waiting periods, caregivers completed the CIS, the MCTQ, and the M-CRPR. In the presence of their caregivers, children were asked to answer verbally to the CHILDIS, R-FSSC, and CMFS. A baseline heart rate was obtained after each child had rested for 15 minutes in a sitting position. Throughout all phases of the procedure, children's behavioral responses were measured using the OCDS, and heart rate was monitored with a pulse oximeter. Data obtained during the third phase of the venipuncture, which is associated with the experience of pain, is reported in this study. Only one caregiver was absent during the venipuncture. Within 10 minutes following the procedure, children completed the APPT.

● RESULTS

Examination of the distribution of the pain-related variables (Table 1) led to the exclusion of pain location scores from further statistical analyses due to limited variability. Since the distributions of pain intensity and quality scores were skewed, square root transformations were performed. Though the majority of children reported minimal pain intensity, 20% of the children regarded venipunctures as very painful procedures. Most children (98%) described their pain experiences using sensory descriptors, 75% chose evaluative words, and 40% selected affective qualities. Children's behavioral responses associated with the insertion of the needle were minimal; however, heart rate changes were of greater magnitude. For most children (96.7%), magnitude in heart rate change was within two standard deviations. For 3.3% of the sample, important changes in heart rate were recorded (< or > 3 SD).

As presented in Table 1, data about children's past experiences with venipunctures were not normally distributed. Following transformation, the majority of children (64%) were found to have prior experience with venipunctures. The distributions for the temperamental dimensions of distractibility, intensity, and threshold were found to be normal. Children's scores on general fears were normally distributed; however, medical fear scores required square root transformation. Parental restrictiveness and nurturance scores were not normally distributed and were dichotomized into high and low groups. About half of the caregivers (43.6%) scored low on parental restrictiveness and 46.8% scored low on nurturance.

TABLE D-1	Summary of Children's Scores on Dependent and Independent Variables			
	N	M	(SD)	RANGE
Pain location	94	1.2	0.5	0–3
Pain intensity	94	29.4	24.0	0–100
Pain quality	94	8.0	6.3	0–41
Behavioral responses	93	1.7	1.4	0–6
Magnitude in heart rate change (%)	90	18.9	28.7	−40 to 101.3
Age	94	10.3	1.4	8–12
Past experiences with venipunctures	84	5.1	8.9	0–40
Temperament				
Distractibility	94	4.07	0.9	1.5–6
Intensity	94	3.69	0.9	1.6–6
Threshold	94	3.85	0.8	2–5.5
General fears	90	137.9	24.3	94–212
Medical fears	90	27.6	6.8	17–49
Child-rearing practices				
Restrictiveness	84	64.2	19.2	32–130
Nurturance	86	93.3	11.9	21–107

Correlations were computed between all independent and dependent variables. Threshold was correlated with pain quality ($r(94) = .25, p < .05$)—that is, low sensory threshold was associated with more pain descriptors. Age, $r(93) = -.48, p < .001$, and threshold, $r(93) = .24, p < .05$, were correlated with behavioral responses, suggesting that with age, children manifest fewer behavioral responses, and that low sensory threshold is associated with more behavioral responses. Distractibility, $r(90) = .33, p < .05$, threshold, $r(90) = .23$, $p = .03$, general fears, $r(87) = .27, p < .05$, and medical fears, $r(86) = .26$. $p < .02$, were correlated with magnitude in heart rate change. Children with high distractibility, low threshold, and high general and medical fears had greater changes in heart rate. None of the independent variables were related to pain intensity. Consequently, pain intensity was excluded from the main analysis.

Examination of the correlations between the independent variables revealed multicollinearity for general and medical fears, $r(87) = .83, p < .001$. Consequently, general fears were excluded from the main analysis.

The correlation matrix for the dependent variables revealed low to moderate correlations between pain quality, intensity, behavioral responses, and magnitude in heart rate change. Specifically, pain quality correlated with pain intensity ($r(94) = 0.59, p < 0.001$), behavioral responses ($r(93) = 0.41, p < 0.001$), and magnitude in heart rate change ($r(90) = 32, p < 0.05$). Lower correlations were found between pain intensity and behavioral responses

($r(93) = 0.26$, $p < 0.05$) and magnitude in heart rate change ($r(90) = 0.22$, $p < 0.05$). As expected, behavioral responses were correlated with magnitude in heart rate change ($r(90) = 0.31$, $p < 0.01$). Together, these findings suggest that as children select more pain descriptors, they report higher pain intensity and exhibit more behavioral responses and greater heart rate responses.

Of the initial variables, only the independent and dependent variables that correlated significantly were retained for the canonical analysis. They were age, distractibility, threshold, medical fears, pain quality, behavioral responses, and magnitude of heart rate change. As can be seen in Table 2, two canonical variates were found to be significant. The first canonical variate (.526) was found for age and threshold, and correlated with pain quality, behavioral responses, and magnitude of heart rate change, explaining 12% of the variance. The second canonical variate (.411) revealed that age, medical fears, distractibility, and threshold correlated with pain quality and magnitude of heart rate change, explaining 5.7% of the variance. Overall, 17.7% of the variance was accounted for. Inasmuch as all variables did not enter the analysis, the study hypothesis was not supported.

TABLE D-2 *Canonical Correlation Analysis**

	CANONICAL VARIATES	
VARIABLES SETS	*I*	*2*
Set 1: independent variables		
Age of child	0.884[a]	−0.328[a]
Medical fears	−0.146	−0.582[a]
Distractibility	−0.251	−0.793[a]
Threshold	−0.572[a]	−0.504[a]
Set 2: dependent variables		
Pain quality	−0.463[a]	0.414[a]
Behavioral responses	−0.944[a]	0.055
Magnitude in heart rate change	−0.308[a]	0.912[a]
Canonical correlations	0.526	0.411
	$p < 0.001$	$p = 0.014$
Variance explained	12.0%	5.7%
Total variance explained	17.7%	

*Summary table is between age, distractibility, threshold, and medical fears (Set 1) and pain quality, behavioral responses, and heart rate magnitude (Set 2)

[a]Structure coefficients ≥ 0.30.

A closer examination of the first variate in the set of independent variables supported an association between age and threshold. That is, with age, children learn to become less sensitive to environmental stimuli. In the set of dependent variables, pain quality was found to be associated with behavioral and heart rate responses. The second variate of the canonical analysis suggested that younger and fearful children tend to be more distractible and have low sensory thresholds.

Additional findings from t-test and chi-square analyses showed no differences on most independent and dependent variables between subjects from the preoperative clinic and those from the gastroenterology and nephrology clinics. However, children from the preoperative group had less experience with past venipunctures, X^2 (1, $N = 84$) = 4.24, $p < .05$, and reported higher pain quality, $M = 2.7$, $SD = 1.1$, $T(93) = -2.1$, $p < .05$. In the total sample, girls had higher general fears than boys, $T(90) = -2.0$, $p < .001$, but no difference was found with regard to medical fears. Finally, girls had higher temperamental intensity than boys (girls, $M = 3.9$, $SD = 0.8$ vs. boys, $M = 3.5$, $SD = 0.9$; $T(94) = -2.05$, $p < .05$).

On all dependent variables, children were found to be homogeneous except that girls cried significantly more than boys during the venipuncture, X^2 (1, $N = 93$) = 4.22, $p < .05$. No differences were noted in children experienced and inexperienced with venipunctures with regard to temperament, general and medical fears, pain intensity and pain quality scores, behavioral responses, and heart rate magnitude. Regardless of children's health problems, family income, and race, there were no differences in children's responses to pain.

DISCUSSION

Although the study hypothesis was not supported, the results from the canonical correlation revealed several important relationships. Data from the first variate showed that with increasing age and in children with high sensory threshold, fewer words are used to describe pain, fewer behavioral responses are manifested, and a lower magnitude of change in heart rate is observed. With increasing age, children are more emotionally and behaviorally organized (Maccoby, 1983). Moreover, school-age children's greater understanding of the procedure, increasing awareness of socially acceptable behaviors, and competency in controlling behaviors may account for the restricted body movements. Finally, children less sensitive to sensory stimuli were less upset by the venipuncture and showed fewer behavioral responses and changes in heart rate.

Findings from the second variate suggest that younger, highly fearful, distractible, and sensitive children report higher pain quality and have higher heart rate reactivity. Lack of familiarity combined with a limited repertoire of coping skills may account for the younger child's increased vulnerability to stressful events. These findings support the need for the implementation of interventions for young children before and even during such relatively brief and simple medical procedures as venipunctures.

Correlations between the dependent variables as shown in the correlational matrix and in the first canonical variate support a relationship between the perceptual and sensory dimensions of pain. However, the relationship is low in magnitude. Gross motor responses may be less relevant in school-age children, suggesting that a focus on muscular rigidity and/or facial activity might be more appropriate for this group. In this study, no relationship was found between the independent variables and pain intensity. It may be that the venipuncture did not evoke enough variability in children's pain intensity or that no relationship can be established with pain intensity since it is essentially a subjective and unpredictable characteristic of pain.

The study results provided limited support for the Roy Adaptation Model. Based on the proposition that focal and contextual stimuli influence responses, empirical support was found for the contextual stimuli of age, medical fears, and the temperamental dimensions of distractibility and threshold. Only the contextual stimuli that affect developmental stage (age), self-concept (medical fears), and interdependence between parent and child (temperamental dimensions of distractibility and sensory threshold) were supported. The lack of a relationship between gender and subjective pain responses, though unexpected, is consistent with prior work on gender and pain intensity (Fowler-Kerry & Lander, 1991; Fradet et al., 1990; Manne et al., 1992). Limited support was found for the relationship between gender and behavioral responses, in that girls cried more than boys. The influence of parental child-rearing styles on responses to venipunctures was not noted in this study.

Contrary to prior research (Fradet et al., 1990; Jacobsen et al., 1990) but consistent with the work of Manne et al. (1992), the findings showed no relationship between experience with venipunctures and children's pain-related responses. This suggests that experienced children did not habituate to the procedure. It may also be that frequency of exposure is not sufficient information for understanding children's responses to pain. Rather, as the RAM suggests, children's coping abilities with procedures need to be taken into account.

Most importantly, findings from the correlational and canonical analyses support the multidimensionality of pain as conceptualized by the RAM. This empirical evidence is consistent with the need for clinicians and researchers to use a comprehensive approach to assess pain by integrating valid and reliable subjective, behavioral, and physiological measures. Such a global approach to understanding pain is in accordance with the RAM.

Several instruments used in the study need further evaluation. The Revised Fear Survey Schedule for Children should be revised to be more sociohistorically appropriate for children. Low scores obtained by the Child Medical Fears Scale suggest a need to reexamine the relevancy of several items with a school-age population. In view of the fact that there was no relationship between behavioral responses and pain intensity, more attention needs to be paid to the meaning of behavioral responses. For example, it is important to understand which behavioral responses are reflective of the pain experience in different age groups. This information is particularly critical in the care of children unable to express their needs verbally.

This study supports the need to assess children's pain and to identify the factors that may aggravate the pain experience. Research on helping children cope with aversive medical procedures has produced somewhat equivocal results (Dahlquist, 1992). While certain strategies may be helpful to some children, others may have no or negative effects. In order to individualize the care of children undergoing procedures, future research may be directed toward matching interventions with children's age, fears, and temperament. The findings of this research have contributed to the extension of the knowledge base on school-age children's pain to venipunctures.

Acknowledgment

This study was supported by a doctoral fellowship from the Canadian National Health Research and Development Program (# 6605–4006–47), the Canadian Nurses Foundation, a Sigma Theta Tau Xi Chapter research grant, the University of Pennsylvania, and the Marion R. Gregory Award from the Faculty of the School of Nursing at the University of Pennsylvania. The author gratefully acknowledges the assistance of Jacqueline Fawcett, PhD, FAAN, Margaret Grey, DrPH, FAAN, and David E. Cohen, MD, during her doctoral work. The helpful comments of Dr. Fawcett on a draft of this manuscript are also acknowledged.

REFERENCES

Andrews, H. A., & Roy, C. (1991a). Essentials of the Roy adaptation model. In C. Roy & H. A. Andrews (Eds.), *The Roy Adaptation Model: The definitive statement* (p. 325). Norwalk, CT: Appleton & Lange.

Andrews, H. A., & Roy, C. (1991b). The nursing process according to the Roy adaptation model. In C. Roy & H. A. Andrews (Eds.), *The Roy Adaptation Model: The definitive statement* (pp. 27–54). Norwalk, CT: Appleton & Lange.

Broome, M. E., Bates, T. A., Lillus, P. P., & McGahee, T. W. (1990). Children's medical fears, coping behaviors, and pain perceptions during a lumbar puncture. *Oncology Nursing Forum, 17,* 361–367.

Broome, M. E., & Endsley, R. C. (1989). Maternal presence, childrearing practices, and children's response to an injection. *Research in Nursing and Health, 12,* 229–235.

Broome, M. E., Hellier, A., Wilson, T., Dale, S., & Glanville, C. (1988). Measuring children's fears of medical experiences. In C. F. Waltz & O. L. Strickland (Eds.), *Measurement of Nursing Outcomes* (Vol. 1, pp. 201–214). New York: Springer.

Cohen, J. (1988). *Statistical power analysis for the behavioral sciences* (2nd ed.). Hillsdale, NJ: Erlbaum.

Dahlquist, L. M. (1992). Coping with aversive medical treatments. In A. M. La Greca, L. J. Siegel, J. L. Wallander, & C. E. Walker (Eds.), *In stress and coping with child health* (pp. 345–376). New York: Guilford Press.

Dekovic, M., Janssens, J. M. A. M., & Gerris, J. R. M. (1991). Factor structure validity of the Block Child rearing practices Report (CRPR). *Psychological Assessment: A Journal of Consulting and Clinical Psychology, 3,* 182–187.

Fowler-Kerry, S. (1990). Adolescent oncology survivors recollection of pain. In D. C. Tyler & E. J. Krane (Eds.), *Advances in pain research therapy* (Vol. 15, pp. 365–371). New York: Raven Press.

Fowler-Kerry, S., & Lander, J. (1991). Assessment of sex differences in children's and adolescents self-reported from venipunctures. *Journal of Pediatric Psychology, 16,* 783–793.

Fradet, C., McGrath, P. J., Kay, J., Adams, S., & Luke, B. (1990). A prospective survey of reactions to blood tests by children and adolescents. *Pain, 40,* 53–60.

Garrison, W. T., Biggs, D., & Williams, K. (1990). Temperament characteristics and clinical outcomes in young children with diabetes mellitus. *Child Psychology and Psychiatry, 31,* 1079–1088.

Harrison, A. (1991). Preparing children for venous sampling. *Pain, 45,* 299–306.

Hegvik, R. L., McDevitt, S. C., & Carey, W. B. (1982). The middle childhood temperament questionnaire. *Developmental and Behavioral Pediatrics, 3,* 197–200.

Humphrey, G. B., Boon, C. M. J., van Linden van den Heuvell, G. F. E. C., & van de Wiel, H. B. M. (1992). The occurrence of high levels of acute behavioral distress in children and adolescents undergoing routine venipunctures. *Pediatrics, 90,* 87–91.

Jacobsen, P. B., Manne, S. L., Gorfinkle, K., Schorr, O., Rapkin, B., & Redd, W. H. (1990). Analysis of child and parent behavior during painful medical procedures. *Health Psychology, 9,* 559–576.

Jay, S. M., & Elliot, C. (1984). Behavioral observation scale for measuring children's distress: The effects of increased methodological rigor. *Journal of Consulting and Clinical Psychology, 52,* 1106–1107.

Jay, S. M., Ozouns, M., Elliot, C. H., & Caldwell, S. (1983). Assessment of children's distress during painful medical procedures. *Health Psychology, 2,* 133–147.

Katz, E. R., Kellerman, J., & Siegel, S. (1980). Behavioral distress in children with cancer undergoing medical procedures: Developmental considerations. *Journal of Consulting and Clinical Psychology, 48,* 356–365.

King, N. J., Gullone, E., & Ollendick, T. H. (1991). Manifest anxiety and fearfulness in children and adolescents. *Journal of Genetic Psychology, 153,* 63–73.

Lander, J., & Fowler-Kerry, S. (1991). Age differences in children's pain. *Perceptual and Motor Skills, 73,* 415–418.

Maccoby, E. E. (1983). Social-emotional development and response to stressor. In N. Garmezy & M. Rutter (Eds.), *Stress, coping, and development in children* (pp. 217–234). New York: McGraw-Hill.

Manne, S. L., Jacobsen, P. B., & Redo, W. H. (1992). Assessment of acute pediatric pain: Do child self-report, parent ratings and nurse ratings measure the same phenomenon? *Pain, 48,* 45–52.

Maziade, M., Cote, R., Boudrealt, M., Thivierge, J., & Boutin, P. (1986). Family correlates of temperament continuity and change across middle childhood. *American Journal of Orthopsychiatry, 56,* 195–203.

Melamed, B. G., & Bush, J. P. (1985). Family factors in children with acute illness. In D. Turk & R. Kems (Eds.), *Health illness and families: A life-span perspective* (pp. 183–219). New York: Wiley.

Ollendick, T. H. (1983). Reliability and validity of the revised fear survey schedule for children (FSSC-R). *Behavior Research Therapy, 21,* 685–692.

Ollendick, T. H., & Yule, W. (1990). Depression in British and American children and its relation to anxiety and fear. *Journal of Consulting and Clinical Psychology, 58,* 126–129.

Rickel, A. U., & Biasatti, L. L. (1982). Modification of the Block child rearing practice report. *Journal of Clinical Psychology, 38,* 129–134.

Rothbart, M. K., & Derryberry, D. (1981). Development of individual differences in temperament. In M. E. Lamb & A. L. Brown (Eds.), *Advances in developmental psychology* (pp. 37–86). Hillsdale, NJ: Erlbaum.

Roy, C. (1991). Senses. In C. Roy & H. A. Andrews (Eds.), *The Roy Adaptation Model: The definitive statement* (pp. 164–189). Norwalk, CT: Appleton & Lange.

Roy, C., & Andrews, H. A. (1991). *The Roy Adaptation Model: The definitive statement.* Norwalk, CT: Appleton & Lange.

Roy, C., & Corliss, C. P. (1993). The Roy Adaptation Model: Theoretical update and knowledge for practice. In M. E. Parker (Ed.), *Patterns of nursing theories in practice* (pp. 215–229). New York: National League for Nursing.

Savedra, M. C., Holzemer, W. L., Tesler, M. D., & Wilkie, D. J. (1993). Assessment of postoperative pain in children and adolescents using the adolescent pediatric pain tool. *Nursing Research, 42,* 5–9.

Savedra, M. C., Tesler, M. D., Holzemer, W. L., & Ward, J. A. (1992). *Adolescent Pediatric Pain Tool (APPT): User's manual.* San Francisco: University of California, School of Nursing.

Savedra, M. C., Tesler, M. D., Holzemer, W. L., Wilkie, D. J., & Ward, J. A. (1989). Pain location: Validity and reliability of body outline markings by hospitalized children and adolescents. *Research in Nursing and Health, 12,* 307–314.

Savedra, M. C., Tesler, M. D., Holzemer, W. L., Wilkie, D. J., & Ward, J. A. (1990). Testing a tool to assess postoperative pediatric and adolescent pain. In D. C. Tyler & E. J. Krane (Eds.), *Advances in pain therapy* (Vol. 15, pp. 85–93). New York: Raven Press.

Scherer, M. W., & Nakamura, C. Y. (1968). A fear survey for children (FSS-FC): A factor analytic comparison with manifest anxiety (CMA). *Behavior Research and Therapy, 6,* 173–182.

Tesler, M., Savedra, M., Ward, J. A., Holzemer, W. L., & Wilkie, D. (1988). Children's language of pain. In R. Dubner, G. F. Gebhart, et al. (Eds.), *Pain research and clinical management. Proceedings of the World Congress on Pain* (Vol. 3, pp. 348–352). Amsterdam: Elsevier.

Tesler, M. D., Savedra, M. C., Holzemer, W. L., Wilkie, D. J., Ward, J., & Paul, S. M. (1991). The word-graphic rating scale as a measure of children's and adolescents' pain intensity. *Research in Nursing Health, 14,* 361–371.

Thomas, A., & Chess, S. (1977). *Temperament and development.* New York: Brunner and Mazel.

Van Cleve, L., Johnson, L., & Pothier, P. (1996). Pain responses of hospitalized infants and children to venipuncture and intravenous cannulation. *Journal of Pediatric Nursing, 11,* 169–174.

Wallander, J. L., Hubert, N. C., & Varni, J. W. (1988). Child and maternal temperament characteristics, goodness of fit, and adjustment in physically handicapped children. *Journal of Clinical Child Psychology, 17,* 336–344.

Wilkie, D. J., Holzemer, W. L., Tesler, M. D., Ward, J. A., Paul, S. M., Savedra, M.C. (1990). Measuring pain quality: Validity and reliability of children's and adolescents' pain language. *Pain, 41,* 151–159.

Wong, D. L., & Baker, C. M. (1988). Pain in children: Comparison of assessment scales. *Pediatric Nursing, 14,* 9–17.

Young, M. R., & Fu, V. R. (1988). Influence of play and temperament on the young child's response to pain. *Children's Health Care,* 209–215.

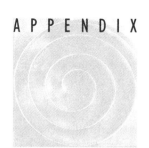

APPENDIX E

Example of a Qualitative Research Report

Bed Rest From the Perspective of the High-Risk Pregnant Woman

Annette Gupton, RN, PhD, Maureen Heaman, RN, MN, and Terri Ashcroft, RN, MN

● ABSTRACT

Objective: To describe the experience of prolonged bed rest from the perspective of women during high-risk pregnancies.

Design: A focused ethnographic study that used interviews, participant diaries, and field notes as data sources.

Setting: Participants were obtained from an acute-care hospital antepartum unit and an antepartum home care program.

Participants: Twenty-four women with complications of pregnancy requiring prolonged bed rest (range, 7–50 days).

Results: A model of the stress process in pregnant women on bed rest emerged from the data analysis. Stressors were grouped into situational (sick role, lack of control, uncertainty, concerns regarding fetus's well-being, and being tired of waiting), environmental (feeling like a prisoner, being bored, and having a sense of missing out), and family (role reversal and worry about older children) categories. Two main mediators of stress were social support and coping. Families, friends, and professionals were perceived as sources of support. Women used coping strategies, such as keeping a positive attitude, taking it 1 day at a time, doing it for the baby, getting used to it, setting goals, and keeping busy. Manifestations of stress were evidenced by adverse physical symptoms, emotional reactions, and altered social relationships.

Conclusions: Prolonged bed rest is a stressful experience for pregnant women at high risk. Understanding the stress process in pregnant women confined to bed rest may assist nurses in developing interventions to reduce stressors and enhance mediators.

Bed rest at home or in the hospital often is prescribed for women experiencing complications of pregnancy (Crowther & Chalmers, 1989). In light of the extensive use of antepartum bed rest, more information is needed about the physical and psychosocial effects of prolonged bed rest on pregnant women (Maloni, 1993). Preliminary studies indicate pregnant women on bed rest experience physiologic deconditioning, dysphoria, and prolonged postpartum recovery (Maloni et al., 1993).

Several studies have delineated stressors associated with high-risk pregnancy and antepartum hospitalization. However, none of these studies has focused specifically on the experience of prolonged bed rest during a high-risk pregnancy, particularly from the perspective of women. Werner (1993) indicates that lack of qualitative research on stressors constitutes a major gap in the literature. The purpose of this qualitative study was to explore the experience of prolonged bed rest from the pregnant woman's perspective. Understanding the experiences of pregnant women on bed rest will assist nurses in improving the quality of care they provide.

● LITERATURE REVIEW

Stressors Associated With High-Risk Pregnancy

Until recently, most research on high-risk pregnancy focused on women undergoing antepartum hospitalization. The effects of long-term antepartum hospitalization are the result of the interaction of the various stressors impinging on the woman (Snyder, 1984). Stress is a broad concept encompassing an entire field of study (Barnfather, 1993), whereas a stressor is defined as "an internal or external event, condition, situation, and/or cue, that has the potential to bring about or actually activates significant physical or psychosocial reactions" (Werner, 1993, p. 15). Stressors associated with antepartum hospitalization include separation from home and family, feelings of helplessness and loss of control, boredom, loneliness, concerns for health of the fetus, and frequent mood swings (Curry, 1987; Loos & Julius, 1989; McCain & Deatrick, 1994; Waldron & Asayama, 1985; White & Ritchie, 1984). Most of these studies do not specify the extent to which pregnant women were confined to bed rest. However, bed rest is frequently an integral component of hospitalization.

Researchers investigating the impact of stressors associated with antepartum hospitalization have found significant manifestations of stress. Hospitalized pregnant women who are at high risk report greater anxiety and depression, lower self-esteem, and less optimal family functioning than pregnant women not hospitalized or at high risk (Becker, 1984; Mercer & Ferketich, 1988; Mercer, Ferketich, DeJoseph, May, & Sollid, 1988). Length of hospitalization also may be a significant variable. In White and Ritchie's (1984) study, women hospitalized for more than 2 weeks experienced increased levels of stress. Significant negative correlations have been found between number of hours hospitalized and self-esteem and between number of hours hospitalized and evaluation of pregnancy (Becker, 1984). Ford and Hodnett's (1990) findings suggest that hospitalized pregnant women's level of adaptation decreases as hospitalization progresses. In addition to immediate manifestations of stress, long-term antepartum hospitalization also has the potential for influencing later maternal-child relationships, family interactions, and future child-bearing (Snyder, 1984).

Effects of Bed Rest in Pregnant Women

Only a few studies have been conducted that examine the effects of bed rest in pregnant women. Curtis (1986) examined the effects of bed rest in two groups of high-risk pregnant women (N = 30): one group was on bed rest for 2 or more weeks and a second group was not on bed rest. The women on bed rest had significantly more somatic complaints, anxiety, and depression. They also reported major concerns around issues of planning and control, family responses and support, opinions of professionals, and emotional lability.

Maloni et al. (1993) studied the type of bed rest and its effect on hospitalized pregnant women. Complete bed rest was defined as confinement to bed with no skeletal weight bearing for 2 or more days, and partial bed rest was defined as confinement to bed for part of the day and never on complete bed rest for 2 or more days (Maloni et al., 1993). Women on complete bed rest (n = 10) had greater weight loss, gastrocnemius muscle dysfunction, and dysphoria than did women on partial bed rest (n = 7) or no bed rest (n = 18). Dysphoria was a composite score of anxiety, depression, and hostility. For women on complete bed rest, the time needed to recover from exercise increased as the length of bed rest increased. Postpartum recovery from the side effects of bed rest was prolonged and included symptoms of muscular and cardiovascular deconditioning, such as shortness of breath on exertion, muscle soreness, and difficulty descending and ascending stairs during the 1st postpartum week.

Pregnant women on bed rest face many stressors common to those experiencing a high-risk pregnancy. Most studies concerning high-risk pregnancy have involved hospitalized antepartum patients experiencing various levels of restricted activity. The purpose of this study was to explore the experience of prolonged bed rest from the perspective of women with high-risk pregnancies and to develop a conceptual model to illustrate their experience.

● METHODS

Design

This focused ethnographic study was designed to discover personal meaning and describe the experience of bed rest. The term "focused ethnography" (Morse, 1991; Muecke, 1994) has been used to describe the topic-oriented, small-group ethnographies found in the nursing literature. The purpose of ethnography is to understand the lives of other individuals, in this case pregnant women on bed rest.

Sample

Pregnant women with complications that required them to be placed on partial or complete bed rest at home or in the hospital were approached to participate in the study. Criteria for participation included being on bed rest for at least 7 days and being a minimum of 26 weeks gestation. A purposeful sample, as described by Morse (1989), in which participants are chosen according to the needs of the study was used. The sample size of 24 women was determined by the focused nature of the investigation. When saturation occurred, data collection was terminated.

Setting

Participants were recruited from two settings. The first was an antepartum unit within a tertiary-care hospital in midwestern Canada with approximately 4,000 deliveries per year. In the second setting, pregnant women with complications received care at home from a team of specially trained public health nurses.

Procedure

Agency access was obtained and ethical approval was received from a human subjects committee. After obtaining informed consent from participants, data were collected through the use of interviews, participant diaries, and field notes. Interviews occurred at the bedside of participants and were tape-recorded. The interview guide began with a general inquiry about the woman's present pregnancy, "I would like to hear the story of your pregnancy and what it has been like for you." This was followed by a broad question about bed rest: "Tell me what it has been like for you to be on bed rest." Additional probes included "What has been the most difficult part of being on bed rest?"; "What kind of emotions have you experienced since being on bed rest?"; "What if anything has made this period of bed rest bearable?"; and "How has being on bed rest affected your family relationships?"

At the end of the interview, participants were asked to keep a diary of their experiences for the duration of their bed rest. Women were given the following instructions:

> The purpose of the diary is to record your feelings and reactions during the time you are on bed rest. We would suggest that you write down the events of each day, how you felt during that day and any other emotional or physical reactions. Your worries, concerns and happy moments are an important source of information to further understand what it is like to be on bed rest.

Participants also completed a demographic data collection form. Unstructured field notes were written at the end of each interview. They included details of the situation, personal insights, and contextual factors at the time of the interview.

Data Analysis

Interviews and diaries were transcribed and entered into a qualitative data management software package, Qualpro (Blackman, 1984–1991). Content analysis as described by Burnard (1991) was used to analyze data and identify themes. Initially, all three investigators coded each line of data conjointly to establish basic codes. Subsequently, the investigators completed coding separately. To examine interrater reliability, the three investigators coded a segment of the same transcript; an 88% agreement rate was achieved. Codes were collapsed and combined, and relationships between the themes were examined. Demographic data were analyzed through the use of descriptive statistics.

⬤ RESULTS

Twenty-four women took part in the study. The majority of participants were white and married; their ages ranged from 18 to 36 years, with a mean of 29 years. Participants were well-educated, with a mean of 14.7 years of education (range, 12–20 years). Gestational age ranged from 26 to 39 weeks at the time of interview, with a mean of 32.5 weeks. Diagnoses varied. Seven women had a diagnosis of placenta previa, four of spontaneous premature rupture of membranes, five of pregnancy-induced hypertension, and eight of preterm labor. Most of the women had planned their pregnancies ($n = 20$, 83.3%). Ten were primigravidae, and 14 were multigravidae. Five of the women had undergone bed rest during a previous pregnancy. None of the participants were receiving tocolytic medications to inhibit labor because tocolytics are used infrequently at the hospital.

At the time of the interview, 12 women had been on bed rest exclusively in the hospital setting, 3 women had been on bed rest solely in the home, and 9 had been on bed rest in both settings. Participants' number of days on bed rest ranged from 7 to 50, with a mean of 20 days. Only four women experienced a period of complete bed rest in which they were not allowed out of bed. Most of the women were on partial bed rest, defined as being allowed out of bed to use the bathroom or allowed to be up for short periods.

Most themes emerging from the data were related to various aspects of the stress process. The investigators examined literature on stress and chose to use Pearlin's (1989) three domains of the stress process to assist in organizing the data and form the basis for development of a model. The domains of the stress process include stressors, stress mediators, and stress outcomes or manifestations. Figure 1 depicts a model of the stress process in pregnant women undergoing bed rest.

Stressors

Themes related to stressors fell into three main categories: situational, environmental, and family.

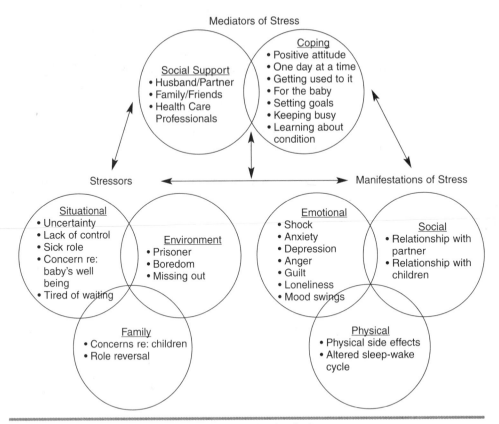

Mediators of Stress

Coping
• Positive attitude
• One day at a time
• Getting used to it
• For the baby
• Setting goals
• Keeping busy
• Learning about condition

Social Support
• Husband/Partner
• Family/Friends
• Health Care Professionals

Stressors

Manifestations of Stress

Situational
• Uncertainty
• Lack of control
• Sick role
• Concern re: baby's well being
• Tired of waiting

Environment
• Prisoner
• Boredom
• Missing out

Family
• Concerns re: children
• Role reversal

Emotional
• Shock
• Anxiety
• Depression
• Anger
• Guilt
• Loneliness
• Mood swings

Social
• Relationship with partner
• Relationship with children

Physical
• Physical side effects
• Altered sleep-wake cycle

FIGURE E-I. Stress process in pregnant woman assigned to bed rest.

SITUATION

Situational stressors refer to the stressors created by the situation of having a complicated pregnancy and being assigned to bed rest. Situational themes included sick role, uncertainty, lack of control, concerns regarding fetus's well-being, and being tired of waiting. Being assigned to bed rest reinforced the sick role and became a stressor because most of the women did not feel sick. One woman was particularly troubled by having to take on the sick role:

> Like I said before, it is very frustrating when you can't feel your sickness inside. I mean, I know it can be pretty dangerous with hypertension; it affects a lot of major organs, but you know when you can't feel it, you can't see it, it is like you feel good half the time. You feel like you can go outside and do all these things, and you are used to doing all these things. It is very frustrating that all of a sudden you can't do anything, you feel like you are a quadriplegic, and all of a sudden life is over and you have to just stay in bed.

Uncertainty and lack of control have been documented as part of the high-risk pregnancy experience (Stainton, McNeil, & Harvey, 1992). In the current study, similar phenomena, heightened by assignment to bed rest, were observed. Women indicated their uncertainty by stating, "You kind of lie here and you are kind of like a time bomb." Lack of control and uncertainty was described as

> . . . not knowing how long I would be on bed rest. I never knew for sure, will I be here another 4 weeks or 2 weeks, what will happen after that? . . . I am not controlling my own life; the doctors and everybody else are in control, my life is in their hands, so is my baby's life. I am totally helpless.

Concern about the fetus's well-being was another situational stressor. Women described spending a great deal of time thinking about the fetus. One woman said she thought about the fetus constantly and was concerned about its health. Lying in bed with nothing to do gave women a great deal of time for such thoughts.

Bed rest often was described as a waiting game. Waiting and being tired of waiting was the final situational stressor. Women got frustrated with the whole experience and wanted it to be over. One woman said, "You get into bed because you know another day is going by. Even though you are waiting for time to go by you lose track of time . . . at one point I said, 'Well, that is it, I want this baby out.' "

ENVIRONMENT

Environmental stressors include those imposed by being confined in the home or hospital environment. These included feeling like a prisoner, being bored, and a sense of "missing out." Women described feeling like a prisoner as, "Well, at first it was like being locked up," "It's boring, confining, and in a sense you feel like a prisoner," and "You can't do anything, you are a prisoner in your own home." One woman referred to her admission date as her "date of incarceration." Boredom, another stressor, was described by the women: "I felt like a slug laying there," and "There has been the odd day where my body would just like to jump out of its skin, I just couldn't stand it, I couldn't occupy myself." Many women felt that because of bed rest they were missing out: "It feels like you are missing out on something," and "Missing the whole summer." One woman in the hospital cried when she described missing out on her child's developmental milestone of starting to walk.

FAMILY

Aspects of family life also were stressors, particularly women's concerns about their children and role reversal. One woman stated, "The first thing that I thought of was the kids, that I wouldn't be at home with them." A woman cared for in the home said, "That has been the most frustrating thing . . . letting somebody come in and pretty much take over everything that I did, especially with Bobby [her son] and now when something goes wrong he screams for Daddy and it has always been me." Role reversals resulting from bed rest occurred and were an additional stressor. Husbands were described as taking on child care and household duties that the women previously had performed. Bed rest often forced role reversal, as the following mother explained:

> He has to learn to take care of a baby 24 hours a day, be a Mr. Mom! It is hard not to contribute . . . just to even keeping the household going, forget about work and everything. Just kind of lying here and watching someone have to do it all.

Mediators of Stress

Themes related to mediation of stress fell into two main categories: social support and coping.

SOCIAL SUPPORT

Social support, which refers to emotional or tangible support provided by the woman's social network, was obtained from the husband or partner, family and friends, and health care providers. Having visitors was important. "The biggest help that I have from them is just visiting," one woman said. Another said:

> I have a lot of family support and my husband is great, he doesn't ever complain. He goes to work and comes home and cooks, cleaning and shopping and doing all that stuff. . . . It has been not a bad experience because I haven't had to worry about anything. I could just worry about laying here and the baby and stuff. If that wouldn't have been the case, I think it would have been more stressful.

Health care providers also mediated the stress associated with bed rest. Women emphasized that nurses should be friendly, take time to sit and chat, make suggestions about things to do, explain things, provide information, and answer questions. A woman in the home care program said, "Having someone to answer my questions has been the biggest thing." One patient expressed the opinion of many women in the hospital: "The nurses go out of their way for you to feel comfortable, especially knowing that you are here that long." Nurses who conveyed a sense of caring were felt to mediate stress, "like they are concerned about you," a woman said. When asked to describe what nursing approaches were most helpful, many of the women replied, "Talking to me as a real person." Having the physician provide explanations and give reassurance also was valued.

COPING

Women used various coping strategies to help mediate the stress. Keeping a positive attitude was described as beneficial. "Your frame of mind has a lot to do with everything," a woman said. Taking it 1 day at a time was another strategy. Just getting used to bed rest and accepting the situation was another approach. Women indicated that telling themselves they were complying with bed rest for the sake of the baby was a good coping strategy: "I realize I am here for my baby and not just myself and that is top priority" was one comment. To cope, women set goals for themselves, such as, "Well, I set little goals when I first came in. I wanted to make it past 32 weeks. . . . So now we are past 32 and we are onto 33 . . . and now I am counting to 35." Women with strong religious beliefs found prayer and reading the Bible helpful. Keeping busy was a frequently used strategy: "I just basically find that if you are going to be stuck in bed, just think of things to do, take up a hobby," a woman said. Education in the form of learning more about their condition was described as helpful. The women indicated that reading material, video tapes, and tours of the neonatal intensive-care unit were positive influences on stress. Hearing the fetal heart rate and having a reassuring ultrasound examination were found to be stress management strategies. A woman said, "The most important thing to me is that fetal heart monitor. I wish I had one; you know, hearing that every day means the world to me."

Manifestations of Stress

Stress in women on bed rest was manifested in emotional reactions, altered relationships with family members, and physical side effects.

EMOTIONAL

Women experienced a variety of emotional reactions to their bed rest experience, including feelings of shock and confusion, anxiety, depression, anger, frustration, guilt, loneliness, mood swings, and disappointment. One woman wrote in her diary:

> It just seemed that I couldn't stop crying. I felt truly disappointed that my pregnancy wasn't "perfect." I wanted to be able to go out, to be able to wear all my maternity clothes, to show off my pregnancy, to go shopping, to do "normal" things, but most of all, to enjoy my pregnancy.

SOCIAL

Families played a central role in the bed rest experience. They were a source of stress and also mediated stress, which was manifested by altered family relationships with the partner and children. The negative effects of bed rest on the couple's relationship were described as:

> I miss our sexual life! I miss the intimacy. Here, all we can do is kiss and hug. . . . It's hard to be centered on one another when you know anyone will waltz into the room at any time. The kisses are too brief!

Another woman said, "It kind of made our visits really tense at first, and I was telling him I don't feel married, it feels like it is just some friend coming to visit me." Women felt guilty about having their partners take on extra responsibilities. One said, "Sometimes [my husband] would get home from work, and he would be just beat and be cooking dinner and then he would have to get groceries, and I would think, 'Oh, God!' " Positive effects on the relationship also were described, including, "I don't think we have grown apart at all. I think we realized more and more how much we need each other."

PHYSICAL

Women on bed rest mentioned physical side effects and changes in their sleep–wake cycles. Difficulty sleeping at night, especially in the hospital, was a common theme. Women tried to avoid taking naps or sleeping during the day in the hope that they would sleep at night. Several other physical side effects were described. Women felt they tired easily and felt weaker than before bed rest. "It kind of zaps your energy," one said. Women reported problems with digestion, constipation, physical aches and pains, sore joints, weight loss, and loss of muscle tone. Women made the following comments: "I feel like I am withering away," "These legs, they just don't have the muscles to carry me the way they used to," and "I find it even hard to climb the stairs now."

● LIMITATIONS

The study consisted of a small, select sample of women in one geographic location. Homogeneity of participants in terms of social class, education, and marital status limits generalization of findings. Results should be considered preliminary because further investigations are needed to expand and explore the applicability of the model to more diverse populations.

● DISCUSSION

A major contribution of this study is the development of a model to describe the stress process in pregnant women on bed rest, which was based on data from the perspective of women living the experience. Although many of the stressors, mediators, and manifestations of stress are similar to those described in the literature about high-risk pregnancy and antepartum hospitalization, the model offers a detailed and specific understanding of the experience of bed rest in home and hospital settings.

The stressors and manifestations of stress reported in high-risk pregnancy are exacerbated and altered by the experience of bed rest. Feeling like a prisoner, boredom, difficulties imposed by having to take on the sick role, lack of control, role reversal, and physical side effects were heightened by assignment to bed rest.

Loss of control has been identified as a stressor in previous studies on high-risk pregnancy (Loos & Julius, 1989; Stainton et al., 1992; Waldron & Asayama, 1985). For women in this study, restrictions on physical activities imposed by bed rest led to a heightened sense of relinquishing control over oneself to others. Women's sense of being a prisoner was an additional stressor not found in other literature, but which is inherent in the bed rest experience in the home and hospital settings. This theme of feeling like a prisoner conveys the strong sense of loss of control associated with the restrictions of bed rest. Antepartum hospitalization also has been associated with feelings of boredom (Curry, 1987; Loos & Julius, 1989). Boredom was compounded by the limits bed rest imposed on activity in the hospital and home. The number of alternative activities, such as taking short walks or going outside, was severely restricted because of bed rest. Stainton et al. (1992) found that pregnant women at high risk were forced into the sick role when they had no sense of feeling ill. This role change was further reinforced by bed rest and in turn contributed to feelings of powerlessness.

In this study, as in May's (1994) investigation of activity restriction for women with preterm labor, family relationships were strained. Partners took on larger amounts of the woman's role activities because of bed rest. Women who had other children found bed rest placed limitations on their ability to care for and interact physically with their children. Consequently, the woman experienced anxiety and frustration.

All women described the physical effects of bed rest, which were similar to those described by Maloni et al. (1993). They frequently mentioned weakness and disturbance in sleep patterns related specifically to bed rest. Lying in bed most of the day fostered frequent napping; the usual patterns of being awake during the day and sleeping at night were altered drastically.

● *NURSING IMPLICATIONS*

Having an in-depth understanding of the experience of bed rest during pregnancy will help nurses improve the quality of care for pregnant women. Study participants emphasized the importance to them of having sensitive and caring nurses. However, women frequently commented that the most important nursing intervention was to listen to their concerns. Being treated like a "person" was particularly important to women during this stressful time. They wanted nurses who were compassionate and who could understand their feelings.

The situational stressors of bed rest may be reduced by allowing women to participate in their care and hence enhancing their sense of control. The sense of the sick role and feelings of being a prisoner may be lessened if women are allowed to wear street clothes or go outside for brief periods. In addition, environmental stressors may be alleviated by planning activities to prevent boredom. Encouraging family visits and fostering clear communication between partners may decrease family stressors, increase social support, and decrease social manifestations of stress. Coping can be enhanced by providing information about the woman's condition and survival tips for how to deal with bed rest, answering questions, and establishing a support group. Physical manifestations may be prevented through referrals to a physiotherapist for a program of exercises for bed rest.

RECOMMENDATIONS FOR FUTURE RESEARCH

Many recommendations for future research arise from this study. This model must be tested in more diverse populations. The experience may be different for women with less education and income than for those in the current sample. Women with small children may have an experience different from those without other children. There is a need for prospective quantitative research on the physiologic and psychologic changes associated with prolonged bed rest during pregnancy. Researchers must differentiate the effects of complete versus partial bed rest and the effects of bed rest at home versus in the hospital. In particular, there is a need to study the extent of physiologic deconditioning that occurs during pregnancy bed rest, and what, if any, interventions are effective in alleviating these symptoms. The effect of bed rest during pregnancy on postpartum recovery and implications for nursing care should be investigated. Given the documented negative physical and emotional effects of bed rest, more clinical trials are needed on the effectiveness of bed rest as a treatment for various pregnancy complications.

CONCLUSION

This study has contributed to the knowledge base on stress during high-risk pregnancy and the role bed rest plays in the experience. Women's perspectives of the experience form the basis for enhanced understanding. Mercer and Ferketich (1988) suggest, "Stress results not from a particular life event per se but from the individual's perception of that event and of his or her ability to control and deal with the event" (p. 26). The model developed in this study provides a clear depiction of women's specific experiences with bed rest within a broader framework of stress. Nursing care of patients may improve when caregivers gain empathic insight into the experience from women's perspectives.

Acknowledgment

This study was funded by the Manitoba Association of Registered Nurses.

REFERENCES

Barnfather, J. (1993). History, overview, and project methodology. In J. Barnfather & B. Lyon (Eds.), *Stress and coping: State of the science and implications for nursing theory, research and practice* (pp. 1–10). Indianapolis, IN: Center Nursing Press of Sigma Theta Tau International.
Becker, C. (1984). *Self-concept of hospitalized gravidas in the last trimester of pregnancy.* Unpublished doctoral dissertation, University of Texas at Austin.
Blackman, B. I. (1984–1991). *Qualpro Text Database and Productivity Tool* (computer software). Tallahassee, FL: Impulse Development Co.
Burnard, P. (1991). A method of analysing interview transcripts in qualitative research. *Nurse Education Today, 11,* 461–466.

Crowther, C., & Chalmers, I. (1989). Bedrest and hospitalization during pregnancy. In I. Chalmers, M. Enkin, & M. Keirse (Eds.), *Effective care in pregnancy and childbirth* (Vol. I: Pregnancy, pp. 624–632). Oxford: Oxford University Press.

Curry, M. (1987). Maternal behavior of hospitalized pregnant women. *Journal of Psychosomatic Obstetrics and Gynaecology, 7,* 65–182.

Curtis, K. (1986). *The psycho-physiologic effects of bedrest on at-risk pregnant women: A pilot study.* Unpublished master's thesis, University of Madison–Wisconsin.

Ford, M., & Hodnett, E. (1990). Predictors of adaptation in women hospitalized during pregnancy. *Canadian Journal of Nursing Research, 22*(4), 37–50.

Loos, C., & Julius, L. (1989). The client's view of hospitalization during pregnancy. *Journal of Obstetric, Gynecologic, and Neonatal Nursing, 18,* 52–56.

McCain, G. C., & Deatrick, J. A. (1994). The experience of high-risk pregnancy. *Journal of Obstetric, Gynecologic, and Neonatal Nursing, 23,* 421–427.

Maloni, J. (1993). Bedrest during pregnancy: Implications for nursing. *Journal of Obstetric, Gynecologic, and Neonatal Nursing, 22,* 422–426.

Maloni, J., Chance, B., Zhang, C., Cohen, A. W., Betts, D., & Gange, S. J. (1993). Physical and psychosocial side effects of antepartum hospital bed rest. *Nursing Research, 42,* 197–203.

May, K. A. (1994). Impact of maternal activity restriction for preterm labor on the expectant father. *Journal of Obstetric, Gynecologic, and Neonatal Nursing, 23,* 246–251.

Mercer, R., & Ferketich, S. (1988). Stress and social support as predictors of anxiety and depression during pregnancy. *Advances in Nursing Science, 10,*(2) 26–39.

Mercer, R., Ferketich, S., DeJoseph, J., May, K., & Sollid, D. (1988). Effect of stress on family functioning during pregnancy. *Nursing Research, 37,* 268–275.

Morse, J. M. (1989). Strategies for sampling. In J. M. Morse (Ed.), *Qualitative nursing research: A contemporary dialogue* (pp. 117–132). Rockville, MD: Aspen Publishers, Inc.

Morse, J. M. (1991). Qualitative nursing research: A free-for-all? In J. M. Morse (Ed.), *Qualitative nursing research: A contemporary dialogue* (Revised ed., pp. 14–22). Newbury Park, CA: Sage Publications.

Muecke, M. (1994). On the evaluation of ethnographics. In J. Morse (Ed.), *Critical issues in qualitative research methods* (pp. 187–200). Thousand Oaks, CA: Sage Publications.

Pearlin, L. (1989). The sociological study of stress. *Journal of Health and Social Behavior, 30,* 241–256.

Snyder, D. (1984). Effects of long-term hospitalization on the antepartal patient. *NAACOG Update Series* (Vol. 1, Lesson 19). Princeton, NJ: Continuing Professional Education Center.

Stainton, M. C., McNeil, D., & Harvey, S. (1992). Maternal tasks of uncertain motherhood. *Maternal-Child Nursing Journal, 20,* 113–123.

Waldron, J., & Asayama, V. (1985). Stress, adaptation and coping in a maternal-fetal intensive care unit. *Social Work in Health Care, 10,* 75–89.

Werner, J. S. (1993). Stressors and health outcomes: Synthesis of nursing research, 1980–1990. In J. Barnfather & B. Lyon (Eds.), *Stress and coping: State of the science and implications for nursing theory, research and practice* (pp. 11–38). Indianapolis: Center Nursing Press of Sigma Theta Tau International.

White, M., & Ritchie, J. (1984). Psychological stressors in antepartum hospitalization. *Maternal-Child Nursing Journal, 13,* 47–56.

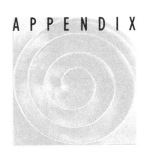

APPENDIX F

Example of a Qualitative Research Report

Nursing Students' Experience Bathing Patients for the First Time

Zane Robinson Wolf, PhD, RN, FAAN

● ABSTRACT

This study describes nursing students' experience bathing an adult patient for the first time. The students feared giving their first patient a bath and voiced concern about harming him or her. They discovered that it was easier when they were paired with another student and acknowledged being supported by fellow nursing students. Beginners were uncomfortable about exposing and touching the patient's private body parts and were surprised when patients helped them through the bath.

Every nursing student is expected to give a bath to a patient early in his or her nursing career. Nursing educators consider the skill of bathing to be fundamental and include it in one of the first nursing courses. The first time students are assigned to bathe a patient is often the second day they have a clinical experience in a hospital.

Students begin to bridge the gap between theory and practice wherever nurses work with patients.[1] By participating in the routines, reports, procedures, and events that make up the practice environment, students learn how to plan and give nursing care to patients. They are expected to practice the skills associated with hygienic care in a campus learning laboratory before the first clinical experience. Subsequently, clinical instructors carefully select the first patient the student will bathe guided by the advice of the nursing staff and with the consent of the patient. Faculty hope that students will become competent when performing bathing activities as they care for real patients, and master the cognitive, affective, and psychomotor abilities associated with this work.[2] Some faculty understand that students are very anxious during clinical experiences, and that a major contributor to their anxiety is fear of harming patients.[3]

Bathing a patient is performed by many nursing personnel.[4] Nurses have tacitly incorporated the bath as a part of their identity. That the bath has therapeutic benefits is seldom doubted.[5] But little literature has been devoted to students' experiences as they learn common nursing procedures, such as bathing patients.

Nursing students will probably bathe adult patients initially, because courses involving the care of children are often sequenced later in a program of studies. The purpose of this study was to describe nursing students' experiences bathing an adult patient for the first time. It was hoped that the essences and meanings of the experience would be revealed so that faculty and others would become more sensitized to this aspect of the nursing student's experiences.

● METHOD

Sixteen junior nursing students who attended a private university described their experiences bathing adult patients for the first time in written accounts produced during a scheduled undergraduate nursing research class. Participants were chiefly young adults (mean age, 23.56; SD, 5.03); 11 were Caucasian, with 4 African American students, and 1 Asian American. All but 1 reported belonging to a Christian religion, whereas 13 were single and 3 married. The students were not identified by name in the narratives. They were guaranteed anonymity and confidentiality, gave verbal consent, and signed their names at the completion of the study, thus consenting to appear as coauthors. No data were linked to a specific student; rather, data were coded anonymously.

The patients whom the students bathed included, in some cases, those of the opposite sex or a different race. Many were elderly. For example, one student cared for an elderly gentleman who was semiconscious and ventilator-dependent and had a lot of tubes. Another patient had great difficulty speaking and moving. One young adult was paraplegic, whereas an elder was recovering from a severe stroke. Yet another weighed approximately 300 pounds; he had a central line and was attached to a ventilator via an endotracheal tube.

Students were asked to write their response to the following: "Tell me what it was like to bathe your first patient." The faculty member teaching the course analyzed the text, identifying common meanings and essential structures (themes) of the experience. She attempted to set aside presuppositions during the analysis and reflected on the bathing experience as she read the written accounts of the students. She read the transcripts three times. Using a word processing program, structures (themes) and indicators (significant statements) were added to a table. Meanings were identified throughout the analysis phase. Themes were grouped with other themes of related meaning and organized into aggregates. The investigator returned to the original accounts as she wrote and revised the exhaustive description of the experience.

The scientific adequacy of the study was established in various ways. First, a doctoral-prepared nurse who was skilled in interpretive research reviewed the audit trail from textual accounts to exhaustive description and confirmed the adequacy of the methods. Second, the professor returned the exhaustive description to the students and requested that they discuss the experience and the adequacy of the portrayal. Seventeen of the students in the class reviewed the description of the phenomenon and verified that it reflected their experience. They discussed their experience and submitted written revisions. Points of discussion were recorded and included in the results.[6,7] Also, the first draft of the description was shared with a senior nursing student and a seasoned nurse. Both confirmed that the narrative included their experience as well. Student responses and suggestions were incorporated into the final draft.

RESULTS

The following is the description of nursing students' experience bathing patients for the first time. The themes and patterns are found in Table 1.

> My reaction was that of unease, because my patient was an elderly male. I have not given anybody, that is, an adult male or female, a bath before.

When nursing students bathe their first patient they bring their past experiences with them. Many have never bathed anyone but themselves, and they are uncertain about bathing a stranger. Previous experience bathing another, such as an infant or toddler, makes bathing an adult easier. For example, a previous job in a day care facility afforded a student an earlier opportunity to give hygienic care. Or, another student worked as a volunteer in a hospital and assisted an intensive care unit nurse to bathe a very sick male patient.

The nursing students who have never bathed a patient find it easier to bathe their first patient when they are paired with another student. When two are assigned to the same patient, they consider themselves fortunate. They work through their fear together and support each other by actual physical help as well as verbal and nonverbal encouragement. It is much easier to give the patient a bath with another student than to go through it alone.

Students are afraid of bathing a patient. Some are horrified. Their state of alarm is characterized by a student's acknowledgment, "I was sitting in the hospital's parking lot at 6:30 in the morning with the fear of giving a bed bath racing through my mind . . . I was scared, I admit it." Somehow they manage to overcome their dread and bathe the patient: "I was so scared beforehand and when it finally came down to it, I just did what needed to be done and it wasn't scary at all. The other thing that was scary was that the patient had a Foley, so I had to show her how to clean around it even though I had never done it."

Some of a student's fear is associated with imaginings about how the patients would react to a stranger, who is also younger, bathing them. "I was mostly scared because of the way the patient would feel being exposed to a 21-

TABLE F-1 *Themes in Nursing Student's Experiences Bathing Patients for the First Time*

Easing Into the Bath
  previous experience with bathing helped make this experience easier
  pairing with another student made it easier sharing fear
Emotional Reactions
  stress response
  neophyte
  shy
  nervous
  self-conscious
  fearful
  horrified
  nightmare
  very anxious, so anxious loses sight of patient's response
  self-absorbed
  avoidance behavior
  self-confrontative
Discomfort about Bathing Patient of Opposite Sex
  student sex/patient sex
Antecedent to Bath Experience
  worry about competent performance
  awareness of standards of care
  procrastinating, avoidance
  pretends to be self-assured and in control
  was nervous as she filled basin with water
  more difficult if female student bathes male patient
  easier if bathing same sex patient
  time assigned to bathe patient
Bath as Chore and Endeavour to Carry Out
  bath as experience to get "under your belt"
Preparations Before Getting Started
  type of bath
  collect linen
  assemble equipment

How Student Performed Bath
  skill required to bathe patient
  time it took to bathe patient
  what patient does as he or she bathes herself
  other accompanying functions, as helping patient with grooming
Responding When "In" the Experience
  thought situation funny
  felt awkward
  felt clumsy with hands and body position
  fear of exposing and touching stranger's genitals
  fear of rejection
  doing good, causing pain
  performing dirty work with other agendas in mind: comforting and cleansing
  awareness of genitals invading personal space, exposing patient, seeing what few people see
  student actions flowed after he or she started
Cautious about Privacy of Patient
  invading patient's privacy
  providing for patient's privacy
  student places herself in patient's situation
  observing that patient was incontinent of stool
  concern and respect for patient
  keeping patient safe
Meeting the Challenge and Exceeding Expectations
  teaching others allays nervousness
  taught another how to bathe patient
  courage bolstered by need to appear knowledgeable and competent
  confidence grew during bathing
Aftermath
  presently confident
  wasn't as embarrassed as anticipated
  still fearful
  still embarrassed
  did what needed to be done
  satisfied with teaching

(continues)

TABLE F-1 *(Continued)*

Open to Patient, Situation, and Responses

    sensitive to patient discomfort

    male patient uneasy with being bathed by female nurse

    afraid of hurting patient

    fear of bothering or annoying patient

    recognizing that patient in a lot of pain

    patient limitations

    personal profiles and sociodemographic characteristics of patients

    patient challenging to new student

Thinking Critically

    sought experienced nurse

    sought help of another student

Joining the "Club": Invitation to Become Insider experienced nurse tells student her plan for patient

Bathing Made Difficult or Easy by Patient Characteristics

    patient dementia makes bathing easier

cooperative

    accepted nurse

    patient pleasant

    patient wasn't overly nice

    patient makes bath easy for nurse: patient comfort related to student comfort

    patient thankful for student's company (presence)

    patient helped nurse

Aftermath

    success at performing bath

    comparison to subsequent bathing experiences

    student relief that bath finished

    judging bath experience

    gains confidence as result of first bath so that second bath is easier to perform

Reciprocity

    bath mutually enjoyable to patient and nurse

    patient invites student to visit her later

year-old nursing student." Others label the experience a nightmare, they are so upset about the situation.

Even though some students complete the bath alone and for the first time, they are still fearful about future expectations when they bathe other patients. Nonetheless, they find that their hesitation and insecurity wanes. They are more prepared to bathe patients the next time, because they proved themselves by having done it once.

A student is often relieved when the first time he or she bathes a patient that the person is of his or her same sex. One student admits that the first bath she gave a patient wasn't difficult at all. "I was glad my patient was female too (I am female also)."

If, on the other hand, a female student bathes a male patient, such as a 34-year-old male patient who is close to her age, this is a difficult experience. One student agrees that such a scenario was one of the most uncomfortable of her life.

However, it is imperative that every nursing student learn how to bathe a patient by actually doing it. It is a skill to get under his or her belt, something that has to be performed. Students can't wait to get it over with. They get through it even though they are shy or uneasy. They envision the bath as a chore, even though the experience turns out later to be less of one than anticipated.

In spite of the fact that students prepare to carry out the actual bath procedure in a campus learning laboratory, they are often nervous when confronted with a patient. The preparations help to get them set for the experience but do not eliminate their fear. One states, "Sure, I practiced on dummies, but the fact that dummies do not talk makes all the difference in the world."

Nevertheless, whatever the students' preparation for giving the bath has been, the time comes when they cannot avoid it. "I pretended to look in the chart, I was so nervous." This procrastination works for only so long. "I put the bath off as long as I could. I also remember checking her chart and asking the nurse if she really needed a bath, over and over. I finally realized that there was no getting around it. I would have to do it sooner or later." If the patient is "self-care," the student is able to put off the bath experience for another day. Nevertheless, he or she will eventually have to deal with it.

According to students, the nervousness persists as they begin to fill the basin with water. Some delay starting the bath, finding it necessary to refill a basin. "I finally decided to start the bath, but by that time the water was cold, so I went and got some warm water." Reluctantly they confront themselves with the fact that they have "to get used to bathing people."

Students thoughtfully get ready to give a patient a complete or partial bath by collecting bed linens and towels from the closet, and assembling equipment. They discover in person the extent that the patient is able or allowed to participate in bathing activities. They figure out the differences in types of baths as they rehearse the following: some patients require total care (complete bath) because they are unable to take care of themselves; others need minor assistance with bathing (partial bath or bath with assistance). One student explains, "I bathed her back and areas she couldn't reach. She bathed the rest."

After their experience they may understand that some patients require the assistance of more than one nurse because they are large or are otherwise considered heavy care. The first patient may be challenging, in that he or she tries to pull tubes out or requires heavy physical exertion. Some situations necessitate that a student call another student into the room to help. One student describes her solution: "She was a large woman so the toughest thing was keeping her on one side to do her back. I needed another student to help so the student could hold my patient." The student also relies on other coworkers, such as experienced nurses. In solving the problem he or she discovers that there are other healthcare personnel who can be relied on.

Moreover, having a patient assignment and carrying it out brings the student into the nursing profession. Students are gradually included as nurse colleagues. Staff nurses invite them into the profession implicitly by discussing plans for patient care.

Often, the patient participates in bathing activities; the student needs to be attuned to this and encourages the patient to assist. Thus the student waits for the patient to "bathe the rest," including genitalia and perianal areas. Other personal care functions are accomplished in concert with the bath as the student helps the patient, "It was a total grooming day for her. She combed her hair with my assist[ance]."

Students are acutely aware that it takes them longer than seasoned nurses to give their first bath. "I also know that her bath took probably twice as long as it should have." Also, they are already cognizant of the time pressures that shape nurses' work.

Additionally, students are mindful of a nurse's fundamental responsibility to keep patients safe. In the middle of bathing a patient, one recognized that a patient could hurt himself and ensured that another student or nurse stayed with the patient. "I grabbed another student to help hold him in position and make sure his hands stayed clear of his tubes (he was restrained because he had been pulling out his tubes the night before)."

Students are so afraid of being rejected by patients that they have physical symptoms. For example, "When I entered the room, I thought my heart was going to jump out of my chest." Or, their anxiety is manifested by thinking the situation amusing. They call the whole situation "funny" and laugh nervously.

Students are apprehensive, self-conscious, and shy as they broach the topic of beginning the bath to the patient. They are especially anxious as they start the bath, feeling ". . . somehow shy, not only for me but also for my patient." Some are so upset that they act clumsily or feel clumsy as though they are tripping on their own feet. It is difficult to think of what to say or where to start. The nervousness is compounded by lack of skill in handling the washcloth. They position their bodies awkwardly in relation to the patient in the bed. They are also afraid of hurting patients and worry about how competent they will be.

> But as old as she was, made me worry that I would somehow hurt her by just moving her. I was worried about the temperature of the water and how hard I was washing/rubbing her with the wash cloth. She just seemed so fragile that I could not help but worry."

They are troubled about not doing a good job: "I was also worried about . . . forgetting something or some part of the body."

A student's anxiety might be so profound that she or he loses sight of the patient's response to the bathing. The beginner is very self-absorbed, and in some cases projects on the patient the personal discomfort that the student feels.

New nursing students are afraid of exposing and touching a stranger's genitals. The fear does not abate after they manage to do this for the first time. A female student admits, "I was worried about my first complete bath being a male but in the end I think it was better. I was cautious about a male, but now that I've done it (bathed the genitalia), the next time won't be a problem." They know intuitively that they are invading another's privacy by contact with body surfaces that are generally considered the most private and secret parts. By invading the patient's personal space, the student sees what very few strangers see. Furthermore, patients can be weak, confused, and incontinent of urine or stool. This adds another dimension to a student's fear. Contact with the unclean and potentially dangerous aspects of personal care, such as excreta, is alarming, even repugnant. "When I uncovered his genital area, I noticed he had severe scrotal edema and he was lying in a pool of his own stool." Students are very attuned to the fact that their presence and access to the patient might cause the patient to feel very uncomfortable. A student is certain of her male patient's embarrassment. "I guessed (he) was somehow uneasy also by being bathed for the first time by a female. I know this because he verbalized it."

Students make sure they cover body parts during the bathing and remember to close the curtain around the patient's bed. They share that they are dismayed that more seasoned nurses seem unconcerned to some extent about exposing patients. They can easily place themselves in the patient's situation, being closer to that role than they are to the role of the nurse at this point in their career. "I thought about how it would feel being exposed to a male nursing student. I would absolutely hate it!"

In spite of fears and concerns, students manage to do what needs to be done. Some find that it is not as scary as they imagined. They rise to the occasion. For example, a student taught a spouse how to bathe her husband at the same time that she gave a bath for the first time. She was satisfied with her performance: "I felt good about the whole thing because I, a student, got to teach someone something." Teaching the wife how to bathe her husband helped the student to become less apprehensive. "I was showing her what to do and didn't want to sound like I had no idea what to do or that I was scared." Her courage was bolstered by her need to appear knowledgeable and competent.

Students' confidence grows as they bathe the patient. "As I worked my way down his body, my confidence grew. By the time I got to his back I was relaxed and was attempting to talk to him."

A student's self-assurance also grew as she realized her patient was enjoying being bathed. "Once I realized how enjoyable the bath was to my patient, my perspective made a 180 (degree turn)." Slowly, giving the bath seems less upsetting. One student reports that after she started the bath she moved smoothly: "By doing this we forgot it was our first time and the subsequent actions flowed as if we had done this before."

Some patients help students realize an easy first bath experience: "He was comfortable and subconsciously helped me through my first patient's bath." "She made me very comfortable in being there." Patients cooperate by moving in concert with the students' actions as the bath ensues. Also, when patients are pleasant, the bath goes smoothly. When patients accept the student, this makes it easier for the beginner to wash all areas of the body. "His acceptance made it extremely easy for me to wash all areas of the body. It made the bath a bit easier to administer."

The more comfortable the patient is with the bath situation and the student, the more comfortable the student is with bathing the patient. "She made me very comfortable in being there, and was glad to have my company."

Another student admits, "Fortunately he was very nice and didn't mind the bath, which helped a lot. He made me feel comfortable because he was comfortable." The patient may even be very thankful for the student's presence. "She thanked me for helping her and wanted me to come back and see her."

Furthermore, while giving the bath the student realizes that he or she is not as embarrassed as anticipated. "What I recall the most was not being as embarrassed as I thought I would when it came to washing the vaginal and anal area." The student may always be embarrassed, but gets on with it: "I get over the embarrassment I feel and realize (I need to meet) the needs of the patient." That the patient would find the bath comforting surprises the beginner. The patient's appreciation helps the student's perspective to change. His or her fear of bothering the patient disappears. The patient wasn't annoyed, so the student relaxes.

After bathing a patient for the first time, students reflect on their performance. If the first bath goes well it paves the way for the success of the next. They label the experience a success especially if they remember the steps of the bath procedure.

Gradually, students become more comfortable as they bathe more patients. Having passed the first hurdle, the skills continue to develop. "Now I don't feel as conscious of every stroke I make."

The characteristics of the patient and his or her situation shape the student's experience. The first patient may be a very challenging one:

> I was accidentally assigned to a ventilator-dependent patient, which we were not supposed to have until next semester because of the care involved. He was an elderly gentleman who was only semiconscious. He was in very bad shape and had a great deal of different tubes and devices hooked up to him.

The physical limitations of the patient and the severity of his or her illness soon convince the student of the necessity of the provision of complete care, including the bath. "I had to give her a complete bath because she was recovering from a CVA [cerebrovascular accident] and she had limited mobility on her right side." Another student recognizes a patient's need for assistance; a patient who is weak, confused, and incontinent needs help.

The bath experience becomes more difficult if the patient displays some problems, such as having a lot of pain with movement or not being able to communicate clearly. In such cases, the student manages to get through it, slowly developing more communication skills that are used simultaneously with the bath procedure. Additionally, the students realize that what they do to help can also result in patients having pain. "I felt bad because the patient was in severe pain but I knew I had to get him clean."

Students admit that they would prefer their first patient being "totally comatose." Having a confused patient could make a bathing episode easier as compared with an oriented one. "She wasn't completely oriented and basically had no problems with me helping her."

They see that doing dirty work accomplishes other outcomes for the patient. The patient is comforted as well as cleansed. "I found that throughout the procedure of bathing him I did not really focus on the feces, which I had feared would sicken me. I was more concentrated on getting the patient as clean as possible and with the least amount of pain."

DISCUSSION

The first bathing experience was stressful for the baccalaureate nursing student, as evidenced in the description of the phenomenon. Patients represented a challenge for the students in that they had to "fish or cut bait" to prove that they could manage a quintessential nursing skill. Students feared harming the patient, touching genitalia, and handling stool and other potentially dangerous bodily fluids. They put off the bath as long as they could. Students recognized that they lacked skill in performing a fundamental nursing procedure, having never bathed a stranger in most cases. At the same time they were aware that some patients were as uncomfortable as the students when the body was exposed.

Students became more confident as the bath progressed; some appeared to be comforted by the bathing and found it enjoyable. Reciprocally, patients seemed soothed by the ministrations. Furthermore, students recognized that patients appreciated their presence at the bedside.

Teaming students with other students and assigning them to bathe patients of the same sex, at least for the first time, reduced anxiety. Practicing the removing and replacing of a patient gown and bathing a mannequin with a Foley catheter and a wound would also help, because the nursing laboratory at the university is a less threatening place than the hospital to practice.[8] Students could more readily learn what to do and what not to do as a result of such simulations by handling equipment and being careful with dressings.

Rather than being thrown into the hospital and bathing situation, students might benefit from being teamed at first with a primary nurse who bathes a patient. Also, being with an experienced nurse for a day could help reduce student fear. Students suggested that they might feel less anxious if the first day they perform the bath there are no other procedures to be demonstrated.

Faculty should reconsider how they make assignments for students who bathe patients for the first time and recognize the extent to which their selections could affect the nursing student's experience. Mozingo and Brooks[9] believed that students require more positive feedback when learning skills during clinical experiences. Perhaps such feedback would also serve to reduce students' fear. In addition, the results support Windsor's[10] conclusions that fellow students are important people in the clinical setting. It may also be helpful for faculty to hold preclinical conferences and discuss some of the students' fears before the actual performance of critical skills. Providing more opportunities for students to discuss their feelings about clinical educational experiences may enable students to progress more easily through the various phases of professional development. The gradual development of assertiveness, information seeking, decision making, problem solving and technical skills is challenging for the beginner.[11] Faculty may find it useful to reflect on the rapid and complex transition from student to professional stranger[12] as students practice the skills that are part of the professional nurse's repertoire.[13]

Acknowledgments

The author thanks the following Junior Nursing Students from the School of Nursing, La Salle University, for their contributions: Christine Biddington, Catherine M. Branconi, Kathryn A. Cioffi, Donald Chiappini, Barbara A. Colligon, Christine M. Copestake, Michelle D. Emilio, William J. Donahue, Anita L. Dudzek, Mary K. Fitzgerald, Pamela L. Foster, Aron M. Gordon, Jimmie L. Harmon, Tammy L. Hartman, Hoa T. Huynh, Michelle Murrill, Cynthia A. Operacz, Michelle R. Peralta, Jill C. Putro, Jennifer A. Repchak, Stella C. Scott, Ellyn C. Taylor, Adriano Vitale, Jennifer A. Warwick, Melissa A. Watkins, and Stephanie L. Willis.

REFERENCES

1. Frizzell J. Successful recruitment tool: A nurse extern program. *Nurs Management.* 1993; 24(9):112.
2. Sheetz LJ. Baccalaureate nursing student preceptorship programs and the development of clinical competence. *J Nurs Educ.* 1989; 28(1):29–35.
3. Wilson ME. Nursing student perspective of learning in a clinical setting. *J Nurs Educ.* 1994; 33(2):81–86.
4. Verderber A, Gallagher KJ, Severino R. The effect of nursing interventions on transcutaneous oxygen and carbon dioxide tensions. *West J Nurs Res.* 1995; 17(1):76–90.
5. Wolf ZR. The bath: A nursing ritual. *J Holistic Nurs.* 1993; 11(2):135–148.
6. Colaizzi PF. Psychological research as the phenomenologist sees it. In: Valle RS, King M (eds). *Existential-Phenomenological Alternatives for Psychology.* New York: Oxford University Press; 1978:48–71.
7. Lincoln YS, Guba EG. *Naturalistic Inquiry.* Beverly Hills: Sage; 1985.
8. Haukenes E, Halloran CS. A second look at psychomotor skills. *Nurs Educ.* 1984; 9(3):9–13.
9. Mozingo J, Brooks E. Factors associated with perceived competency levels of graduating seniors in a baccalaureate nursing program. *J Nurs Educ.* 1995; 34(3):115–122.
10. Windsor A. Nursing students' perceptions of clinical experience. *J Nurs Educ.* 1987; 26(4):150–154.
11. Bennett SJ. Seeking-out behavior: Criterion for success in clinical learning experiences. *Nurse Educ.* 1992; 17(2):13–15.
12. Rosenberg CE. *The Care of Strangers: The Rise of America's Hospital System.* New York: Basic Books; 1987.
13. Melosh B. *The Physician's Hand: Work, Culture and Conflict in American Nursing.* Philadelphia: Temple University Press; 1982.

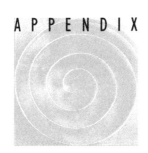

Guidelines for Evaluating a Quantitative Research Report

A. Problem Statement
   1. The problem is clearly identified.
   2. Background information on the problem is presented.
   3. Rationale for selecting the problem is clear.
   4. The problem is timely in terms of current trends in nursing.
   5. The problem is significant to nursing in that the results could benefit nursing practice and/or contribute to nursing knowledge.
   6. The quantitative approach is appropriate for investigating the problem.
B. Literature Review
   1. The review is relevant to the study.
   2. References are well documented and current (unless relevant classical studies are cited).
   3. The relationship of the problem to previous research is clear.
   4. There is a range of opinions and varying points of view about the problem.
   5. The review identifies important gaps in the literature.
   6. Documentation of references is clear and complete.
   7. The organization of the review is logical.
   8. The review concludes with a brief summary of the literature and its implications for the problem.
C. Theoretical or Conceptual Framework
   1. Is the research isolated rather than theory-linked?
      a. Is this appropriate or should the research have been theory-linked?
   2. If the research is theory-linked:
      a. Does the report describe a theoretical or conceptual framework?
         i. Is the framework appropriate for the research problem?
         ii. Is the framework clearly developed?
         iii. Is the framework useful for clarifying pertinent concepts and relationships?
D. Purpose of the Study
   1. The statement describing the purpose is appropriate for the study (declarative statement, research question(s), statement of hypothesis or hypotheses).

2. The purpose statement is clear as to:
   a. what the researcher plans to do.
   b. where the data will be collected.
   c. from whom the data will be collected.
3. If hypotheses are being tested:
   a. Each hypothesis is logically related to the research problem.
   b. Each hypothesis specifies an expected relationship among variables.
   c. Each hypothesis is clearly and concisely stated.
E. Definition of Terms
   1. Relevant terms are clearly defined, either directly, operationally, or theoretically.
F. Statement of Significant Assumptions
   1. Significant assumptions are stated clearly and are logical.
G. Subject Selection
   1. The target population is clearly described.
   2. The method for selecting the sample is appropriate.
   3. The sample size is adequate for the problem being investigated.
   4. The sample size is adequate for the number of variables in the study.
H. Ethical Considerations
   1. The procedure for obtaining informed consent is described.
   2. Monitoring by an institutional review board or committee is described, if appropriate.
   3. If the study poses any potential risks to subjects, does the researcher describe these risks and evaluate them?
I. The Research Design
   1. The design is clearly identified.
   2. The design is appropriate for the purpose of the study.
   3. If a pilot study was conducted, the results are discussed.
J. Data-Collection Instruments
   1. Instruments are appropriate for the study design.
   2. The rationale for selecting each instrument is discussed.
   3. Each instrument is described as to purpose, content, strengths, and weaknesses.
   4. Instrument validity is described in terms of type and coefficients (if appropriate).
   5. Instrument reliability is described in terms of type and size of reliability coefficients (if appropriate).
   6. If the instrument was developed for the study:
      a. Rationale for development is discussed.
      b. Procedures in development are described.
      c. Validity and reliability are addressed.
      d. A pretest is discussed, if appropriate.
K. Data-Collection Procedures
   1. Steps in the data-collection procedure(s) are clearly described.
   2. The data-collection procedure(s) is appropriate for the study.

L. Data Analysis
   1. The choice of statistical procedures is appropriate (descriptive/inferential or both).
   2. Statistical procedures are correctly applied for the level of measurement of the data.
   3. Data are analyzed in relation to the purpose of the study.
   4. Each hypothesis was tested and the results are reported accurately.
   5. Tables and Figures:
      a. Information in the text is consistent with each.
      b. Reflect reported findings.
      c. Are clear and well labeled.

M. Discussion
   1. Interpretations are based on the data.
   2. Finding are discussed in relation to the study's purpose.
   3. Findings are discussed in relation to the theoretical or conceptual framework and/or previous studies.
   4. Generalizations are warranted by the results.
   5. A distinction is made between statistical significance and clinical relevance and discussed, if appropriate.
   6. Conclusions are based on the data.
   7. Conclusions are clearly stated.
   8. Limitations of the study are appropriately discussed.
   9. Implications for nursing are plausible and relevant.
  10. Recommendations are clearly formulated and appropriate.

N. Additional Components
   1. The investigator(s) is qualified.
   2. The title is appropriate, accurately reflecting the problem.
   3. The abstract presents an accurate and concise summary of the content.
   4. The report is well organized and flows logically.
   5. Grammar, sentence structure, and punctuation are correct.
   6. References are accurate and complete.

RATE THE SCIENTIFIC MERIT OF THE REPORT ACCORDING TO THE FOLLOWING SCALE:

  4 Critique indicates that overall, the study satisfies the basic requirements of scientific research.
  3 Critique indicates that overall, the study satisfies the basic requirements of scientific research, with the following exceptions: (state the exceptions)
  2 Critique indicates that overall, the study does not satisfy the basic requirements for scientific research, with the following exceptions: (state the exceptions)
  1 Critique indicates that overall, the study does not satisfy the basic requirements of scientific research.

RATING FOR SCIENTIFIC MERIT: _____.

APPENDIX H

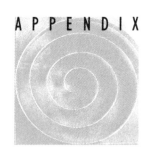

Guidelines for Evaluating a Qualitative Research Report

A. Problem Statement
1. The problem (phenomenon of interest) is clearly identified.
2. Background information on the problem is presented.
3. The rationale for selecting the problem is clear.
4. The problem is timely in terms of current trends in nursing.
5. The problem is significant to nursing in that the results could benefit nursing practice and/or contribute to nursing knowledge.
6. The qualitative approach is appropriate for investigating the phenomena of interest.
B. Literature Review (report may not have a literature review)
1. The documentation of references is clear and complete.
2. The organization of the review is logical.
3. The review is relevant to the study.
C. Purpose of the Study
1. The statement describing the purpose is clear as to what the researcher plans to do.
2. Significant assumptions are clearly stated and logical.
D. Selection of Subjects (Participants)
1. The selection of subjects (participants) is clearly described.
2. If sampling methods were used, are these clearly described? Are they appropriate for the study?
E. Ethical Considerations
1. The procedure for obtaining informed consent is described.
2. Monitoring by an institutional review board or committee is described, if appropriate.
3. If the study poses any potential risks to subjects, does the researcher describe these risks and evaluate them?
F. Data Collection and Data Analysis
1. The research method is appropriate for the purpose of the study (phenomenology, ethnography, grounded theory or other).
2. Data Collection
   a. How/why was the study setting selected? Is the setting appropriate for the study?
   b. Data-collection strategies are described (personal diaries, observation, interviews).
   c. Data-collection strategies are appropriate for the research method and problem.
   d. Steps in the data-collection process are described.

3. Data Analysis
    a. Each data-analysis strategy is logically discussed and is appropriate for the purpose of the study.
    b. Data-coding procedures are described.
    c. The themes and hypotheses are related to the purpose of the study.
    d. If narrative data are cited, do the themes capture the essence of the narratives?
4. Evaluating the Confirmability of the Findings
    a. Credibility: Did the participants validate that the reported findings truly reflect their own experiences?
    b. Auditability: Can another individual follow the documentation of data collection and analysis that led to the researcher's conclusions?
    c. Transferability (Fittingness)
        i. Are the findings transferable—that is, applicable outside the research situation?
        ii. Would the findings have meaning to others in a similar situation or situations?
G. Discussion
    1. Interpretations are appropriate for the phenomena of interest.
    2. Findings are discussed in relation to the research question or problem.
    3. Findings are discussed in relation to relevant literature and the findings of other studies.
    4. Conceptual categories are appropriately described and true to the data.
    5. Theoretical formulations, if developed, are supported by the data.
    6. Conclusions are logically consistent with the phenomenon of interest and with the context of the study.
    7. Conclusions are clearly stated.
    8. Limitations of the study are appropriately discussed.
    9. Implications for nursing are plausible and relevant.
    10. Recommendations are clearly formulated and appropriate.
H. Additional Components
    1. The investigator(s) is qualified.
    2. The title is appropriate, accurately reflecting the problem.
    3. The abstract presents an accurate and concise summary of the content.
    4. The report is well organized and flows logically.
    5. Grammar, sentence structure, and punctuation are correct.
    6. References are accurate and complete.

RATE THE SCIENTIFIC MERIT OF THE REPORT ACCORDING TO THE FOLLOWING SCALE:

4 Critique indicates that overall, the study satisfies the basic requirements of scientific research.

3 Critique indicates that overall, the study satisfies the basic requirements of scientific research, with the following exceptions: (state the exceptions)

2 Critique indicates that overall, the study does not satisfy the basic requirements for scientific research, with the following exceptions: (state the exceptions)

1 Critique indicates that overall, the study does not satisfy the basic requirements of scientific research.

RATING FOR SCIENTIFIC MERIT: _____.

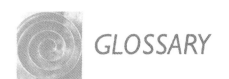

GLOSSARY

Abstract A concise summary of a study that communicates the essential information about the study.

Accidental sampling See *convenience sampling*.

Action research A research approach in which researchers pursue action and research outcomes at the same time.

Alpha error See *type I error*.

Alternate forms reliability Method of determining reliability in which at least two different forms of an instrument are administered to the same individuals and the scores are then correlated. Also called *equivalent forms reliability*.

Analysis of covariance (ANCOVA) Parametric statistical test to determine the differences between the means of two or more groups by removing the effects of one or more confounding variables.

Analysis of variance (ANOVA) Parametric statistical test to determine the differences between the means of two or more groups.

Anonymity Protection of the rights of study subjects so that their identity is not disclosed and their responses are not linked to them.

Applied research Research conducted to generate new knowledge that can be immediately applied to solve practical problems directly related to clinical practice.

Assumption A statement based on logic or reason whose correctness or validity is taken for granted.

Attrition Loss of subjects during a research study. A consideration related to internal validity in experimental studies.

Auditability In qualitative research, asks the question, "Can another individual follow the documentation of data collection and analysis that led up to the conclusions of the researcher?"

Audit trail In qualitative research, used in connection with auditability; refers to the systematic process by which an investigator records all activities that are related to the investigation so that an outside individual can examine the data and draw independent conclusions.

Basic research Research concerned primarily with establishing new knowledge and developing and refining theories rather than being immediately applied to practical problems.

Beta error See *type II error*.

Blind study See *single-blind study* and *double-blind study*.

Broad-range theories "Systematic constructions of the nature of nursing, the mission of nursing, and the goals of nursing care" (Meleis, 1997, p. 18). Broad-range theories in nursing deal with the scope, philosophy, and general characteristics of nursing (also called *grand theories*).

Case study Intensive and in-depth investigation of a single unit of study.

CD-ROM Compact disk–read only memory.

Chi-squared (χ^2) A statistical technique used to determine whether observed frequencies differ from expected frequencies. Also known as *chi square*.

CINAHL (Cumulative Index to Nursing and Allied Health Literature) A data base available either in print or on CD-ROM or on-line.

Cluster random sampling A probability sampling procedure that progresses in stages from larger sampling units to smaller sampling units. Also called *multistage sampling*.

Cohort A group of persons who share a common characteristic, such as age, occupation, or a delineated area of residence.

Compact disk—read-only memory See *CD-ROM*.

Complex hypothesis A statement of the predicted relationship between three (or more) variables.

Concept An idea or complex mental formulation of a specific phenomenon.

Conceptual framework Discussion of the relationship of concepts that underlie the study problem and support the rationale (reason) for conducting the study.

Concurrent validity A measure of how well an instrument correlates with another instrument that is known to be valid; a type of criterion-related validity.

Confidentiality Protection of research subjects so that the researcher will safeguard not only their identities but also their responses from public disclosure.

Confirmability In qualitative research, the trustworthiness of the findings as an indicator of the extent to which the researcher conducted the investigation in a rigorous manner.

Confounding variable Variable outside the purpose of the study that could influence the study's results. Sometimes called *extraneous variable* or *intervening variable*.

Constant comparative method Characteristic of the grounded theory method in which data collection and data analysis occur simultaneously so that all the data being collected are compared to all the data previously collected in order to determine their importance and position in the hierarchy of data analysis.

Construct An abstract phenomenon that is deliberately invented (constructed) by researchers for scientific purposes.

Construct validity An approach for establishing the validity of a quantitative measuring instrument that represents the degree to which a measuring instrument measures a specific hypothetical trait or construct, such as intelligence.

Content analysis (1) In qualitative research, a process to analyze the content of qualitative information gathered from the study participants by "categorizing the observations into themes and concepts emerging from the data." (2) In quantitative research, "a method to make inferences based on systematic, objective, and statistical analyses of written text or oral communication and documentation" (Doordan, 1998, p. 47).

Content validity An approach for establishing the validity of a quantitative measuring instrument that determines the extent to which the instrument represents the phenomena under study.

Continuous data Data that can be located at some point along a continuum or scale and are characterized by fractional values of a whole unit.

Control Process of eliminating or reducing the influence of confounding variables that could interfere with the findings of a research investigation.

Control group The group in which the experimental treatment is not introduced.

Convenience sampling Nonprobability sampling procedure in which the sampling units are selected because they are available to the investigator at the time of data collection; also called *accidental sampling*.

Correlation coefficient The number that represents the strength of the quantifiable relationship between two or more variables.

Correlation The strength of the quantifiable relationship between two or more variables.

Correlational research design Nonexperimental quantitative research design that measures the relationship between two or more variables.

Credibility In qualitative research, asks the question, "Are the reported findings true?"

Criterion variable See *dependent variable*.

Criterion-related validity An approach for establishing the validity of a quantitative measuring instrument. Refers to the relationship of the measuring instrument to some already known external criterion or other valid instrument. The term includes both concurrent validity and predictive validity.

Cross-sectional research design A research design in which data are collected from subjects at one point in time.

Data Units of information (singular: datum).

Debrief To provide subjects of the study with information about the study after the study has been concluded.

Deductive reasoning Method of reasoning that moves from the general to the specific.

Delphi technique A research methodology for predicting or emphasizing the main concerns of a group.

Demographic variable A characteristic or attribute of a study subject, such as age, gender, marital status, ethnicity, educational level, employment status, and family income.

Dependent variable The variable that changes as the independent variable is manipulated by the researcher; sometimes called the *criterion variable*.

Descriptive research Nonexperimental research designed to discover new meaning and to provide new knowledge when there is very little known about a phenomenon of interest.

Descriptive statistics Statistics used to describe and summarize data.

Diffusion The process of spreading an innovation through a social system.

Direct definition Definition of a term taken from a dictionary.

Directional hypothesis A hypothesis that specifies the predicted relationship between the independent variable (or variables) and the dependent variable (or variables).

Discrete data Data that exist only in distinct units expressed as whole numbers that are precise and definite: 6 beds, 5 hospitals, 6 patients (not 6-1/2 beds, 5-2/3 hospitals, 6-1/4 patients).

Diversity sampling A nonprobability sampling procedure used when the investigation requires that subjects with a wide variety of opinions and views be included in the sample. Also called *heterogeneity sampling*.

Double-blind study Research design technique in which neither the subjects nor those who collect the data know which subjects are in the experimental group and which subjects are in the control group.

Emic In ethnographic research, the interpretation of the data from an insider's point of view.

Empirical evidence Data gathered to generate new knowledge. It must be rooted in objective reality and gathered directly or indirectly through the human senses.

Empirical generalization A principle derived from empirical evidence.

Empiricism A characteristic of the scientific method in which evidence gathered to generate new knowledge must be rooted in objective reality and must be gathered directly or indirectly through the five human senses.

Equivalent forms reliability See *alternate forms reliability*.

Ethnographic research Qualitative research approach for in-depth investigation of a culture or subculture in which data related to the members of the culture are collected, analyzed, and described.

Ethnomethodology Literally, "people's methods." A qualitative research approach that attempts to understand how people see, describe, and explain the world in which they live. Ethnomethodology focuses on the tacitly held knowledge that people use to function in a familiar situation.

Ethnonursing A term unique to nursing, used by Madeline Leininger in connection with her theory of culture care diversity and universality.

Ethnoscience A qualitative research approach that analyzes the language used by a study's participants in order to determine how things are connected or recognized as belonging to the same categories.

Ethology The observation and measurement of behaviors in animals.

Etic In ethnographic research, the interpretation of data as an outsider looking in.

Event sampling A nonprobability sampling procedure in which the investigator is concerned only with sampling from those specific occurrences and/or events that are relevant to the study.

Evidence-based practice Professional practice based on the use of well-established research findings as well as other valid and relevant evidence.

Ex post facto **research design** See *retrospective research design*.

Experimental group The group in which the experimental treatment is introduced.

Experimental research design Quantitative research design in which the independent variable(s) is manipulated by the researcher, subjects are randomly assigned to groups, and the experiment is conducted under controlled conditions.

Experimenter effect Consideration related to internal validity in experimental studies. Experimenters can unconsciously bias subjects by the tone of their voice, facial expressions, or other behavioral mannerisms.

Expert sampling A nonprobability sampling procedure in which the researcher selects study participants based on the need to ascertain how experts in a field would react to or judge the phenomena of interest for the study.

Exploratory study Study conducted when relatively little is known about the phenomenon. Sometimes called a *pilot study*.

External criticism The evaluation of the validity of a historical data source.

External validity The ability to generalize the results of the study.

Extraneous variable See *confounding variable*.

Face validity A subtype of content validity that is determined by inspection of the items to see whether the instrument contains important items that measure the variables being studied.

Fatigue Consideration related to internal validity in experimental studies. Subjects or researchers can become tired, bored, or inattentive during the course of an experiment, thus affecting the results of the study.

Fittingness See *transferability*.

Focus group research design A method that allows the researcher to examine the points of view of a number of individuals in a group as they share their opinions/concerns about a topic. Usually consists of a small number of individuals who share a common bond.

Friedman two-way analysis of variance by ranks Nonparametric statistical test using ordinal-level data to determine whether related samples have come from the same population by determining mean ranks. Symbolized by χ_r^2.

Generalizability A characteristic of the scientific method in which information from a sample of a population can be said to be representative of the entire population from which it was drawn. The findings from the sample of a specific study can then be inferred to the entire population.

Generalization See *generalizability*.

Grand theories See *broad-range theories*.

Grounded theory research A qualitative research approach that uses inductive reasoning to generate the theoretical underpinnings of the research by "grounding" or basing the theory in the data being collected.

H See *Kruskal-Wallis one-way analysis of variance by ranks*.

Hawthorne effect Consideration related to external validity in experimental studies; the psychological reactions to the presence of the investigator or to special treatment during a research study, which may alter the responses of the subjects.

Heterogeneity sampling See *diversity sampling*.

Historical factors Consideration related to internal validity in experimental studies. If an experiment is carried out over a period of time, factors that are extraneous to the experiment, such as maturation or increased knowledge on the part of the subjects, may affect responses.

Historical research Qualitative research approach that deals with what has happened in the past and how these events affect the present.

H₀ See *null hypothesis*.

Human subjects review board See *institutional review board*.

Hypothesis A statement of the predicted relationship between two or more variables in a research study; an educated or calculated guess by the researcher (plural: hypotheses).

Independent variable The variable that is purposely manipulated or changed by the researcher; also called the *manipulated variable*.

Inductive reasoning Method of reasoning that moves from the specific to the general.

Inferential statistics Statistical tests used to make inferences (generalizations) to the larger population from which the sample was drawn.

Informed consent Voluntary agreement by a study subject to participate in a research study after being fully informed about the study.

Innovation Change perceived as new, such as new ideas or methods.

Institutional review board (IRB) A committee appointed by an agency to review proposed research and monitor ongoing research within the agency to ensure protection of the rights of subjects participating in a research study. Also called *human subjects review board*.

Internal criticism Evaluation of the reliability (authenticity and consistency) of what is stated in a historical document.

Internal validity In an experimental study, refers to whether or not manipulating the independent variable(s) really does make a significant difference on the dependent variable.

Internet An international electronic network that allows computers to communicate regardless of where the machines are located.

Interrater reliability Method for determining reliability in which the strength of agreement between the observations made by two or more observers is determined. Also called *interobserver reliability*.

Intervening variable See *confounding variable*.

Interval data Data based on a scale that has equal intervals but has no absolute zero starting point.

Interview Verbal questioning of respondents by the investigator in order to collect data. Requires interaction between people.

IRB See *institutional review board*.

Isolated research Research that is not linked to the theory-development process.

Judgment sampling See *purposive sampling*.

Key informants Individuals who are willing to participate in a study and whose positions or roles in a society or institution place them in a position to know what is really taking place.

Kinesics The study of physical activity exhibited by individuals.

Kruskal-Wallis one-way analysis of variance by ranks (H) A nonparametric statistical test that ranks ordinal-level data to determine whether independent samples were drawn from the same continuous population.

Likert scale A self-report measure in which each statement usually has five possible responses, such as strongly agree, agree, uncertain, disagree, strongly disagree. Five responses is typical, but up to seven responses may be provided.

Limitation Restriction identified by the researcher that may affect the outcome of a study but over which the researcher has little or no control.

Link-tracing sampling See *snowball sampling*.

Longitudinal research design A research design in which data are collected from the same subjects at different points in time.

Manipulated variable See *independent variable*.

Mann-Whitney U Nonparametric statistical test that uses ordinal data (ranks) to determine whether two independent samples have been drawn from the same population.

Mean The arithmetic average.

Measures of central tendency See *mean, median, mode, standard deviation*.

Median The number that divides the sample in half so that 50% of the sample falls above the median and 50% falls below the median.

Meta-analysis A synthesis of the findings of many separate investigations relating to the same general phenomena.

Microtheories See *narrow-range theories*.

Middle-range theories Theories that have a narrower focus than broad-range theories. "Middle-range theories are more precise than grand theories and focus on developing theoretical statements to answer questions about nursing" (Marriner-Tomey & Alligood, 1998, p. 11). Also called *midrange theories*.

Modal instance sampling Type of nonprobability sampling procedure that identifies subjects who represent the typical case that is constructed by the researcher for purposes of the study.

Mode The most frequently occurring score or number value.

Model A symbolic representation of reality used to demonstrate the interrelationships among a set of concepts or phenomena that cannot be directly observed but that do represent reality.

Mortality threat Loss of study subjects; a consideration related to internal validity in experimental studies, especially when the dropout rate is much different between the experimental and the control groups.

Multiple analysis of variance (MANOVA) Parametric statistical test to determine interaction effects between two or more independent variables and two or more dependent variables.

Multistage sampling See **cluster random sampling**.

N See *population*.

n See *sample*.

Narrow-range theories Theories that deal with a limited range of discrete phenomena of concern to a discipline; also called *microtheories*.

Naturalistic paradigm An approach to scientific inquiry in which reality is subjective as mentally constructed by individuals.

Network sampling See *snowball sampling*.

Nominal data Data that can be separated into only two mutually exclusive categories.

Nominated sampling See *snowball sampling*.

Nondirectional hypothesis A hypothesis that predicts a relationship between the independent and dependent variables but does not specify the direction of the relationship.

Nonparametric statistics Inferential statistics that do not require the same rigorous assumptions as parametric statistics. Nonparametric statistics are most often used when samples are small and/or when the data are measured on the nominal or ordinal scales.

Nonprobability sampling Sampling approach in which the investigator cannot estimate the probability that each element of the population will be included in the sample, or even that it has some chance of being included.

Normal curve A theoretical bell-shaped curve with most measurements clustered about the center and a few measurements at the extreme ends.

Null hypothesis (H₀) See *statistical hypothesis*.

Nursing research Research conducted to answer questions or to find solutions to problems that fall within the specific domain of nursing.

Observation Watching and noting actions and reactions.

Odd/even reliability See *split-half reliability*.

Operational definition The researcher's definition of a term that provides a description of the method for studying the concept by citing the necessary operations (manipulations and observations) to be used.

Opinionnaire A questionnaire designed to elicit data about a subject's opinions.

Order A characteristic of the scientific method that uses a series of systematic steps: (1) identification of a problem to be investigated; (2) precise definition, measurement, and quantification of the phenomena related to the research problem; (3) collection and analysis of data (information) that bears on the solution to the problem; and (4) formulation of conclusions regarding the problem being investigated.

Ordinal data Data that are ordered but for which there is no zero starting point; the intervals between individual datum are not equal. Big, bigger, and biggest are ordinal data.

p In inferential statistics, the symbol *p* stands for probability.

Paradigm "A way of looking at the world or a perspective on phenomena that presents a set of interrelated philosophical assumptions about the world. The perspective guides research and practice" (Doordan, 1998, p. 91).

Parametric statistics Inferential statistics that assume a normal distribution of the variables and the use of interval or ratio measures.

Participant observation Observation technique in which the observer becomes a participant in the situation being observed. Used in ethnographic research.

Pearson *r* Pearson product-moment correlation coefficient. A parametric correlation statistic.

Percentile rank Descriptive statistic indicating the point below which a percentage of scores occurs.

Phenomena Facts or events that can be observed and scientifically described because they are known through the senses rather than by thought or intuition (singular: phenomenon).

Phenomenology Research approach based on the philosophy of phenomenology, which proposes to understand the whole human being through "the lived experience."

Pilot study A small-scale version of the actual study conducted with the purpose of testing and potentially refining the research plan. Sometimes called an *exploratory study*.

Population The total group of individual people or things meeting the designated criteria of interest to the researcher. Typically shown as N. Also known as the *target population*.

Positivist-empiricist paradigm See *positivist paradigm*.

Positivist paradigm The traditional scientific method in its approach to research—that is, a scientific, objective view of the world. Also called the *positivist-empiricist paradigm*.

Power analysis A statistical procedure that allows the researcher to estimate how large a sample should be in order to determine the likelihood of accepting a null hypothesis that should actually be rejected or determining that a relationship does not exist between variables when a relationship actually does exist.

Predictive validity The ability of an instrument to predict an individual's behavior in the future; a type of criterion-related validity.

Pretest (1) The process of testing the effectiveness of a measuring instrument in gathering appropriate data. (2) In an experimental study, the data-collection procedure before the experimental phase of the study.

Primary source First-hand information obtained from original material; not interpretive or hearsay information.

Principle of beneficence Ethical principle that requires that a researcher should do no harm to the individual or, if risks cannot be avoided, that the benefits of research should be maximized while the possible harm should be minimized.

Principle of justice Ethical principle that requires that subjects be treated in a fair and equitable manner and that the resulting benefits of research must be equitably applied to all members of society rather than just to those who can afford them.

Principle of respect for human dignity Ethical principle that requires that individuals be treated as autonomous agents who are capable of self-determination that allows them voluntarily to take part in activities that may harm them when they are made fully aware of the potential dangers of such activities.

Probability sampling Sampling approach in which the investigator can specify, for each population element, the probability that it will be included in the sample—that is, there is a known probability of each element being included in the sample.

Problem-solving process A process to find an immediate solution to a practical problem in an actual setting.

Projective test Psychological test that requires the subject to project a meaning into essentially ambiguous or meaningless materials.

Proportional sampling A sampling technique that requires that the researcher be able to identify the percentage of the population that each stratum contains. The researcher then samples the population proportionately, based on these percentages.

Proposition A statement of a relationship between two or more concepts in a theory.

Prospective research design A nonexperimental research design that identifies the independent variable(s) in the present and looks to the future to identify potential effect(s) (the dependent variable).

Protocol See *research-based clinical protocol*.

Proxemics The study of body language, such as facial expressions, proximity to one another, touch, and gestures, all of which can be analyzed to determine patterns of behavior accompanying various tasks.

Purposive sampling Nonprobability sampling procedure in which subjects are selected because they are identified as knowledgeable regarding the subject under investigation. Also called *judgmental sampling*.

Qualitative data Data characterized by words rather than numbers.

Qualitative research A research method in which the investigator seeks to identify the qualitative (nonnumerical) aspects of the phenomenon under study from the participant's viewpoint in order to interpret the meaning of the totality of the phenomenon. Usually conducted in the natural setting.

Quantitative data Data characterized by numbers.

Quantitative research A research method in which the study variables are preselected and defined by the investigator and the data are collected and quantified (that is, translated into numbers), then statistically analyzed, often with a view to establishing cause-and-effect relationships among the variables.

Quasi-experimental research design Quantitative research design in which there is always manipulation of the independent variable(s) and control measures are employed, but the other element of a true experiment, random assignment of subjects, is absent.

Questionnaire A paper-and-pencil data-collection instrument that is completed by the study subjects.

Quota sampling Nonprobability sampling procedure in which study subjects are selected in such a manner that each stratum of the population is proportionately represented.

r See *Pearson r*.

r_s See *Spearman's rho*.

Random route sampling A probability sampling procedure that is useful in conducting research when the investigator intends to conduct interviews in households, businesses, or other such premises that need to be sampled.

Random sampling Selection of subjects based on chance alone. Also see *simple random sampling* or *stratified random sampling*.

Randomization Random assignment of subjects to the groups in an experimental study on the basis of chance alone.

Range The difference between the lowest and the highest score on a measuring instrument; the high score minus the low score.

Rating scale A type of data-collection instrument designed to allow respondents to place their responses on a scale that has a range of potential responses.

Ratio data Data based on a scale that has equal intervals and an absolute zero starting point.

Refereed journal A journal that uses the process of having three or more experts independently review and judge the merits of a manuscript before acceptance for publication.

Regression toward the mean Consideration related to internal validity in experimental studies; the tendency for changes in scores of individuals when given the same test several times to come closer to the mean scores of the group.

Reliability (1) In quantitative research, the stability of a measuring instrument over time. (2) In qualitative research, "the measure of the extent to which random variation may have influenced stability and consistency of results" (Morse & Field, 1995, p. 243).

Replication Repeating a study using the same methods in order to determine whether the results will be the same as or similar to the original study.

Research An orderly process of inquiry that involves purposeful and systematic collection, analysis, and interpretation of data (units of information) in order to gain new knowledge or to verify already existing knowledge.

Research critique An objective and critical evaluation of the strengths and weaknesses of an entire research study.

Research design The overall plan for a research study.

Research hypothesis Method of stating a hypothesis so that it specifies the relationship between the variables that the researcher expects as the study's outcome.

Research process A guide for deriving systematic information (new knowledge) concerning the phenomena of interest to the researcher.

Research proposal A detailed written description of a proposed research study; sometimes called a *prospectus*.

Research utilization (RU) A systematic process by which the scientifically valid results of research are transferred for use in practice.

Research-based clinical protocol A written document that organizes and transforms research-based knowledge so that it can be used to direct clinical practice activities.

Research-based document A written document that transforms research-based knowledge so that it can be used in practice.

Retrospective research design A nonexperimental research design in which changes in the independent variable have already occurred before the research due to the natural course of events. Also called *ex post facto research design*.

Risk-benefit ratio Anticipated benefits to subjects should outweigh the risks to the subjects, and knowledge to be gained should be of sufficient importance to merit any risks to which subjects might be subjected.

Sample A smaller part of the population selected in such a way that the individuals in the sample represent (as nearly as possible) the characteristics of the population. Typically shown as n.

Sampling frame The list of all of the members of the population from which the sample is taken.

Sampling Process of selecting a sample from the target population.

Science A unified body of systematized knowledge concerned with specific subject matter obtained by establishing and organizing facts, principles, and methods.

Scientific merit The degree to which the study is both methodologically and conceptually sound.

Scientific method "An orderly, systematic, controlled approach to obtaining precise empirical information and testing ideas" (Doordan, 1998, p. 112).

Secondary data analysis A research technique in which the investigator uses existing data either to design research studies to answer new questions and/or to test new hypotheses, or to reinterpret the existing data.

Secondary source An interpretive or hearsay source of data.

Self-report A subject's response to a survey instrument, such as a questionnaire or interview.

Semantic differential scale A scale consisting of a listing of bipolar adjectives with a five- to seven-point scale between them that may describe a setting, object, profession, or any other variable of interest.

Serendipitous findings Important and unexpected discovery of significant results in a research study not related to the purpose of the study.

Simple hypothesis A statement of the predicted relationship between two variables—that is, a single independent variable and a single dependent variable.

Simple random sampling A probability sampling procedure in which the required number of sampling units is selected at random from the population in such a manner that each population element has an equal chance (probability) of being selected for the sample.

Single-blind study Design technique for achieving control in a research study carried out in either of two ways: (1) The study subjects know whether they are in the experimental or control group, but the data collectors do not know; (2) the data collectors know whether subjects are in the experimental or control group, but the subjects do not know.

Snowball sampling A nonprobability sampling procedure in which study subjects are asked to provide referrals to other study subjects. Also called *nominated sampling* or *network sampling*.

Sociometric technique A quantitative research technique used to determine social interaction and leadership patterns within a group.

Spearman's rho *(r₍ₛ₎)* A nonparametric measure of correlation.

Split-half reliability Method for determining reliability in which responses to a measuring instrument are divided in half, scored separately, and then correlated. Also called *odd-even reliability*.

Standard deviation The general indicator of the dispersion or spread of scores from the mean.

Standard score A number reflecting the distance that an individual score is from the mean in standard deviation units. Reported as z, Z, or T.

Statistical hypothesis A statement of no statistically significant difference or relationship between the variables of a study. Also called the *null hypothesis*.

Stratified random sampling A probability sampling procedure that is a variation of the simple random sample. The population is divided into two or more strata or groups with different categories of a characteristic. A simple random sample is then taken from each group.

Subject sensitization Subjects become knowledgeable about or sensitized to the procedures used during a research study.

Survey research The collection of data directly from the study subjects, usually by questionnaire or interview.

Systematic random sampling A probability sampling procedure in which subjects are randomly selected from the population at fixed intervals that are predetermined by the researcher.

T score See *standard score*.

*t **test*** A parametric statistical measure to determine the differences between the means of two groups. Symbolized by *t*.

Target population See ***population***.

Test-retest reliability Approach to estimating reliability that indicates variation in scores from one administration to the next, resulting from measurement errors. The same instrument is administered to the same individuals at different times and the two sets of scores are then correlated.

Theoretical definition Definition of a variable using the specific language of the theory or conceptual model that serves as the framework for a research study.

Theoretical framework Discussion of one theory or interrelated theories being tested in order to support the rationale (reason) for conducting the study.

Theoretical sampling A nonprobability sampling procedure most often associated with qualitative research, primarily the grounded theory method.

Theory A set of logically interrelated statements that is "a creative and rigorous structuring of ideas that project a tentative, purposeful, and systematic view of phenomena" (Chinn & Kramer, 1995, p. 72).

Theory-generating research A type of theory-linked research that is designed to develop theory.

Theory-linked research "Research designed with reference or linkage to theory" (Chinn & Kramer, 1995, p. 141).

Theory-testing research A type of theory-linked research that is designed to test how accurately a theory depicts phenomena and their relationships.

Time sampling A nonprobability sampling procedure used by researchers who are concerned with collecting data on activities that take place at specific times of the day or night.

Transferability In qualitative research, asks the questions, "Are the results applicable outside the research situation; would the findings have meaning to others in a similar situation or situations?"

Triangulation (1) The use of both quantitative and qualitative methods in the same research study. (2) In quantitative studies, the use of three or more techniques to collect data.

Trustworthiness See *confirmability*.

Type I error The rejection of the null hypothesis when it should have been accepted; also called *alpha error*.

Type II error The acceptance of the null hypothesis when it should have been rejected; also called *beta error*.

U See *Mann-Whitney U*.

Unobtrusive measure The researcher decides what needs to be measured and then determines how to measure it without direct intervention.

Usability The practical aspects of using a measuring instrument.

Utilization See *research utilization*.

Validity (1) In quantitative research, the ability of a data-gathering instrument to measure what it purports to measure. (2) In qualitative research, "the extent to which research findings represent reality" (Morse & Field, 1995, p. 244).

Variable An attribute or characteristic that can have more than one value, such as height, weight, and blood pressure.

Visual analog scale (VAS) A self-report paper-and-pencil scale that consists of a straight line that has the extreme limits of the variable being measured at each end of the line. The straight line may be either vertical or horizontal. The scale is designed to have the respondent indicate a point on the line that indicates where the intensity of the specific attribute being measured is located.

Voluntary sampling A type of nonprobability sampling procedure in which volunteers either offer or are actively recruited to participate in a study.

World Wide Web See *Internet*; also called *www*.

χ^2 See *chi-squared*.
χ_r^2 See *Friedman two-way analysis of variance by ranks*.

z score See *standard score*.
Z score See *standard score*.

REFERENCES

Chinn, P. L., & Kramer, M. K. (1995). *Theory and nursing: A systematic approach* (4th ed.). St. Louis: Mosby.

Doordan, A. M. (1998). *Research survival guide*. Philadelphia: Lippincott-Raven.

Marriner-Tomey, A., & Alligood, M. R. (1998). *Nursing theorists and their work* (4th ed.). St. Louis: Mosby.

Meleis, A. F. (1997). *Theoretical nursing: Development and progress* (3rd ed.). Philadelphia: Lippincott-Raven.

Morse, J. M., & Field, P. (1995). *Qualitative research methods for health professionals* (2nd ed.). Thousand Oaks, CA: Sage.

INDEX

Page numbers in *italics* denote figures; those followed by a "t" denote tables; those followed by a "b" denote boxes; those in **bold** denote glossary entries.